VASCULAR SPIDERS

AND RELATED LESIONS OF

THE SKIN

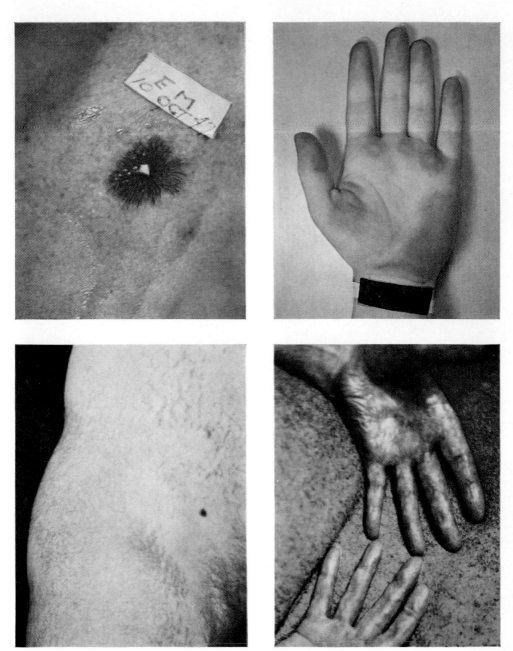

Frontispiece—*Upper left*—Vascular spider of the skin covered with oil to reveal the details of the numerous branches. The triangular area is a highlight. One should notice details of small satellite lesions and the paper money skin are emphasized. *Upper right*—The acquired palmar erythema of pregnancy illustrating the intense reddening of the hypothenar area, the discrete spots between the regions where the fingers and the palms join, the red surface of the distal phalanx of the fingers, and the roughly triangular area in the center of the palm retaining its usual color. *Lower left*—Striate atrophy of the skin of the hip, thigh, and lower abdomen, illustrating the irregular linear pattern, the relation to skin folds, and the varying degrees of intensity. *Lower right*—Palmar varix. The increased size and accessibility of veins on the palmar surface of the fingers and the palm and the thin, almost parchment-like, quality of the skin are illustrated.

VASCULAR SPIDERS
AND RELATED LESIONS OF
THE SKIN

By

WILLIAM BENNETT BEAN, M.D.

Professor of Medicine

Head of the Department of Internal Medicine

The College of Medicine

State University of Iowa

Iowa City, Iowa

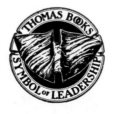

CHARLES C THOMAS • PUBLISHER

Springfield · Illinois · U.S.A.

CHARLES C THOMAS · PUBLISHER
BANNERSTONE HOUSE
301-327 East Lawrence Avenue, Springfield, Illinois, U.S.A.

Published simultaneously in the British Commonwealth of Nations by
BLACKWELL SCIENTIFIC PUBLICATIONS, LTD., OXFORD, ENGLAND

Published simultaneously in Canada by
THE RYERSON PRESS, TORONTO

Library of Congress Catalog Card Number: 58-12146

With THOMAS BOOKS *careful attention is given to all details
of manufacturing and design. It is the Publisher's desire to
present books that are satisfactory as to their physical qualities
and artistic possibilities and appropriate for their particular use.*
THOMAS BOOKS *will be true to those laws of quality that
assure a good name and good will.*

Printed in the United States of America

For "Abigail, . . . a woman of good understanding and of a beautiful countenance."

— I Samuel, 25, III.

INTRODUCTION

The writer of a book should tell the reader his purpose. Then a reader or critic can say whether the purpose has merit and, if he chooses, wherein the writer has failed or succeeded. If a book consists largely of original personal observations it becomes a diary of sorts and the introduction is modified autobiography. How did I get interested in spiders and such things and why must I write about them? This I have detailed elsewhere (53, 61, 62, 63). Suffice it to say here that I was discouraged and a little disillusioned that none of my splendid clinical teachers at Johns Hopkins, Harvard or Cincinnati could answer my annoying questions about spiders. I began to collect data, studying spiders wherever I found them, approaching them from all sides and in all places. I ignored the boundaries between the sundry sundered specialties of medicine. Thus I learned of the comings and goings of spiders, something of their natural history, and their ecology. The observations served as stimulus for hypotheses. These led to studies which still have not answered many of the questions old or new. Interest in spiders led me to look at a host of other vascular lesions, some related, some not. It is my purpose in this book to describe and discuss this large miscellany of vascular lesions of the skin and to point out their significance within the limits of my present understanding. I shall try to relate my observations to those made by others, comment on historical items, and keep within the always tentative boundaries of clinical science.

Anyone's review of his own motives is apt to be distorted by conscious or unconscious shifts of emphasis as well as the subtle reinterpretations which time brings. In any work going on over the years, we assume that we must have had the same urges and insights all along that we have now. We tend to look upon ourselves and our accomplishments as substantial if not indeed remarkable. This book has the faults and merits of personal observation and narrative. Much of it deals with observations independent rather than necessarily original. If clinical trivia and ephemera illustrated no general principles in medicine I would not care. I have never been able to stimulate or simulate interest in popular medical problems just because they were popular. Nevertheless small lesions may help us understand larger ones and lead to generalization bearing directly on practical medicine. Thus they may have importance for patients and so for society out of proportion to their small size. If we really understood the significance of spiders or any other vascular lesion of the skin it would be a large achievement.

In every specialty in medicine, blood vessels play a central part. In normal function and in disease, blood vessels, large and small, can be examined easily by direct inspection of the surfaces of the body. With little difficulty we examine with various scopes through natural apertures the retina, much of the alimentary canal, the genito-urinary tract and the larger respiratory passages. By slightly more formidable procedures such as thoracoscopy and peritoneoscopy, we look at serosal surfaces. Surgical operations may now lay bare all the secret chambers of the body. Even the interior of the heart stunned into asystole by chemical means, or bypassed by mechanical pumps, or torpid and idling in a chilled body, lies before the surgeon in repose while he repairs its wrongly built or spoiled interior partitions or rearranges large or small vessels.

No part of development, growth, normal function, disease, aging or death is without its intimate vascular context. In spite of these truisms and in spite of much desultory and concerted study there are large chasms of ignorance which disfigure and Balkanize in separate, mutually excluding systems our knowledge of blood vessels. Though the notion developed in retrospect rather than as part of the motivation for the studies constituting the theme of this book all medicine stands to gain from a better understanding of blood vessels. A truth demonstrated under certain peculiar circumstances for small vessels may illuminate a distant and seemingly unrelated obscurity. Running as a persistent motif through all medicine is the problem of structure and action of blood vessels. On this theme are hung somewhat loosely the diverse observations and thoughts of the several chapters of this book.

The organization and plan of the book need some comment. By far the longest chapter deals with spiders and palmar erythema. Thereafter the vascular lesions of the skin are grouped about a common etiologic mechanism or process, a region of the body, or a common clinical complication. Since several might have been put in more than one place the Table of Contents contains redundant headings in several chapters. For instance, hereditary hemorrhagic telangiectasia, which I call Osler's disease, appears in the chapter on congenital lesions but might have appeared with vascular lesions which increase with aging, or the chapter on enteric bleeding with diagnostic skin lesions. The index should help in orientation.

A few nonvascular syndromes or processes are discussed. Fascial hernias, nails, melanosis with intestinal polyposis and the masque biliáre have crept in, because they illustrate a point and because they interest me. With the exception of Fabry's syndrome and epidemic dropsy, I have observed all the lesions and disorders under discussion. My own personal contributions to natural history include the first relating of spiders and palmar erythema to both liver disease *and* pregnancy, the use of infrared photography to produce vascular obliteration of red lesions as well as to accentuate the appearance of blue ones, an elaboration of the dermovascular changes in the syndrome of metastatic carcinoid, the demonstration of secular changes in the lesions of Osler's disease and the dynamic state of changing patterns of small vessels in normal skin, too. I have brought together the congenital dysplastic angiectases showing a tangential relation to Maffucci's syndrome while trying to escape the anachronistic errors of eponyms by avoiding many but using some. Naming a characteristic lesion the blue rubber-bleb nevus may be just as bad. I am not aware that others have described venous lakes, palmar varices, striate atrophy of the skin, dysautonomia in the adult or the combination of vascular lipomas, ophthalmoplegia, steatorrhea and phlebectasia into a possible syndrome, but I have not searched all possible repositories, or even many textbooks of dermatology. The history of medicine reveals that very few people really discover anything new and many whose names are tacked onto a lesion or syndrome may be embarrassed to learn that others not only have described it before, but better. I could not care less. At least I have resuscitated if not discovered many interesting vascular lesions.

The inclusion of lesions has been arbitrary and though my interests are eclectic the main reason for including anything was that it interested me. I have said very little about nerves though they may be crucial to the solution of many of the problems of etiology. I have said almost nothing about treatment. Other books contain little else. The role of aging has been emphasized in a number of lesions, and a few ancient heresies buried, though their talent for survival is a natural cause for pessimism. I have left several hypotheses dangling in mid air, not knowing how to claw them down or to fasten them where they belong. The observations may stimulate others to solve my problems, or even to study for themselves the array of enchanting vascular lesions Nature has put before us.

WILLIAM B. BEAN

Iowa City

ACKNOWLEDGMENTS

In a work of this sort much of which consists of individual observations and tests it is well to recognize the tremendous amount of help I have had from others at one time or another during the study of spiders which is now in its third decade. I owe a debt to Louis Hamman and Warfield T. Longcope for giving me the information that there was some relationship of spiders to liver disease. Over an intermittent period of eleven years in Cincinnati and Birmingham, the late M. A. Blankenhorn encouraged what so many people looked on as a pursuit of a will-o'-the-wisp. Donald Forster and Morton Hamburger were early partners in the enterprise while we were together in Cincinnati, and the review of case notes with them was a strong stimulus to me to continue the study. Seaton Sailer did much work with me on histopathology early in this study. His death in France and loss of our serial section material discouraged me from taking up this problem again. I am greatly indebted to G. A. Martini for the use of his material and many profitable discussions about his observations. I had much stimulus in Fort Knox days from Ludwig Eichna, William Ashe, Arthur Friedman, and Steven Horvath who criticized one or another of the drafts of the monograph on spiders which appeared in *Medicine*. A whole series of friends, associates, and colleagues at Iowa have been of invaluable help. Harold Schedl and Murray Franklin worked with me on the steroid hormone problem for a time continuing work I had done in association with Arthur Mirsky in Cincinnati. Innumerable students, undergraduate students, interns, and residents have made helpful contributions. Richard Eckhardt, Margaret Vance Siems, and David Olch were very helpful in keeping records on innumerable patients studied for all manner of vascular lesions. My colleagues in dermatology, Leon Goldman in Cincinnati and Ruben Nomland, C. E. Radcliffe, and Robert Carney in Iowa have been of great help in many ways. George Easton provided me with material about the gums in pregnancy. A long correspondence with Parkes Weber has increased my admiration for him as a natural historian of disease and I marvel at his activity still continuing briskly as he approaches his hundredth year. I must express particular thanks to the Study Sections and

Staff of the National Institutes of Health. They gave me liberal support of a project to study spiders in pregnant women at a time when otherwise it would have been impossible for me to continue in academic medicine. Joseph Homan, Frederick Kent, Jack Davis and many others have been of invaluable assistance in obtaining a series of excellent photographs. Morris Dexter, Robert Cogswell, and James Embick will long remember our pursuit of spiders in the obstetrical clinic and wards of the Cincinnati General Hospital where our curious studies amused and amazed the obstetricians who were extremely cooperative. Nurses and members of hospital and administrative staffs have provided assistance in too many ways to recall. I have had editorial assistance from many people and continue to get free and enlightening criticism about matters of style in writing from George Day in England to whom and to many others I am most grateful. The almost endless problems of typing and retyping, checking bibliographies, and attending to the busy routine of departmental typing and administration have gained for Mrs. Charlotte Fell, Miss Eula Van Meter and Mrs. JoAnn Drevets my admiration and thanks. How they manage to get the job done while putting up with my extravagant demands is a marvel. Rex Jamison and Norman Rinderknecht were extremely helpful in collecting and analyzing data when they worked for me during several summers while they were undergraduate medical students. I must thank Charles C Thomas for his forbearance in receiving a manuscript some years after I thought I would be able to get it to him and for courteous help in many other ways. I have had a great deal of help from Miss Nina Frohwein in the Medical Library in checking references and obtaining photostats. I would be remiss not to mention the many dozens of physicians who have written me about interesting problems, asked questions, and in general stimulated my interest and provided information about spiders and related lesions. For permission to employ illustrations already used elsewhere I am indebted to the editors and publishers of *Medicine; Surgery, Gynecology, and Obstetrics; The A.M.A. Archives of Internal Medicine, Journal of Laboratory and Clinical Medicine, American Journal of the Medical Sciences, Quarterly Bulletin of the Northwestern University Medical School, American Heart*

Journal, Journal of Clinical Investigation, Geriatrics, Journal of the Iowa State Medical Society, Ciba Foundation Symposia, The American Practitioner and Digest of Treatment, Surgery, and *Springer-verlag.* And finally I must thank the innumerable patients who have provided the substance for my investigation and the theme of these endeavors. It has been a happy and fruitful partnership, and not a unilateral relationship.

W. B. B.

TABLE OF CONTENTS

xvi

xvii

VASCULAR SPIDERS

AND RELATED LESIONS OF

THE SKIN

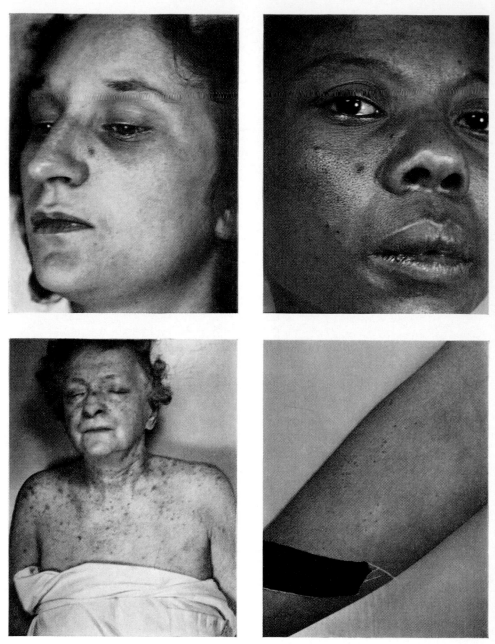

Figure 1. Four Kodacromes. *Upper left*—Spider on the side of the nose which developed in a woman during pregnancy, revealing the elevated central punctum and the diffuse erythema. *Upper right*—Spider which developed on the cheek of a negro woman during pregnancy. *Lower left*—Extensive spider proliferation and vascularization of the skin over the upper portion of the chest, shoulders and face in a woman with cirrhosis. *Lower right*—Clusters of spiders appearing in the center of the pale areas of skin in a pregnant woman.

I

SPIDERS AND PALMAR ERYTHEMA

THE ARTERIAL SPIDER

"His cheek displays a second spring of roses
taught by wine to bloom."

1. Introduction

Outward and visible signs of internal disease have been fundamental to the art and science of medicine from ancient times. Nonetheless until recently students of internal medicine and dermatology have evinced only sporadic and casual interest in the acquired impermanent arterial lesion in the skin variously termed *nevus araneus, nevus arachnoideus, nevus arachnoides, spider angioma, spider telangiectasis, spider nevus, spider cancer, spiderweb nevus, stellate nevus, stellar nevus, star nevus, tâche stellaire, étoile vasculaire,* and more simply, *vascular* or *arterial spider.* They are called "spiders" or "devils" by barflies who have long been familiar with their connotation as occupational hazards of their craft. The lesions will be referred to as spiders hereafter. Many years ago this disorder of the small vessels of the skin and its relationship to hepatic disease was brought to my attention by Louis Hamman and Warfield T. Longcope. Since that time, I have studied the vascular spider in a variety of abnormal conditions as well as in apparently healthy persons. Many curious lesions have been seen in formal consultation and in curbstone or al fresco review. Instead of approaching the problem in relation to cirrhosis only, or hepatic diseases, or pregnancy, or in persons seemingly normal, I have pursued the study wherever spiders were encountered. This has given a panoramic rather than specialized point of view. One of the byproducts of the investigation has been the realization that in some persons the spider is the specialized form of a general disorder of

3

the blood vessels of the skin, sometimes accentuated locally as palmar and plantar erythema and even occurring in mucous membranes. Data have accumulated upon many kindreds of persons in the several categories of disease and apparent health in which the spider and associated vascular change have been observed.

An interest in spiders has led to an interest in many similar lesions of the skin. From this it has gone on to include a number of vascular lesions, blushes, nevi, moles and other conditions rather remote in appearance and in meaning from the spider. Their vascular structure has been the common denominator. They have sufficient clinical interest to be included in the miscellaneous list of vascular lesions I have collected.

2. Material and Procedures

I have notes and records of more than one thousand persons with vascular spiders, and I have looked for them in several thousands of patients and more than two thousand "normal" persons. This study has gone on for more than twenty years. The patients and normal persons were seen under conditions so diverse that except for those with liver disease and pregnancy they reflect no regular samples of the general population. The details of the various groups have been set forth in several papers and will be referred to at appropriate places. Subsequent observations have led to the inclusion of patients with B-complex deficiencies in the normal group. They had no manifest liver disease and were not pregnant. I have not found any connection with any deficiency disease. I have detailed notes on nearly two thousand other patients referred for consultation, with very little preselection into narrow diagnostic categories. These patients were searched for most of the skin lesions discussed in the book, and data on the incidence of various lesions are based on this experience, supplemented with records made on many hundreds of ward patients from the Medical Service of the University Hospitals at Iowa City.

3. Description

The numberless variations in the size and shape of the cutaneous arterial spider make generalizations difficult. Nevertheless, certain oft repeated features permit the description of a generic norm. Such terms as *tâche, étoile,* and spider indicate the basic pattern so frequently seen. The typical example is characterized by three main features: body, legs, and surrounding erythema, plus various lesser attributes.

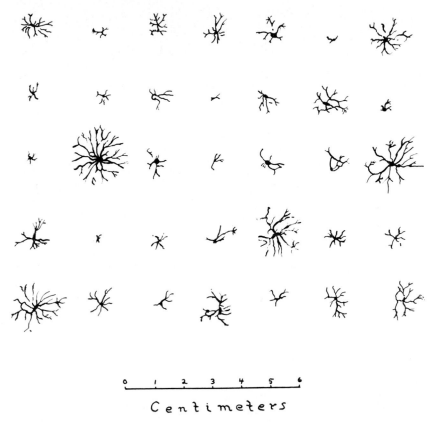

Figure 2. Scale drawing of actual spiders made by direct tracing on transparent paper to reveal the great variety of size, shape and pattern.

A. BODY

First, the *central point* or *eminence* constitutes the body. This may be so small as to escape detection without magnification, or so large as to command instant notice. Ordinarily there is a direct relationship between the size of the center or punctum and the size of the entire spider. Exceptions occur. There is a tendency for the body of the larger ones to be elevated, sometimes as much as 5 mm. above the adjacent skin surface. When the central point is large and elevated, it may be *seen* to pulsate. Palpable pulsation is found more frequently. The larger the center, the more apt it is to be symmetrical, and nearly hemispherical in silhouette. In the sketches and pictures, a variety of forms is shown.

B. LEGS

Secondly, branching vessels, the *legs* or *radicles*, radiating from the central hub spread out parallel to the plane of the skin, just below the surface. These may occur as a few well-seen vessels of fairly large caliber or as a large number of clearly defined smaller ones; or the vessels may be hidden beneath the skin, the only indication of their existence being the erythematous area surrounding the central point. They may appear to overlap in crisscross pattern (Figure 1). It is not uncommon to see microscopic connections; and if oil is placed on the skin and magnification of twenty diameters is employed, small inter-connecting loops are seen very often. With this technic branches of the sixth order may be counted in some lesions. In many instances, branches are not apparent to the unaided eye. The legs of the spider are irregular in direction and may twist, branch, coil, disappear for a millimeter or two, and emerge distally. These features are clear in the illustrations. When the spider occurs in a fold of skin, or in a place where there are wrinkles, there is a tendency for many legs to follow the lines in the skin. Isolated single vessels may appear as strands which resemble the scattered silk threads in American paper money; or they may unite to form a loosely or closely knit reticulum which in advanced stages becomes a telangiectatic mat. On close inspection, some of the isolated vessels exhibit one or more branches. When the fork is bulbous or beaded, the simplest form of spider occurs (Figure 2).

C. ERYTHEMA

Thirdly, the *area of erythema* surrounds the central punctum. It may be roughly circular, or may be star or cog-shaped. Usually it extends several millimeters beyond the clearly visible legs but in some cases the legs extend beyond the perimeter of the erythema. When the branches are not readily seen, the spider may appear as a circular area of erythema with a central red punctum or pulsating papule. Sometimes the central punctum may also be hard to find, and the lesion may simulate the early stage of an acne pustule (46, 628). A pale ring may surround the blush area of the lesion, but this anemic halo is not very common unless the patient is in a cool or cold place.

D. Color

Distinctive of the lesion is its fiery red color, which results from the rich supply of arterial blood brought abundantly in very thin-walled vessels towards the surface of the skin. This color may be seen even when jaundice or pigmentation gives an abnormal hue to the background.

E. Temperature

The region encompassed by the vascular ramifications of the arterial spider is warmer than the adjacent skin. This may be explained by the fact that a large amount of rapidly moving blood is brought near the surface. The elevation in temperature above that of the neighboring uninvolved skin is roughly proportional to the size of the spider. It may amount to as much as 2°-3° C.

F. Direction of Blood Flow

Blood flows from the central body through the legs towards the periphery. This has been observed many times (53, 265, 422). It may be demonstrated by the application of pressure to the center, which causes fading of the whole area; or by enclosing the spider in a transparent capsule fixed to the skin, and gradually increasing the pressure. The erythema fades and recedes from the border towards the center, the whole being obliterated by adequate pressure.

G. Collecting Veins

In Figure 3 may be seen the arrangement of superficial veins in the skin surrounding the territory occupied by the vascular spider. It appears that the return of blood from the capillary bed is effected by a system of collecting vessels about the periphery of the spider legs. Nothing like *venae comites* for the central arteries have been seen in our histological sections. It is well to emphasize here that the vascular spider is emphatically not an arteriovenous shunt in the sense of a glomus body, nor is it similar to the arteriovenous aneurysm which may follow injury to an adjoining artery and vein. Arterial blood is contained in the spider legs, however much they may resemble veins in their histological characteristics.

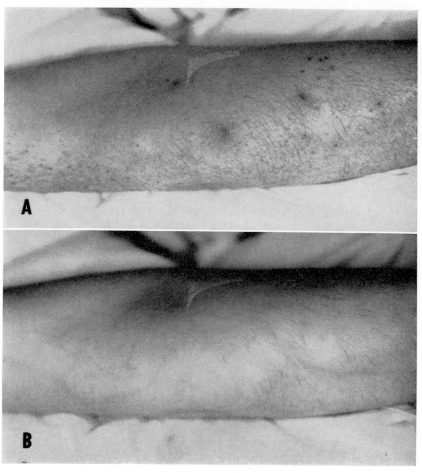

Figure 3. Spiders in a patient with cirrhosis of the liver. The upper photograph is an ordinary black and white picture showing several spiders. The lower photograph shows the same site employing infrared photography. The spider fails to appear when this technique is used. This and other photographs demonstrate that the spider tends to occupy an area away from large veins.

H. Pulsation

If the location is favorable or their size is large, spiders can be felt to pulsate. This is particularly noted when the lesion overlies bone, as over the forehead, sternum, or clavicle. Pulsation can be seen if a capsule is attached to the skin and the pressure within it is adjusted so that a stream of blood flows and ebbs to and from the central point into and out of the legs. Pressure with a glass slide or the lens of one's spectacles reveals pulsation in most spiders. Rarely a large one may be seen to pulsate.

I. Variations in Appearance in Different Types of Skin

The superficial appearance of the spider is modified by the texture, elasticity, pigmentation, and thickness of the overlying skin, as well as by its nearness to the surface. This may be seen to best advantage in a person who has many lesions scattered over the body. When the skin is atrophic, much of the finer structure can be observed by the use of magnification. Examination of the lesion by means of a slit lamp permits visualization of the deeper structures in favorable cases. The erythematous macule, the large round pulsating boss, and other variations are included in the photographs and diagrams.

J. Absence of Hair

It is unusual for a spider to occur where hair is heavy. Rarely does it appear in the scalp, axilla or pubic regions. It may, however, occur on the face in the beard area, or on a hairy chest. Usually the territory which is erythematous has no obvious hair (Figure 3), although hair follicles are commonly seen in the microscopic sections.

K. Distribution

The pattern of distribution is treated in detail under Physiology. Figure 4 portrays the essential features.

L. Associated Changes in Cutaneous Vessels

An indication of the widespread alteration in cutaneous vessels associated with spiders is the *paper-money skin*. This type of change has been emphasized by Steinmann and by Patek, Post and Victor who were struck by the ubiquity of vascular disturbances which rendered many vessels visible in regions of the skin where they are not seen normally.

Large vascular tumors, pulsating hemangiomas 5-25 cm. in diameter have arisen in two patients with severe liver disease both being described to me by physicians who know of my interest in vascular phenomena. In one case it is not absolutely certain that the vascular tumor was not present before the development of ser-

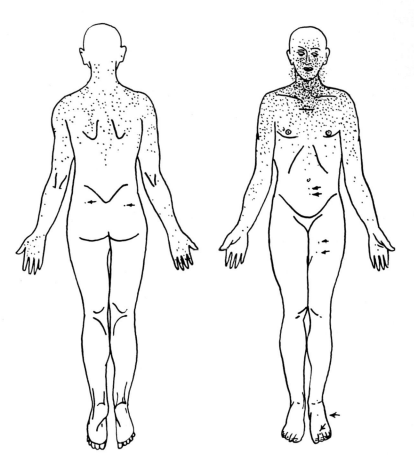

Figure 4.   Distribution of spiders in cirrhosis of the liver. Each mark represents a single spider.

ious liver disease but in the other a compressible pulsatile mass almost as large as the hand arose near the top of one buttock during an outcropping of spiders in a patient with worsening cirrhosis. Whether this represents an extravagant eruption of a structure like a spider but of giant proportions, or whether some stimulus to vascular new growth produced a different lesion, a neoplasm, is speculative.

In addition to the typical spider formation and the scattered strands of vessels in the skin, other characteristic phenomena are associated in many cases. Perhaps the most familiar is vascularization of the external aspect of the nose. Large vessels, firmly imbedded in or just beneath the skin, course over the nose from the nasomalar junction or emerge in front of the alae, imparting a livid appearance. Change in the degree of redness of the nose often proceeds *pari passu* with change in vascular spiders in other parts of the body.

M. TELANGIECTATIC MATS

Persons with spiders may have large or small areas where the skin has blotches, networks, or mats composed of telangiectatic ves-

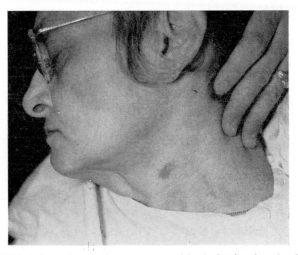

Figure 5.   Telangiectatic mat in a woman with cirrhosis who also had spiders. The area on the neck below the angle of the jaw was slightly warmer than the adjacent skin. Its red color faded completely on pressure, refilling from several different foci when pressure was released.

sels (Figure 5). These are bright red, blanch with pressure and pulsate when compressed with a glass. They may go and come in association with spiders and palmar erythema. In two patients with cirrhosis I have seen these mats but no spiders and no palmar erythema.

N. Vascularization of Mucous Surfaces

Similar vascular changes in the mucous membranes of the body may occur in association with cutaneous spiders. This fact has been emphasized by French clinicians, who attribute much of the bleeding in chronic hepatic disease to these lesions. The mucosal telangiectasis often does not follow the spider-pattern so prominent in the skin, but may occur in any form from a short strand to a complex mat. In my experience mucosal vascularization is not common though I have seen spider lesions of the hard and soft palate, buccal mucosa, of the rectum by proctoscopic examination and of the stomach by gastroscope. Photographs are not satisfactory for publication.

4.   The Vascular Spider in Hepatic Disease

A. Historical Review

It is impossible to decide whether or not certain vague descriptions found in ancient medical writings concern the vascular spider. There is no clear description of them in the works ascribed to Galen or Hippocrates. The latter does not include them in his classical description of that aspect of hepatic disease to which posterity has given the name Hippocratic facies. In some of his case histories he referred to lesions resembling flea bites, which appeared in crops, but there is no hint to help us distinguish them as spiders rather than lesions of purpura, scurvy, vitamin-K disorders, or typhus. Various angiomas are referred to casually in medical writings of the Middle Ages but the interest was often centered on a suspected relationship to witches rather than to disease. Nothing can be made out of the large body of literature on the nevus maternus or mother's marks, which has been of interest chiefly to the gullible as grounds for their fanciful belief in maternal gestational influences on the offspring.

It is related that William Harvey, the discoverer of the circulation of the blood, had an interesting part to play in a hunt for witches' marks, in July 1634. He was called in to give an expert opinion in the case of the famous Lancashire witches. The official report reads as follows:

"Surgeons Hall in Monkwell Street, London.

2 JULY A.D. 1634.

"We in humble obedience to your Lordship's command have this day called unto us the Chirurgeons and midwives whose names are hereunder written who have by the direction of Mr. Dr. Harvey (in our presence and his) made diligent search and inspection on those women which were lately brought up from Lancaster and find as followeth, viz.:——

"On the bodies of Jennett Hargreaves, Frances Dicconson and Mary Spencer nothing unnatural nor anything like a teat or mark or any other sign that such a thing hath ever been.

"On the body of Margaret Johnson we find two things which may be called teats. The first in shape like to the teat of a bitch but in our judgement nothing but the skin as it will be drawn out after the application of leeches. The second is like the nipple or teat of a woman's breast, but of the same colour with the rest of the skin without any hollowness or issue for any blood or juice to come from thence."

The report was signed by ten midwives, by Alexander Reid, M. D., lecturer in anatomy at the Barber-Surgeons' Hall whom Harvey must have gotten to take his place and by six surgeons from among the most noted in London. As a result, the four women were pardoned, an act of justice which, says Mr. Aveling, 'may have been due to the enlightened views and prompt and energetic action of Dr. Harvey.' I have no idea what a witch's mark really was.

I can find no reference to vascular spiders in the writings of Morgagni, Laennec or Bright, who understood many of the clinical relationships of disease of the liver. No description occurs in the works of Addison, Frerichs or Fagge upon hepatic disorders. It has not been possible to make a comprehensive search of the very old German and French dermatological and medical writings, but if any knowledge existed about the vascular spider it has not been handed down to modern writers. Therefore we may conclude that only in relatively recent times have these blemishes in the skin effectually aroused the curiosity of the physician. Perhaps this is not strange when we recall that the striking entity of hemorrhagic telangiectasia was not generally recognized and was certainly not defined until Osler's papers brought out its interesting natural history (628-629).

Very clear mention of spiders, and a fair plate depicting one are contained in Bateman's text of dermatology in the Second American edition of 1824. There is so little general commentary that one wonders whether they were very widely known, or more probably treated as insignificant. I have not searched the earlier texts exhaustively and an ancient lore which has been referred to by Hutchison (422).

More than a century ago Erasmus Wilson, an early English physician and philanthropist, a devotee of dermatology, discussed "spider marks" and spider nevi as banal red spots in the skin (918, 919). This was well before he gave what I believe was the first clearly identifiable description of spiders erupting in alcoholic cirrhosis. This classic note, published in 1867 is given here in full:

"A publican, aged thirty years, had for some time yielded to the temptation of his calling, and had thereby injured his health, when he was suddenly attacked with epistaxis and to the epistaxis succeeded copious bleeding from the gums. After some time, and subsequently there appeared on the face, the neck, the hands, and the arms, an eruption of red papulae with a diffuse areola. On presenting himself for consultation there were six of these papular spots on the face, chiefly on one cheek, two on the neck and three or four on the hands and forearms. It was evident, on careful examination, they were angiomata; the central prominence was vascular, and around this was a plexus of venules spreading out to the breadth of a quarter or half an inch. In one or two of the spots the central prominence was absent and a plexus alone existed, resulting from angiectasia, or multiplication and hypertrophy of the venous capillaries of the skin. The case is very rare, a sudden eruption of angiomata, and its association with hemorrhage from the mucous membrane of the nose and mouth is very instructive. We are unaware of the conditions of the economy which may tend to the sudden hypertrophy of blood vessels, but we can easily understand how such an occurrence, taking place upon the mucous membrane, might lead to serious hemorrhage; and there is no reason to suppose that the cause of the epistaxis in the instance before us, and the bleeding of the gums may not have been a sudden hypertrophy of blood vessels such as we have just described as appearing on the skin. And it appears to us that as a result, to the well-known hemorrhagic diathesis as a cause of hemorrhage there must also be added a sudden hypertrophy of blood-vessels and rupture of their coat as exemplified in the case before us."

This excellent picture has remained buried. The lesion was characteristic and very well described. Association with over-indulgence in alcohol and presumably with cirrhosis is of great interest. The hemorrhages probably arose from the nasal mucosa. These observations led to no investigation to ascertain the validity of the speculations aroused in the mind of their author.

The second reference to vascular spiders in hepatic disease, and the first study devoted to the problem, came from the French clinicians, Hanot and Gilbert in 1890. They described the *étoile vasculaire* and must have realized the arterial nature of the vessels, referring to them as *"tâches érectiles véritables."* In addition they observed that these *étoiles* were not necessarily permanent, disappeared in one patient with cirrhosis who was much improved when he was seen again four years after his initial examination. They showed that cutaneous vascular spiders have some relation to cirrhosis, are arterial in nature, and may disappear with amelioration of the hepatic disorder. Their findings have not been known to many subsequent writers on the subject.

In his classical study of hemorrhagic telangiectasis in 1901, Osler made some interesting remarks about spiders. He believed that the dilated vessels forming the radicle were veins converging upon the "central bright red nodule projecting a little beyond the skin." He commented on the superficial resemblance to the cutaneous lesion of acne. In his own words:

"Angiomata have a curious relationship with affections of the liver. In cirrhosis, in cancer, in chronic jaundice from gallstones spider angiomata may appear on the face and other parts. They may be of the ordinary stellate variety like the stars of Verheyen on the surface of the kidney, or the entire area of the star may become diffusely vascularized, so that there is a circular or ovoid territory of skin looking pink or purple, owing to the small dilated veins. A dozen or more may appear on the trunk or even large ones may disappear. And lastly, in a few cases of disease of the liver I have seen large mat-like telangiectases or angioma involving an inch or two of skin, and looking like a very light birth-mark, but which had appeared during the illness. The skin was not uniformly occupied with the blood vessels but they were abundant enough in the deep layers apparently to give a deep change in color and to form very striking objects. The dilated venules on the nose, and the chaplet of dilated veins along the attachment of the diaphragm are not infrequently accompaniments of the spider angiomata in cases of diseases of the liver. I have recently seen the spider angiomata appear in the face in a case of catarrhal jaundice."

Later students have added little to these early descriptions, although the belief that the vessels were venules has been discarded.

Bouchard made a significant contribution to the subject in 1902. He stressed the fact that the affected vessels were on the arterial side of the capillaries. He was apparently the first to see spiders erupt, fade away, and return during the varying clinical course of cirrhosis and he put great emphasis upon their direct relationship to the severity of the disease. It was his opinion that they appeared in areas in the skin which had been subjected to some trauma. He described similar lesions in the mucosa of the mouth and pharynx. Perhaps some of his patients with bleeding lesions were suffering from Osler's disease although hemorrhage from mucosal spiders has been described by others (46, 374, 494, 918).

In 1903, Gilbert and Herscher reported the occurrence of vascular spiders in one hundred and seven persons with hepatic and biliary disease, including Laennec's (alcoholic) cirrhosis, tuberculosis of the liver, Hanot's (biliary) cirrhosis, familial jaundice, and other forms of hepatic disease. They thought that the characteristic vascular spider should always excite the suspicion of liver disease, even though the disease be latent clinically. Upon grounds not exactly clear they concluded that on the hands and face, spiders were arterial in nature, while on the trunk they were composed of capillaries. Pulsation was specifically noted. It had previously been implied by Hanot and Gilbert.

In 1904, Parkes Weber expressed his belief that they were "in-duced by a small inflammatory papule of the skin." Subsequent observers have expressed a similar opinion.

The vascular spider was noted by Sir James Galloway in 1908. He stressed its evanescent character, its appearing and fading with relapses and remissions in cirrhosis. Somewhat later he described and pictured an advanced stage of this vascular phenomenon occur-ring in a soldier with syphilis, tuberculosis, a large liver and anal fistula. He called attention to the palpable pulsation in the larger lesions and to the bleeding that occurs with mild trauma.

Castaigne and Chiray in the 1910 edition of their text re-marked that patients with Laennec's cirrhosis "have arterial vari-cosities and it is not uncommon to encounter one or more arterial nevi of recent date." They did not, however, remark on the spider form, although the concept of arterial varicosities suggests that they were well acquainted with it.

Frick, in 1912, reported an atypical example in a man suffering from carcinoma of the liver. It is possible that a disorder of a dif-ferent kind was present since the lesions remained clearly discern-ible after death. They may even have been cherry angiomas!

In 1914, Sibley described a woman who had vascular spiders showing a more or less symmetrical distribution. It is not clear that she had hepatic disease. In any event the vascular spiders faded while the patient was still under observation.

The nature of Adamson's case (1918) is by no means clear but it may have been of the same variety.

In the volume of Contributions to Medical and Biological Re-search dedicated to Sir William Osler (1919) there is a report by Gwyn of a patient with Weil's disease in whom vascular spiders developed. I have seen no other example referred to and this lesion is not mentioned in the review of Weil's disease by Ashe, Pratt-Thomas and Kumpe.

A general consideration of angiomas by Emile-Weil in 1927 gave a good account of the occurrence of the spider-like lesion in cirrhosis. He implied but did not describe differences between the acquired vascular spider and other angiomata.

In 1928, Roles reported a case of multiple telangiectasia with splenomegaly. From the description it seems probable that this represented the acquired vascular spider of cirrhosis rather than an unusual complication of Osler's disease, although others have interpreted it differently.

Rolleston has written of the clusters of dilated vessels or stigmata on the face. He said that when cirrhosis in advancing, small angiomas may crop up all over the surface of the body, and in exceptional instances may unite to form areas of considerable extent. Elsewhere (717) he remarked that "small angiomas, probably due to toxemia and sometimes appearing in crops when the disease is advancing, are common in the skin generally, and when on mucous surfaces may account for epistaxis and for false hemoptysis and hematemesis."

In French medical writings there are many articles on the vascular spider. Laffitte believed that it was similar in nature to other arterial nevi of the skin. Steinmann wrote two excellent reviews on the subject and was the first to discuss the morphology of the vascular lesion in detail. He called attention to the irregularities of the legs of the spider which dipped down in places so as not to be visible at the surface, giving the impression of an elongated spiral. He stated that pressure applied to the center caused the peripheral portion of the lesion to disappear. Arterial pulsation was readily detected in some spiders, especially the larger ones with elevated centers. Steinmann was one of the first to stress their curious distribution; their rarity or absence from the legs and lower part of the body; their frequency in the exposed areas of the face, cheeks, nose, brows, forehead, forearms, palms, fingers and upper aspect of the chest. He emphasized their close relationship to the functional state of the liver, fading with remissions and developing or recurring with exacerbations in the severity of the disease. This was correlated in his patients with changes in the rose bengal test of liver function. He saw spiders appearing two or three years before ascites first occurred, at a time when the only indication of hepatic disease was digestive disturbance, sometimes with slight icterus. Hemorrhage from mild trauma to a lesion, especially on the mucous membranes, often called attention to its presence. Finally he noted that after death no traces of the lesion could be found unless it was very large and was angiomatous in character. Fiessinger arrived at similar conclusions. He believed that the arterial spider was of prognostic significance since he observed instances of its fading in patients who recovered, but it is not clear that he was able to predict future improvement in cirrhosis on this basis. He was the first to call attention to similar vascular changes throughout the skin without typical star formation. Loeper, Loew-Lion and Netter stressed the sudden explosiveness of the eruption and the prognostic as well as diagnostic value of the *tâches stellaires*. They were impressed by the association of these lesions with the ascitic and splenomegalic phase of cirrhosis, rather than with any particular type of cirrhosis. They emphasized the occurrence of submucosal lesions in the nose, mouth and pharynx and their rôle in hemorrhage. In some autopsy specimens the liver had extensively dilated portal spaces which were thought to be similar in nature to the vascular change in the skin. Finally, these authors observed that an increased level of tyramine in the blood and ascitic fluid seemed to parallel the advent or enlargement of the subcutaneous *tâches*.

Eppinger summarized his rich experience with the cutaneous spider in his comprehensive monograph on hepatic disease published in 1937. He had been struck by the distribution of these lesions, never having observed them in regions not drained by the superior vena cava. Perhaps he did not look carefully at the legs.

Eller, in 1937, reported an example in a forty-five year old white woman addicted to alcohol. The lesions developed first on the knees, later on the face. The discussion following his article gives a good example of the prevailing confusion about the nature and significance of angiomata in general and acquired vascular spiders in particular.

Bloomfield, in 1938, observed vascular spiders in 39 per cent of 18 patients with chronic hepatitis who were studied for long periods of time. In one instance most of the spiders had faded after a two-year interval during which the manifestations of cirrhosis subsided. There was no single factor in the reported clinical or laboratory findings which was directly correlated with this change.

In 1938, Williams and Snell published an excellent description of pulsating angiomas in hepatic disease. They suggested that the spiders of hepatic disease were related to the glomus body and indeed their sections of a large pulsating lesion revealed the same tissue in the arterial wall that is found in the typical arteriovenous connection so elaborately described and reconstructed by Masson and by Popoff. In their discussion, Williams and Snell described the well known and clearly dissimilar vascular changes in the cutaneous vessels and overlying skin in Osler's disease, although earlier they assumed the identity of the two types of lesions.

Comment on spider nevi is included in Watson's article on regurgitation jaundice. He emphasized the distribution in the upper portions of the body, connecting this phenomenon, as did Eppinger, with the drainage area of the superior vena cava. He had not seen typical multiple nevi except in the presence of hepatic disease. Since that time he has observed spiders in the skin of the lower part of the body.

An extensive study of the vascular spider associated with cirrhosis of the liver, one which combined an excellent analysis with histological sections and descriptions, was reported by Patek, Post and Victor. These authors have added greatly to knowledge of this abnormal vascular structure. In their papers is the clear statement that "the acquired type of spider does not conform to descriptions of the congenital lesions" (i.e., Osler's disease). They found that 76 per cent of 63 patients with cirrhosis of the liver exhibited spiders. They reviewed some of the previous reports and demonstrated beyond cavil that spiders fade on pressure, pulsate and so are arterial in nature. By using a blood pressure cuff they showed that they have a pressure around 85 mm. of Hg.—somewhat lower than pressure in the brachial artery, but distinctly higher than capillary pressure in the fingers. The direction of blood flow is centrifugal, from the body through the radicles to the periphery. Their pharmacological investigation revealed that the smaller branches of the spider reacted to adrenalin and histamine in the same manner as the minute skin vessels. Such observations had been made years before by Lewis and his colleagues, but the connection with liver disease eluded Lewis completely. As might be expected from the arterial structure, lesions fade and may disappear after death, although the larger ones may leave a tell-tale region of increased lividity. Patek emphasized the point that the skin elsewhere was apt to exhibit dilated vessels not arranged in the typical spider pattern. He did not, however, mention any similar changes in the mucous membrane. His histological studies indicated a distinction between two types of spiders. One was an enlarged and dilated artery with branches from the stem going on to merge with the capillaries. The other variety was composed of a central stem artery which resembled the arterial side of an arteriovenous glomus shunt but had this significant difference, that it broke up into radiating branches which continued to the capillary bed at the periphery and did not empty directly into veins. The branches were thinly covered vessels which in structure more closely resembled veins than arteries, but contained arterial blood. This may account for the difference in opinion about the structure of the vascular spider. This difference may have resulted from studying one of the several parts rather than the whole, or perhaps only one of the two types.

Another detailed study of these lesions, one of the few illustrated with photographs, was published by Cicovacki. He found the lesions in 56 per cent of 46 patients with cirrhosis. He noted their distribution, their variation with the changing stages of cirrhosis, and their occurrence in non-alcoholic cirrhosis. Curiously enough he believed that spiders were pathognomonic of cirrhosis and permitted the exclusion of other hepatic disorders. He brought out evidence for associated endocrine disorders, hairlessness, changes in the hypophysis, and atrophy of the testes, phenomena which have been described as occurring in the cirrhosis of hemachromatosis (496). In discussing the nature of these phenomena he called attention to *Chvostek's habitus* in cirrhosis and speculated upon a common constitutional cause for cirrhosis and vascular spiders.

A similar suggestion has been advanced by Parkes Weber in several of his notes on vascular spiders, although he is inclined to attribute the eruptive phenomenon, the provoking force, to an inflammatory reaction. If read aright, he considers the spider to be a mycotic aneurysm of the terminal cutaneous artery of Renaut which may disappear when the infecting organism dies.

Ratnoff and Patek in their classic monograph on Laennec's cirrhosis, reported that spiders had been described in only 15 per cent of 386 cases and "liver palms" in slightly more than 4 per cent. The data were incomplete, which probably accounts for the lowness of these figures as compared with those in the earlier study by Patek, Post and Victor. This underscores the necessity of judging the incidence of such lesions from a study centered upon them rather than from one that deals with the underlying disease where the spider may have been neglected or overlooked.

My own contribution to the subject of spiders, prepared during some months of "spare time" in Army life during World War II, was published at war's end when few monographs of any sort had been gestating and when the epidemic waves of hepatitis had startled the unsuspecting medical profession poised ready to do battle with influenza. Instead of sinking in silence to the bottom of the pool, the paper made such a splash that small eddies are still stirring. The essence of the contribution was to connect vascular changes of the skin in chronic liver disease with their counterparts in normal pregnancy and to search for common denominators. The speculative threads proposed to string together the ideas and observations have proved to be elusive and tenuous. The popularity of spiders is indicated by the fact that I have collected nearly six hundred references to them since 1943. They have achieved the status of clinical acceptibility.

B. Physiology

There has been much confusion about the nature of the vascular spider. Palpation, pressure with a pencil point, or the use of a glass slide at once reveals the pulsation and direction of the blood flow. The bright red color suggests arterial blood. Nevertheless, there has been disagreement as to the nature of the lesion, whether it is essentially arterial, or venous, or both. Some of the difficulty is doubtless a consequence of the histological picture which may include thick muscle-coated artery as well as thin-walled vessels resembling veins. The observations to be recorded here for the most part simply confirm and amplify those of an earlier generation of French clinicians (118, 147, 374, 815, 816) which were extended by Patek, Post and Victor.

a. Pulsation. The pulsation imparted to the palpating finger by the central point or eminence is strong in the large lesion but may be felt with difficulty, if at all, in the smaller ones. If a glass slide is placed over even small spiders, the pulsating center may be seen. By varying the pressure, the erythematous region may be made to contract from, or expand towards the blanched periphery. In very large lesions visible pulsation of the central eminence may be observed. The coiling and angulation of the little artery which has outgrown its normal bounds imparts a whiplash effect which magnifies the pulsation. The artery springs up just as a garden hose will do when the water is suddenly turned on and the coil makes an effort to straighten out. Thus the pulsation is much more vigorous than would be found in a straight vessel of the size of a spider. Reynolds has discussed physiological aspects and philosophic implications of a coiled artery.

b. Direction of Blood Flow. The centrifugal flow is demonstrated by placing point pressure on the center, causing the legs to blanch. When the pressure is released the radicles fill instantly and the skin regains its red color.

c. Pressure. Patek and his associates published the first figures on the intravascular pressure of spiders. They found that compressing the brachial artery with a pneumatic cuff caused obliteration of pulsation in a spider on the arm when the pressure was raised to 85 mm. Hg. Pulsation returned when the cuff pressure, after further elevation, was lowered to the same level.

My studies on more than one hundred separate spiders in twenty-seven persons gave results in substantial agreement with these findings. The method used was also indirect but allowed observations to be made on the several component parts of the lesion. To the skin surrounding the spider a transparent plastic capsule was attached firmly with collodion or rubber cement. A tube from a mercury manometer was connected to a glass rod communicating freely with the interior of the capsule. Pressure could be altered at will by a rubber bulb connected to the manometer. The most satisfactory observations were obtained when the spider was situated over a flat bony surface, such as the sternum or fore-head, although similar results were obtained in other areas if the capsule could be kept in place firmly with counter pressure. The deformity produced in the skin included within the capsule and at the attached edge sometimes introduced artifacts and obscured the changes.

When the spider was exposed to gradually increasing external pressures, fading began in the marginal part of the erythematous skin at a pressure between 10 and 30 mm. Hg. In many cases this fading spread throughout the whole red area, causing the radicles to be silhouetted against a pale background. Into the newly blanched areas the larger legs of the spider pointed like fine red spokes. An ebb-and-flow pulsation was noted. Centrally, where the skin was unblanched, it manifested the same change after the manner of an opening and closing iris. As the pressure was raised by slow incre-ments, the skin was flattened against the underlying bone and the entire blush disappeared. There remained only the center and some of the large branches. These exhibited pulsatile ebb and flow as if small snake tongues were flicking in and out from the central eminence. When the pressure was between 30 and 50 mm. of Hg. the vessels were progressively obliterated centrally and generally empty when the pressure was raised above 50 mm. Hg. At this point, the body of the spider appeared as a rising and falling boss, its red color contrasting brilliantly with the pallid background from which the blood had been squeezed. It called to mind Har-vey's *punctum saliens*. Further increases in the pressure caused the body to be obliterated intermittently, but between 50 and 70 mm. of Hg. there was usually a systolic appearance which faded with diastole. Between 70 and 90 mm. of Hg. the entire vascular pattern was obliterated. The reverse sequence occurred as the pressure was reduced slowly.

The flexibility and elasticity as well as hydration of the skin, and the texture of the subcutaneous tissue had some influence on the pressure determinations. As a general rule the larger the spider, the higher the pressure required for the several stages of oblitera-tion. In two instances in which the spiders had a central elevation of 3-5 mm., the boss was not flattened and blanched until 100 mm.

of Hg. was reached. Pressure above this level usually distorted the skin and caused the capsule to ride up or break loose. With the subject supine, there were no differences in the pressure in spiders at various sites on the body (forehead, cheek, chin, clavicle, sternum, chest, shoulders, forearms, wrists, hands, and knees). No tests were made on mucosal spiders. The pulsations were more vivid and the range from beginning to complete fading greater when there was a high pulse pressure in the large arteries. The pressures in spiders in persons with liver disease, pregnancy, and deficiency diseases, and in normal persons were the same. This indicates that more than a superficial similarity exists among the several classes of spiders.

In three cases, observations made on the same lesions at intervals of ten months to a year gave identical pressures. In one instance, when a spider had faded and after several months returned with a relapse in the cirrhosis, the pressures were the same as before. In two instances pressure readings were made at short intervals during the phase of evanescence. In one, the pulsation could be noted three days after the first measurement, and the radicles disappeared two days later; after two weeks, no mark was left. It seemed that the central artery had become occluded. In the other instance there was a gradual decline in the pressure required to obliterate the spider. Three determinations made over a two-month period revealed a fall in pressure of 20 mm. of Hg per month. Pulsations could not be detected six weeks later, when the only mark was a tiny red spot. I have no observations during the stages of enlargement.

d. Lack of Fluorescence. Because fluorescence is a characteristic of certain lesions of the skin, notably the ulcerated epidermoid carcinoma exposed under the Wood light as Ronchese has demonstrated, I undertook to examine a number of vascular spiders in normal subjects, in pregnant women, and particularly in patients with cirrhosis of the liver under the Wood light. No fluorescence was observed in any of the vascular lesions of the skin. I have occasionally examined other lesions too and have found no fluorescence in any of the vascular lesions discussed in this book including cutaneous lesion found in persons with metastatic carcinoid tumor and hyperserotoninemia.

e. Temperature. Determinations of cutaneous temperature over vascular spiders have been made with a dermotherm, both on the wards and in a constant temperature room at $20°$ C. Tests were made on seven patients and more than fifty lesions. As was to be expected with arterial blood so near an exposed surface, the temperature of the skin over the spiders was higher than that of the adjacent skin. The difference was greater when the environmental temperature was cool. The difference showed variations, ranging from a barely perceptible increase in small spiders to as much as $3°$ C. in large ones. The gradient of temperature difference between spider and adjoining skin was somewhat greater in the extremities than on the face or body.

f. Local Injection of Adrenalin and Histamine. The intracutaneous or subcutaneous injection of these substances near a spider evoked the usual reactions found in normal skin. Blanching with adrenalin did not close down the larger vessels, whereas the erythema produced by histamine was more pronounced in the red area of the spider than in the adjacent skin. Similar results had been reported previously (639).

g. Changes with Menstruation. Several patients have been observed whose spiders increased in size three days before the menstrual period and remained large for two or more days of the period. In three women the same event had been noted by the patients themselves but they believed that the change coincided with, rather than preceded menstruation. Many puzzling relationships of menstruation and skin disease have been reviewed by Bulkley. He made no reference to changes such as we have seen in vascular spiders, although similar periodic variations were reported in many dermatological conditions. No studies were made to see whether the pressure within the spider underwent any variations during the menstrual cycle.

h. Hemorrhage. Bleeding from spiders is unusual; but if it occurs may be exsanguinating. It results usually from mechanical injury rather than from associated liver disease and hypoprothrombinemia. A spider bleeds with a pulsing jet of bright red arterial blood. It is not so rare for a woman during pregnancy to believe that she is dealing with a pimple, squeeze the top off a spider, and be alarmed by the spurting hemorrhage thus released.

i. Fading. Unless the site of a spider is marked the lesion may be impossible to find after death. Fading is invariable, although some of the larger spiders may remain as ghosts, recognized by a fainter tracery than is seen in life. A similar fading occurs abruptly when one is removed during life. Fading and even complete disappearance may occur when severe hemorrhage or shock with intense peripheral vasoconstriction occur. Thus a spider may disappear from view and reappear rapidly when the patient is transfused and recovery ensues.

j. Distribution. Vascular spiders of the skin have a predilection for certain sites; and their distribution presents a regularly recurring pattern with minor variations. This has been discussed only in recent years (53, 639) although case reports indicate that the observation has been made ever since the first writing on the subject (919). In general, spiders occur in largest number on the face and neck, and in decreasing frequency over the shoulders, thorax, upper arms, lower arms, backs of hands, and fingers. They are rare on the lips, ears, nail bed, palms, and very uncommon below the umbilicus where less than 1 per cent have been found. They do, however, occur on the abdomen, foreskin, thighs, knees, feet, and toes. I have not found them in the scalp, whether bald or hairy. No differences in general distribution have been noted between men and women. A better idea of their locations can be gained from Figure 4 than from Table I showing the percentage distribution, since the regions are not comparable in area. Thus they appear most thickly on the neck and face, but the total number occurring on the upper chest and shoulders is larger.

Only after some time of painstaking search did I find spiders below the level of the umbilicus. They were unmistakable, however, and pulsation could be detected in them. The cause of this arrangement has excited much speculation. Two investigators (249, 876), not having seen spiders in the lower regions, suggested that the drainage of the superior vena cava somehow determined their location. This seems improbable. There is no association of collateral circulation and the occurrence of spiders over the abdomen. It may be suggested more logically that the gradient of vascular tonus and temperature in the skin is in some way responsible. The number of spiders is greatest in areas where blushing is most intense. This territory responds most vigorously, by vasodilatation, following the intravenous injection of histamine (898) or nicotinic acid (74). The vasomotor gradient of vascular tone in the subcutaneous arteries is high where the lesions are rare, and it is lower and very labile where they are numerous. If one suspects a humoral cause, the circulating agent might be in contact with the affected vessels for longer periods in areas where the tone was not so high and the flow of blood less rapid.

Why the body is affected by spiders in so uneven a distribution is not known since lesions may occur almost anywhere in the skin. I have seen them everywhere but in the soles of the feet and high in the scalp. The factors which give rise to them are relative and not absolute. Local injury may obviously cause alteration in the skin and its blood vessels which favors the development of the spider. In one instance when a biopsy was made, healing occurred in the vascular wound and a new spider appeared having usurped the location of the old one and having its body exactly in the site of the well-healed scar. Several tiny spiders were appearing elsewhere. In the numerous charts and photographs I have accumulated have

TABLE I

DISTRIBUTION OF SPIDERS IN HEPATIC DISEASE

	Percentage
Face	10.0
Ears	0.2
Neck	12.0
Shoulders	18.0
Upper arms	18.0
Lower arms	3.0
Hands (dorsum)	2.0
Hands (palms)	0.3
Fingers	0.4
Thorax (front)	28.0
Thorax (back)	7.6
Abdomen	0.2
Lower extremities	0.3

been many examples of a single lesion fading, disappearing and re-curring at the original site. One area of the skin may have a peculiar propensity for reacting to the causative process. I have seen a spider develop at the site of abdominal paracentesis in a patient with cir-rhosis but in only one among a very large number in which para-centesis was done. A very observant patient who first had spiders during pregnancy noticed at a time when she was not pregnant that she developed spiders in a very unusual way. Following donation of a pint of blood at which the usual rubber tourniquet had been employed, a new crop of spiders appeared on the arm distal to where the tourniquet had been for about twenty minutes. They did not arise as petechiae but were characteristic spiders when seen three days after onset. Perhaps this may help explain what has oc-curred in some instances of spontaneous unilateral lesions or those confined to a single arm. I have not seen the spider occur in a pus-tule but there are comments from time to time about bee stings, spider and insect bites, and local minor injury being predisposing causes. I have never been able to produce them by repeated minor injury. I have repeatedly punctured the skin with a needle, injected histamine or nicotinic acid into the skin or by other means pro-duced local injury. The observations of Clark and Clark on the stimulating effects of inflammation on the development of arterio-venous shunts may have a bearing on the problem.

Martini has discussed at some length the problem of localiza-tion of spiders and he has been inclined to believe that the major factor responsible for their accumulation on the face and upper part of the body is exposure to sunlight, everyday wear and tear, wind, rain, cold, and heat. In my experience there has been a considerable concentration of these lesions on the chest and back in men and women who had never had much exposure to sunlight either at work or play. One of Martini's amusing observations concerned a patient who had a good many spiders in the lower part of the body as well as the upper part. This patient had been an actively prac-ticing nudist and it was Martini's contention that exposure of the lower part of the body to the sunlight and weather had conditioned the skin so that when the spiders developed, they appeared in pro-fusion where they are not ordinarily seen. The patient's sudden shyness prevented Martini from getting a photograph. I have had no chance to examine fan dancers, striptease artists, or models for the more exotic calendars to see whether nudity under klieg lights would have such an effect. This problem will have to be attacked experimentally by exposing susceptible persons to sunlight during pregnancy. Cirrhotics should have various parts of the body exposed to the sunlight before and after liver function deteriorates.

The influence of nerves in localization has been suspected in persons with all the spiders confined to a single arm or one side of the body. At times several spiders will be arranged in a row along the axis of a custaneous nerve. These are exceptions. There is no consistent pattern of distribution along nerves such as has been suggested in angiomatosis in the trigeminal area.

I have pondered the question of whether spiders are ever internal structures in various organs besides appearing along the lumen of hollow and tubular organs as on the outside of the body. It is well established that, though uncommon, they may occur along the lining of the alimentary canal. We do not have any indication that they exist elsewhere. Some suggestions of a vascular alteration in the liver have been cited. I have observed unusual dilatations of the smaller portal vessels within the liver but nothing like the angiomatous change which Martini and his colleagues have observed in some patients with Osler's disease.

The relation of the distribution of these lesions to exposure to repeated minor trauma must be considered also, for their occurrence in the skin of the face, neck, and the back of the hand is frequent. Exposure to weather and to radiant energy may be a factor. This is strongly suggested by Broq's work. If the metabolism were high in warmer parts of the skin, it might influence the segregation of spiders in warmer areas. Whether histamine plays any part is uncertain. Evidence that local infection is frequently responsible for the production of spiders has not been substantial.

By an ingenious method of photoelectric plethysmography, Hertzman has estimated the richness of the arterial supply of the skin in the following descending order—finger pad, ear lobe, toe pad, palm or hand, skin of forehead and face, dorsum of finger, dorsum of hand, dorsum of foot, forearm, knee, and tibia. It is apparent that the localization of spiders has no exact connection with vascularity of different regions as measured by this technique. Altogether, the suggestions so far adduced are not impressive. The most promising speculation appears to be the one which relates the distribution pattern to the constant variations in vascular tone near the surface of the body. The pattern of density would thus be a function of the arterial vasomotor tone in the skin. The pattern of regional blood flow may have some contributing effect, but it is probably small.

C. GROSS AND MICROSCOPIC STRUCTURE

Systematic study of the histology, histopathology and histophysiology of the vascular spider was neglected for a long time although some texts on the histopathology of the skin offer brief remarks on the subject (579). There has been much disagreement over the kind of vessel mainly implicated, also differences of opinion as to whether the spider is fundamentally an angioma, implying neoplasia, a telangiactasis, or both, and whether the affected vessels are veins or arteries, or both. The confusion was reduced greatly by the work of Patek, Post and Victor. Real advance in this field has come with the brilliant studies of Martini, Staubesand, Nödl, and their associates.

Any effort to understand the aberrant structures under consideration must be based on knowledge of the normal blood vessels of the skin. One of the early students of this problem, Joseph-Louis Renaut, described and pictured a very characteristic nutrient artery supplying the skin, in his treatise on histology which appeared in 1889. He noted the frequent occurrence of a small end-artery in the subcutis which branched in radial fashion in one or more planes at right angles to the axial trunk and parallel to the skin surface. From the smaller branches nutrient arterioles spread in profusion, finally distributing the blood to the capillaries. This small artery supplied a blunt cone-shaped region of skin and subcutaneous tissue. Blood from the region thus supplied was collected into venules in a meshwork surrounding it. The over-all architectural plan was similar to that in Mall's stellate arteries in the stomach and the stars of Verheyen in the kidney. Some such arrangement is usual wherever the blood supply to any surface is abundant. Stellate arteries were pictured by Krogh. It may be concluded that a stellate artery is a normal structure in the skin, but that it cannot be detected by inspection because of its small size.

According to Spalteholz the skin is supplied with blood from numerous arteries with well developed muscle coats which make their way to the epidermis. They divide into small branches and anastomose with each other. They are so arranged that ultimately three or four anastomotic nets are formed parallel to the skin surface, the fascial, the cutaneous, the subpapillary net and eventually the subcutaneous net. From the subpapillary net the small arterial branches originate, form end arteries and break up into capillaries. The cutaneous network of vessels supplies a system which regulates the amount of circulation in the skin. Spalteholz explained the small white spots in the skin as cone-shaped areas, each supplied by a single, terminal artery. Thus he believed that the skin could be divided according to arterial supply into numerous autonomous regions, each supplied by an end artery.

Other observers believe that such cone shaped regions must be microscopic and that the spots in the skin are the result of certain arrangement of the vascular and nervous system and that the white spots on the skin can be explained only on the basis of changes in the caliber of many of the vessels. There is no doubt that the central artery of the spider originates in the subcutis and winding ascends to a point directly under the epidermis where it branches into its end "arteries." The same holds true for the very earliest lesions, the punctate vessel which appear in white spots. When one observes the phenomena of a white spot, and all its transitions, the appearance of a small punctum, central vessel with small branches, and finally large vascular spider with a white halo, it appears that we are dealing with various forms of the same basic structure. By using fine techniques it can be demonstrated that the temperature in the center of the white spot is a few tenths of a degree higher than the periphery, (557). Thus we have to assume that under abnormal conditions of blood flow, changes in the pressure or other factors change vessels which ordinarily are invisible into visible ones. It would appear that the basic change is ectasia of preexisting vessels.

The clinic provides two demonstrations of the pattern of circulation in the skin. Both are accentuations of the normal vascular mottling which may be seen in exposed portions of the arms and legs, especially in young persons, during cold damp weather. In *livedo recticularis,* a disturbance in vascular function makes the paler islands stand out against a cyanotic background (Chapter IV, Section 4). The other condition, in which the reticulated network is pigmented, *cutis marmorata* or *erythema ab igne,* develops in regions exposed for long periods to heat. Vascular spiders often begin in the pale center surrounded by the darker reticulum of slightly mottled skin in normal persons or those with hepatic disease, but exceptions to this arrangement have been noted also.

Although Gilbert and Herscher reported some histological details, Williams and Snell appear to have been the first to suggest a relationship between the spider and the glomus body. In their review they presented excellent photographs of the large elevated pulsating spider, and in histological sections they demonstrated glomic tissue in the basilar angiomatous portion of the lesion. Their photomicrograph displays an example of a blood vessel whose wall shows on one side a mass of "epithelioid" cells and on the other a nearly normal muscular coat. The dilated, thin-walled, superficial vessels—the telangiectatic legs—may be seen clearly. It is unfortunate that they confused the spider with the vascular lesion characteristic of Osler's disease with its atrophic, attenuated arterial wall.

Patek, Post and Victor enlarged upon these observations. They stated that "the acquired type of spider * * * does not conform to descriptions of the congenital lesions," and ably demonstrated this fact in histological sections cut serially. Of interest was their discovery of two types of lesions. One consisted of an abnormally large artery rising from the subcutis, branching into arterioles, and terminating in capillaries. Except for its size it was identical with the artery of Renaut. Two of their seven lesions fell into this class. The others were of the "glomus" type. In it "the afferent artery is of medium size, with a single layer of endothelium resting on an internal elastic lamella, and a media composed of circular muscle fibers. At the junction of this artery with the central vessel of the 'spider' the endothelium and the internal elastic lamella become separated

by a thick layer of cells with elongated oval nuclei, abundant cytoplasm and indistinct cell borders. The nuclei are about as long and
half again as wide as those of the smooth muscle cells of the arterial
media. They have a more diffuse distribution of chromatin and
are more widely separated. From the varying shapes and directions
of the long axes of the nuclei the cells seem to run circularly, longitudinally, and diagonally. The internal elastic lamella and the
media of circular muscle of the afferent artery continue into the
central vessel to form the outer portion of its wall. In the central
vessel the elastic lamella becomes thinner, loses its wavy character
and finally disappears after breaking into delicate threads. The
muscle fibers of the outer media retain the circular direction present in the afferent artery." It was emphasized that this structure
was not a glomus body because there was no arteriovenous shunt.
The lumen became progressively narrower; the many branches
finally emptied into capillaries. Proximal branches retained a
single layer of endothelium and inner cellular layer but lacked the
external layer of muscle. They suggested that this structure was
the result of metaplasia of already existing arteries in the skin, a
process which caused them to resemble glomus vessels, and of their
subsequent hyperplasia.

Walsh and Becker, in their review of erythema palmare and
naevus-araneus-like telangiectases, included a low-power view of a
section of a spider. They stated that "the lesion, reconstructed from
serial sections, seemed to consist chiefly of an arteriole branching
from one of the arteries just within the subcutis. This vessel tra-
versed a somewhat tortuous course to about the subpapillary layer
of the cutis. Here it seemed to change directly into a vein of comparable size without intervening capillaries, which in turn divided
into the network of smaller venules which form the gross spider-like
appearance. It had a muscular wall of about normal thickness for
a vessel of its size (0.25 mm.) and was accompanied by a nerve whose
fibers seemed to end in the vessel wall." Despite this description
they called the lesion a small arteriovenous anastomosis.

Murray and Stout have shown by the tissue culture method that
the "epithelioid" cell of the glomus is derived from Zimmermann's
pericyte, a modified smooth-muscle cell. In their photomicrographs

the various stages of development may be seen in convincing detail. The almost imperceptible graduations in the glomus canal (Suc-quet-Hoyer) from arterial smooth-muscle cell to "epithelioid" cell to venous smooth-muscle cell, as well as the contractile power of each of the three types, speak for an affinity of "epithelioid" cell and muscle cell.

The glomus cell has well defined characteristics which are most pronounced wherever it is most highly differentiated from the smooth muscle of artery and vein. Many gradations occur between the glomus and the muscle cell, and mixed cells with some of the histological characteristics of both may be found. The aspect of the glomus cell varies considerably, depending upon the compactness or looseness of the tissue in which it occurs. These cells are round for the most part, and have large, dark-staining nuclei in the center surrounded by a clear zone of cytoplasm which stains little or not at all. Reticulin fibers appear between adjacent cells. According to Murray and Stout, the usual picture of many tightly packed cells distorts the real character of the individual cell. In their study of tissue cultures of glomus cells the "epithelioid" markings changed into those typical of the pericyte of Zimmermann.

a. Observations. Vascular spiders were studied histologically during my early investigation whenever a biopsy or autopsy speci-men could be obtained. The first few lesions studied in this manner were sectioned only once or twice. A very confusing picture resulted, in part because of the distortion from its living form which occurs in the skin and its nutrient vessels when a small portion is removed from the anchorage of the surrounding tissue. The piece removed shrinks to less than half its normal size and becomes irregularly puckered and wrinkled. The vessels disappear from sight as soon as the incision is made for a biopsy. This source of difficulty has been partly obviated by fastening the specimen to cork with pins so that it retains its proper size, but some distortion persists. It is well to remember Knisely's admonition regarding the size of small ves-sels: "* * * For after the abuse which the tissue undergoes in death and fixation, shrinking and swelling in various reagents, a capillary's diameter has no known or knowable relationship to the size or sizes that it had in life."

Attempts to obtain sections in which the original relationships were not destroyed have not succeeded. Repeated efforts at *intra vitam* injection *in situ* have resulted in profuse spurting hemorrhages, whether the cannula was directed toward the central boss, the stem artery, or one of the larger radicles. If some scheme can be devised which will enable the injection and fixation of the intact vessels and subsequent clearing of the specimen, or dissection, it will reveal the more complex aspects of its structure in their normal relations.

Serial sections of twenty eight individual lesions from eleven subjects with hepatic disease have been examined. This work was done in collaboration with Dr. Seaton Sailer. Unfortunately the entire collection of slides got lost after Dr. Sailer's death in World War II and has never been found. My feelings about all the lost specimens and sections was expressed in another context in Shakespeare's Richard III, "That bottled spider, that foul, hunchback'd toad." Resisting a desire to drop the whole matter, this section was prepared from incomplete notes. Spiders were taken from the skin of the neck, shoulder, chest, back, upper and lower arm. An extension of this phase of the work to include spiders in pregnancy and in normal persons is fundamental to further understanding of the subject. The ensuing discussion is based on observations limited to spiders from persons with hepatic disease. Careful inspection of the vascular spider during life, and subsequent study of the same lesion cut in serial section have elucidated some of the questions not answered by either method when employed alone.

In gross structure the spider may be compared to a branching coral formation whose fronds radiate in a narrow plane parallel to and just below the skin and perpendicular to the main axis of the gnarled or coiled stem. Some lesions call to mind the stump of an uprooted tree. A few spiders with the central eminence elevated reproduce in miniature the caput medusae. A prominent part of the structure, the coiled and tortuous main stem artery, has not received careful study, although it has been noted by others (634, 888, 914). In some instances when the superficial vessels have been scanty, the upper end of this vessel examined during life with retrograde illumination resembled in shape the coiled arteries of the endometrium (46). In the case of both spiral vessels the conclusion is inescapable that the deformity has resulted from an overgrowth of the vessel between two relatively fixed points.

Figure 6 pictures the spider schematically. Many legs or radicles branch from the central punctum or body. The latter may remain below the level of the skin's surface, but large lesions almost invariably elevate the overlying skin in a rounded knob or boss. The structure of the body is very hard to appraise correctly because the irregular contractions of muscle and elastic tissue produce bizarre deformities when the vessels are removed. During life it appears to be an aneurysmal dilatation in some cases, and an irregular knot of branching vessels in others.

The spider legs are large centrally and decrease in size as they branch irregularly toward the periphery. Macroscopic anastomoses

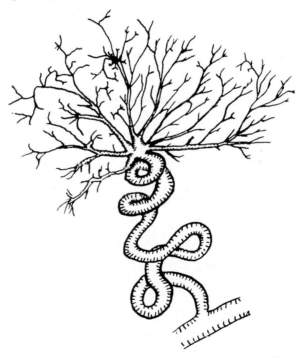

Figure 6. Schematic drawing of an arterial spider showing the coiled artery, the central boss or body, the branches some of which end in secondary knobs or satellite spiders. In addition anastomoses between the small vein-like branches are shown.

may be seen between the larger or smaller vessels but they are uncommon. With a magnification of twenty times, anastomoses not otherwise noticed may be detected. In form the legs may be gracile or knobby, straight or crooked, threadlike or bulbous. It is usual for different forms to exist in a single lesion. Gaps may appear in the course taken by a single radicle as it dips deeper below the surface or when the caliber of the vessel undergoes attenuation, suggesting local irregularities in tonus of the muscle wall or sparsity of muscle fibers. Bulbous dilatations and beading also occur. When the entire area covered by the spider is coated with oil and studied with a dissecting microscope or with a slit lamp, not infrequently one finds connecting legs leading to small satellites which display all the characteristics of the large lesion on a reduced scale.

b. Histology. The most typical spiders consist of a coiled artery with glomus cells in its wall. This artery decreases in size as it gives off branches of similar cellular structure whose walls rapidly lose thickness, although the lumen may increase in diameter as they are traced peripherally. This type of spider differs from the typical artery of Renaut in these respects: the presence of so large an artery so near the skin surface, the presence of glomus cells, and the wide dilatation of the vessels branching from the main artery.

Type I: In only three of our specimens from which many sections were cut did we fail to find glomus cells. In other respects the gross architecture was the same in these specimens as in those with glomus cells. They correspond to the first class of lesions decribed by Patek, Post and Victor.

Type II: Spiders in which the glomus cell, or the pericyte of Zimmermann, is found might be divided into several grades, depending on the prevalence or rarity of these cells. In some of the specimens the finer histological picture corresponded exactly with that reported previously. Others displayed striking differences consisting in the main of irregular distributions of the pericytes or glomus cells.

Serial sections of the stem artery might first cut an area where the muscle and glomus cells were placed in concentric arrangement in symmetrical rings; next would come a sudden or gradual thinning of these cells until the artery did not differ from a normal

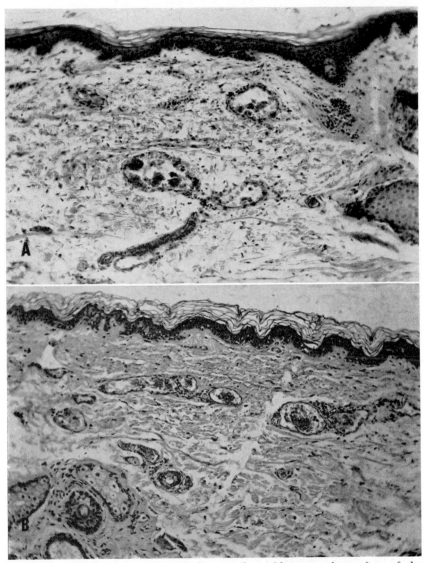

Figure 7.   Histological section of the vascular spider near the surface of the skin.   *A*. Near the center, below the surface, is a thin-walled vessel, a typical leg or radicle.   Smaller vessels are seen at the same level to the left.   Two large thin-walled vessels branching from a narrow, thicker artery cut in longitudinal section which points to the lower left-hand corner where it has been cut transversely.   *B*. Thin-walled vessels of various diameters near the surface including one or more of the radicles.

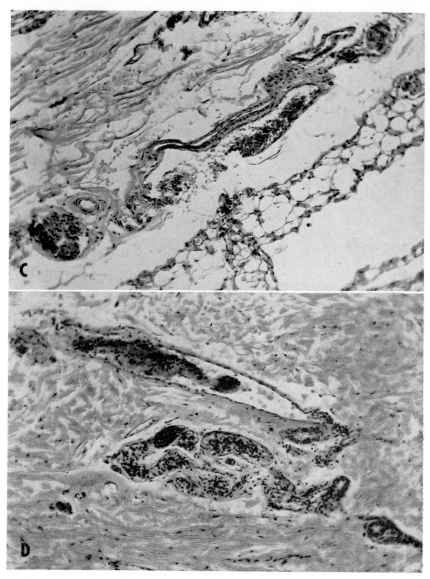

C. Section cut near the end of the coiled artery as it breaks up into "veins," showing both types of vessels in close proximity. This photograph gives an indication of the artifacts introduced by fixing and cutting the sections. *D.* In the upper portion is a spider leg, cut along the long axis seen just as it has emerged from the body or coiled artery. Different varieties of branches may be seen in different areas where the coiled artery is cut.

artery in such a region; then, following a course towards the surface of the skin, the wall of the vessel would continue substantially the same on one side but on the other a great piling-up of glomus cells would appear. This was not the result of cutting at an angle for it occurred on either the acute or obtuse side of a kink. Sometimes in the same main-stem artery, a second cuff of widening in the vessel wall was seen, with the same packing of glomus cells. This gave the impression of a gross beading of the external aspect of the vessel but the lumen remained about the same in diameter. Some of the beads were eccentric, as though strung far from their true center.

In most instances the body or boss seemed to have been de- formed by the contractile forces which acted without counter-pull

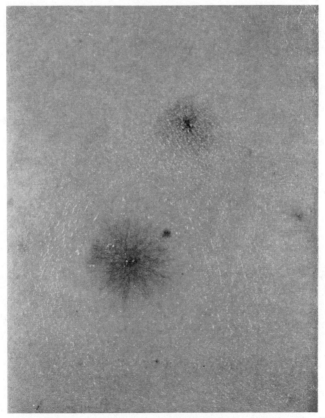

Figure 8. A comparison of the appearance of spiders covered with oil (below), and as they appeared in the untouched skin (above).

after the specimen was removed and before it was fixed. Many contained the same type of cells which occurred in the main arterial trunk. A few had very thin walls without muscle or pericyte cells. Irregularly disposed branches at their proximal attachment usually possessed the same variety of wall as the central punctum. The thick irregular heaping-up of compact pericytes was found in most cases.

Legs of the spider repeated the changing patterns found in the main coiled artery. Near the site of their emergence they usually had thick walls with smooth-muscle cells and pericytes, sometimes commingled, sometimes segregated. As the periphery was approached there was a well marked tendency for the wall to lose both muscle and pericyte. At the point of branching or of a sharp angu-

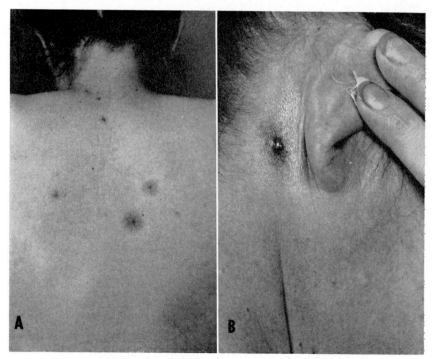

Figure 9. *Left.* Photograph of the back of a patient with cirrhosis revealing large spiders in the relatively unexposed central region of the back and smaller spiders on the exposed upper portion of the back of the neck. *Right.* A large spider projecting 6 mm. above the surface of the skin in the mastoid region. The central body with its red highlight is vaguely suggestive of a *black widow spider.* The area of erythema is apparent.

lation, however, there was more often than not an accumulation of pericytes. Most characteristic of these vessels was their relatively large size and very thin wall, not more than two cells thick. These vessels sometimes arose directly from the central eminence with the thin coat they retained throughout their course. In others there was a gradual transformation from thick-walled artery to thin-walled blood vessel. Some radicles showed the beading phenomenon with regular or eccentric bulges of the vascular coat caused by congregations of pericytes. Just beneath the skin they were uniformly thin-walled and distended with blood.

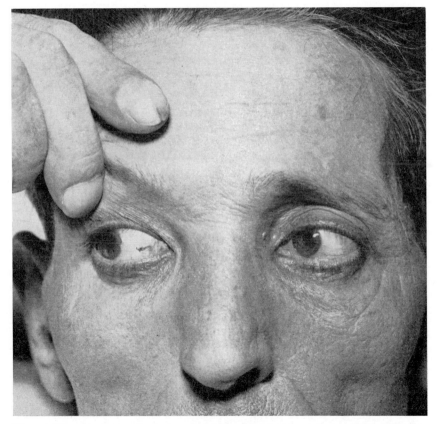

Figure 10.   Angiomatous lesion in the conjunctiva of a patient with far-advanced cirrhosis showing the aneurysmal dilatation of the vessels and clubbing of the fingers.

It should be emphasized that the vascular spider is not an arteriovenous anastomosis in any ordinary sense. The blood flowing rapidly, under high pressure, comes up through the spiral artery to the punctum, whence it flows peripherally through the legs or radicles, which may look like veins or arteries but nonetheless carry arterial blood. From this point the vessels decrease in caliber, their walls become attenuated, and they pass into a capillary bed which is spread throughout the area supplied by the main vessel. Finally, capillaries have a peripheral confluence in small veins tributary to the collecting veins which carry the venous blood back into larger channels. This promiscuous association of veins and arteries is unique. It has given rise to confusion and ambiguity because in the past the arterial spider normally has been categorized as artery or vein, depending on the dominant structure included in a random section.

There is no careful study of the nerves for possible influence in the development of spiders. Vasomotor tone, vascular reactivity, and the neurohumeral control of blood flow as related to spiders are areas of physiology not yet explored.

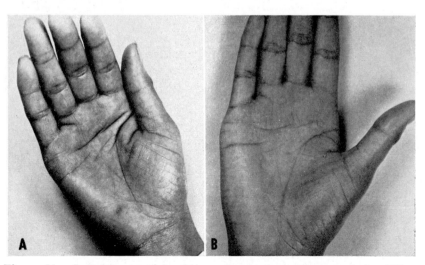

Figure 11. *Left.* An arterial spider and palmar erythema of the diffuse, mottled variety in the hand of a negro woman during pregnancy. *Right.* Follow-up photograph demonstrating the disappearance of the spider and the fading of the palmar erythema after delivery.

Many of the questions left unanswered in our early study of the spider have been clarified by the extensive reconstructions of spiders and other vascular lesions of the skin which have come in recent years from Germany. Martini and Staubesand have made elegant serial sections with reconstruction of the lesions and have expounded the details of the minute structure in a classic study. It is now possible to form a satisfactory opinion of the ordinary structure of the spider along lines which I had hoped to complete years ago. The following discussion is almost a literal translation of appropriate passages in the article of Martini and Staubesand.

While individual variations occurred in the spiders obtained from eighteen persons between sixteen and fifty eight years of age, fourteen with cirrhosis, two pregnant and two normal persons, the standard pattern was constant within narrow limits. There was no substantial variation in the basic structure observed. As far as histopathology is concerned, the subcutis and corium in the areas where spiders occur have no abnormalities to suggest a pathologic process in the connective tissue. The elastic fiber network was normal all the way through to the papillary layer. There was a considerable accumulation of large, closely packed sweat glands in the neighborhood of spiders. Various parts of the spider which were regularly identified included the cutaneous arterial network, the central spider artery, subepidermal ampulla or body, radially arranged efferent vessels and the capillaries. The reconstruction reproduced in Figure 12 was obtained through the courtesy of Dr. Martini. It begins with an artery with a diameter of 350 micra and walls 45 micra thick. It is a normal cutaneous artery with inner elastic layer arranged in typical corrugations. The primary branch of this vessel, the central artery of the spider, has a wall constructed similarly to that of any artery of the vascular type. The other branch in the figure has a large diameter with an eccentric lumen. Studies of many central arteries of spiders reveal characteristic pictures of the vessel wall regardless of whether the section is oblique or longitudinal. The media on one side of the cross section is thick and composed of numerous muscle fibers while on the other side there are only one or two layers of muscle fibers. The thick portion of the wall does not protrude like a cushion into the lumen. In the thick regions most nuclei belong to muscle cells and are oriented with the long axis of the vessel but some are round, drop-like or dumbbell-like. The internal elastic membrane of the central artery of the spider can be made out clearly only in the proximal segment. Distally it thins out and ultimately disappears. There is no evidence

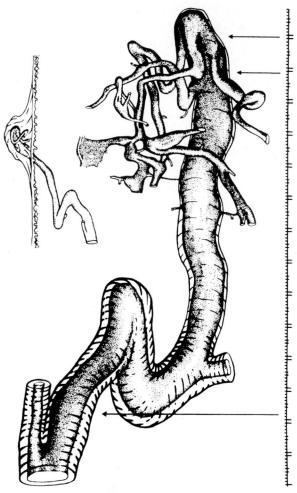

Figure 12. A graphic reconstruction of the spider in a sixteen year old girl, illustrating the large thick-walled artery, and the details of the spider legs, the venous structure, and the satellite lesion. The portion of the lesion which protrudes above the skin is indicated in the small sketch. (Courtesy of Dr. Martini.)

of degenerative changes or sclerosis. The endothelium is completely normal. Small myelinated nerves occur in the adventitia which also contains a network of very thin venules. As the central

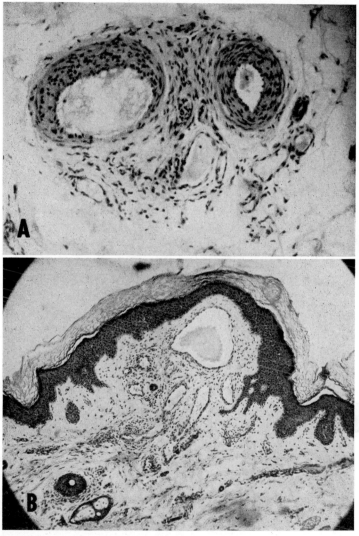

Figure 13.   Two sections from the reconstructed spider with the level of the two sections indicated by the lines in Figure 12.   The lower photograph illustrates the ampullary portion of the body of the spider and several branching, curving legs.   (Courtesy of Dr. Martini.)

artery of the spider progresses in spiral fashion toward the epidermis, the characteristic structure of its walls becomes less and less pronounced, the media thins, the vessel takes on the appearance of a vein, and finally, next to the epidermis it gives the impression of a wide blood sinus (Figure 13). At this level the vessel wall consists merely of an endothelial tube with very few muscle fibers. Ordinarily the ampulla of the spider is collapsed and bloodless; sometimes it contains blood, and the epithelium is flattened. Occasionally in this area there is a homogenous layer of tissue, poor in nuclei, between the endothelial layer and the adventitia of the vessel, comprising mostly connective tissue. The ampullary portion protrudes above the surface of the surrounding skin and the papillae are obliterated so that the contact zone between the epidermis and the corium is smooth. At the peak of the elevation over the spider body the germinal layers of the epidermis are reduced to a thickness of about four cells, and the cornified layer is shriveled and compressed. The legs of the spider branch off the ampulla. In their walls, most muscle fibers run longitudinally but a few are circular though they do not form definite bundles and are rather sparse. The vessels therefore resemble veins rather than arteries. Most of them extend out toward the periphery where they form communications with capillaries and so the blood is returned to the venous system. Contrary to observations that had been made on the material which Sailer and I collected, Martini and Staubesand did not find many epitheloid cells.

In four of the eighteen specimens relatively large arteriovenous anastomoses were found in the subcutaneous tissue in the region of the spider (Figure 14). They were all bridge anastomoses devoid of epithelial cells. In the zone of transition from the arterial branch into the wide and thin-walled venous segment there was a sphincter-like arrangement of the muscle fibers which could produce marked reduction of the lumen. A definitely dilated capillary net was observed in close relationship to the venous segment of the anastomosis and the spider veins. This might account for the diffuse pink background of the vascular spider. The relationship of these anastomoses to the vascular spiders was that they both emptied into the same large cutaneous vein. A valve on the side of the entrance of the venous branch of the anastomosis into the vein assures the flow of blood from the anastomosis into the larger vein.

No differences were found between vascular spiders in the skin of healthy persons, pregnant women, or patients with liver

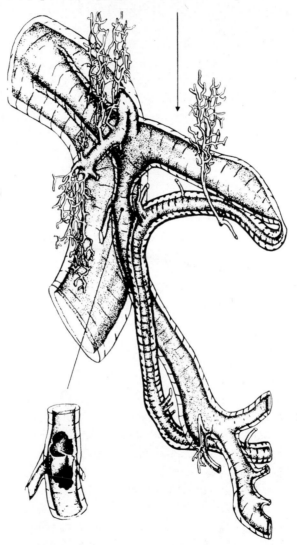

Figure 14. Graphic reconstruction of an arteriovenous anastomosis in the subcutis near a spider, indicating the situation of the sphincter and throttle mechanism described in the text. (Courtesy of Dr. Martini.)

disease. It was Martini's view that the arteriovenous shunt might have an important drainage value for the spider. The thin-walled vessels beyond the central artery of the spider are loaded with a great accumulation of blood which must drain slowly through the corresponding capillary beds. It is well known that the sum of the diameters of skin veins is much larger than ordinarily needed for drainage of the available blood. The circulatory load of the spider introduces a risk of stagnation of blood in the capillaries which would be reduced by an arteriovenous shunt. The speed in the neighboring veins is very rapid owing to great flow. The white halo around spiders thus may result from a rapid drainage of blood produced by the arteriovenous shunt.

D. CLINICAL OBSERVATIONS

It became apparent early in my studies that there was no commonly used test of hepatic function nor any clinical sign of liver disease which was invariably associated with the presence of the vascular spider in a particular patient, at a given instant. This held true for a large series of function tests and for all the diagnostic signs of cirrhosis. There were correlations, however, which showed significant trends. When a comparison was made between a group of persons with hepatic disease and spiders, and a similar group with no spiders, two facts emerged. Spiders were more frequent when the hepatic disease was severe than when mild; and they occurred more often in chronic than in brief diseases. There were enough exceptions to invalidate such a rule in individual cases.

A clinical and laboratory study of particular cases over a long period of time indicated that no sign or symptom heralded the coming of vascular spiders; and when they were established, no change in function or sign anticipated their disappearance. When jaundice was deepening, or ascites accumulating, new spiders were apt to appear, or old ones to return, or existing ones to enlarge, but exceptions occurred often enough to exclude these events as measures of the specific agency which was also responsible for the changes in the vessels of the skin. Likewise clinical improvement often presaged the disappearance of a spider, but occasionally it did not. Moreover, in a particular patient one vascular spider might appear or enlarge while another simultaneously faded or disappeared. This suggested the probability of a dual causation, some local force working on the skin vessels affected, as well as an underlying humoral cause associated with disease of the liver.

In chronic hepatic disease, arterial spiders may develop before other clinical evidence of cirrhosis. The age at onset varies with the epoch at which cirrhosis occurs. Spiders tend to vary in phase with the disease. Explosive bursts of spiders commence as a single tiny red point, often occurring in the center of an island of somewhat pale skin surrounded by a darker region. The tiny red spot then appears to throw out legs. These enlarge and branch. As growth continues the central punctum becomes elevated and the surrounding anemic halo persists, enlarging as its inner edge retreats before the encroaching vein-like legs and erythema of the spider. When spiders disappear, the whole structure may vanish so nearly like the one-hoss shay that one cannot say what part disappeared first. Presumably vasospasm or thrombosis may destroy a spider. Sometimes the radicals lose distal branches and become attenuated, the erythema fades and finally the central red punctum alone remains. Pulsation diminishes, then fails. The center gradually fades, occasionally leaving a faint speck of brown pigment and a suggestion of atrophy of the skin, though often nothing indicates its old site even with photographs to identify the area.

In normal persons, there is a tendency, perhaps dependent on awakening self-consciousness, for spiders to be noted during adolescence.

a. Spiders in Children. I know of no figures obtained from pediatric clinics on the incidence of spiders in well children and well babies, though I suspect that it runs reasonably close to the 10-15% incidence of spiders in "normal" persons. Their natural evolution over a long period of time is unknown.

In several monographs and articles on liver disease in children, spiders are not mentioned at all or it is stated that they do not occur in children with chronic hepatic disorders. It is time to lay this ghost. Spiders and palmar erythema may appear in classic form, even in young children with severe or protracted disease of the liver. Fortunately cirrhosis is not common in children but when

TABLE II

The Occurrence of Vascular Spiders in Persons With Hepatic Disease

Type	White Men		White Women		Negro Men		Negro Women		Totals	
	With Spiders	Without Spiders	With Spiders	Without Spiders	With Spiders	Without Spiders	With Spiders	Without Spiders	With Spiders	Without Spiders
Laennec's cirrhosis	102	27	39	1	3	13	2	4	146	58
Cirrhosis and hepatoma	7	3	2	1	1	1	—	—	10	5
Cardiac cirrhosis	10	21	2	8	1	4	—	1	13	34
"Fatty liver"	4	2	—	3	—	2	—	—	4	7
Hemochromatosis	4	7	—	—	—	—	—	—	4	7
Hepatitis	42	75	5	18	1	7	—	—	48	100
Post-arsphenamine hepatitis	1	1	—	—	1	1	—	—	2	2
Post-bismuth hepatitis	—	—	1	—	—	—	—	—	1	—
Weil's disease	1	6	—	—	—	4	—	—	1	10
Gumma of liver	1	1	1	—	1	—	—	—	3	1
Chronic alcoholism and lobar pneumonia	2	18	—	5	—	11	—	—	2	38
Common-duct stone with jaundice	3	10	1	12	2	5	2	7	6	34
Carcinoma of the head of the pancreas	3	12	2	8	—	7	—	4	5	31
Carcinoma of rectum with hepatic metastasis	—	3	1	3	1	3	—	—	2	9
Felty's syndrome	1	—	—	—	—	—	—	—	1	—
Wilson's disease	2	3	1	2	—	—	—	—	3	5
Total	183	189	55	84	9	58	4	16	261	341

they have cirrhosis the vascular changes in the skin are the same as in adults. Boys and girls are affected equally. While the neglect of the clinical manifestations of liver disease is unfortunate, the positive error of denying that spiders appear in children with serious disease of the liver is an example of casual indifference to facts. As an index of the low esteem of clinical observation, it reflects the contemporary trend away from the natural history of disease.

In Table II are listed all patients with hepatic disease examined for vascular spiders. The numbers do not indicate the relative incidence of the several diseases, since only cases personally observed are included. The proportion of cases with vascular spiders is much higher than would be found in a study primarily based on hepatic disease (687). Because of the cooperation and interest of the house staff, examples were found before the nature of the underlying disease was established, thus weighting my figures on the positive side. In some cases spiders were not found until a later hospital admission, or until repeated tours of inspection had been made.

E. Laboratory Studies

An analysis of routine laboratory tests in persons with chronic liver disease, taken at random times, shows no degree of abnormality invariably associated with spiders nor any inevitable level of normality where spiders never occur. Definite trends in such figures bear out the well established fact that spiders, in incidence of those affected, and in number and size, increase in parallel with the severity and duration of disease of the parenchymal cells. Where serial tests were made over long periods of time changes for the better were associated with a decrease in size and numbers of spiders and in the frequency of persons having them, while the opposite trend of increase in spiders with worsening of the disease is the usual.

Of the first twenty-five patients with cirrhosis and spiders followed for four years, all but eight were known to be dead (two could not be traced). Only three of twenty-three cirrhotic patients with no spiders were dead after the same length of time. This is in keeping with the observation that spiders occur in severe hepatic disease.

These observations on Laennec's cirrhosis were extended by studying patients with other kinds of jaundice and other indications of hepatic failure. Although the spider has been found most often in cirrhosis, and most articles about its relation to disease of the liver are based on this type of hepatic disease (687), its occurrence in a wide variety of affections of the liver becomes obvious from inspection of Table II. In addition to the cases of Laennec's cirrhosis in which spiders were found, they were discovered also in patients with cardiac cirrhosis, fatty liver, and hemochromatosis. Their presence in such a high proportion of the cases of hepatitis was surprising. No spiders were seen to develop during the acute phase in some dozens of cases of hepatitis I observed in soldiers in 1942. Turner had seen them in this condition; not more often, however, than in a similar group of non-jaundiced normal controls. The lesions were less numerous and smaller than in the more protracted hepatic diseases so that many would have been overlooked without careful and repeated search. Among the few patients suffering from toxic hepatitis there were several with spiders. One patient whose illness was diagnosed as Weil's disease (unverified) had spiders. Spiders were rare in persons affected with carcinoma of the head of the pancreas with chronic jaundice. This formed an exception to the rule that prolonged hepatic disease favors the eruption of spiders. The other hepatic diseases associated with spiders are represented by such scanty material that the significance is not clear. No further evidence is needed to demonstrate the nonspecificity of the kind of hepatic lesion which may serve as a background for the spider. Thus it was concluded that neither a special type of hepatic disease, nor the severity nor chronicity of this disease was invariably responsible for the advent of vascular spiders. Nevertheless, chronic and severe cirrhosis was the chief offender.

Case Report

Case 1. C. W., a fifty-year-old white man, had used excessive quantities of spirits during most of his adult life, having taken all available varieties of beverage and non-beverage alcohol. During the recent past his drinking had abated somewhat because he could no longer tolerate his former liberal allowance. Five years before his first admission to the hospital he had jaundice which lasted for ten weeks and kept him in bed. Troublesome nose bleeds had complicated this illness. He recovered with no apparent sequelae and was well for a year. He then had a second attack of jaundice which was associated with abdominal swelling. His family physician warned him against further drinking, but soon after recovery he fell into his usual habits. In spite of his alcoholism he was able to eat an adequate diet until a few months before his *first admission* to the Medical Service of the Cincinnati General Hospital, on January 3, 1939. Here he presented himself in a sorry plight; jaundiced, comatose, and nearly exsanguinated from bleeding esophageal varices. This crisis occurred shortly after a particularly prolonged spree at Christmas time.

Physical examination was notable for the complete picture of hepatic cirrhosis it revealed. The patient was in deep shock, with a rapid, thready pulse, low blood pressure, sweating and cyanotic extremities, which were cold and clammy. The color of the skin, a grey-green-yellow, indicated the presence of jaundice as well as hemorrhagic shock. His breath was strong with the disagreeable mousey odor of hepatic fetor. Careful inspection of the skin disclosed a few small spiders. During a period of transfusions, as his red cells were restored towards normal, many additional spiders could be seen (Figure 15). Other evidences of cirrhosis included a swollen, tense abdomen with demonstrable ascites and many collateral veins. There was edema of the legs and feet. When the ascites had been reduced by paracentesis the liver was found to be small and the spleen palpably enlarged. Even after the hemorrhage had stopped and the hemoglobin was restored, he remained in coma for several days, but finally rallied in spite of what had seemed inevitable disaster.

When he was convalescing his diet was made rich in vitamins and carbohydrate, although he was not given any concentrates or crystalline vitamins. When he was ready for discharge, six weeks after entry, it was found that his spiders had decreased in number from sixteen to seven. Many of the smaller ones had disappeared leaving no trace. Where the larger ones had vanished a small area of atrophic skin, usually with traces of brown pigment, gave the only indication of anything abnormal.

Interval: In spite of the most urgent warning the patient resumed his custom of steady drinking, interspersed with sprees of more pronounced inebriety. This culminated in a relapse; his earlier symptoms reappeared, and he was brought to the hospital the day after the fourth of July in the same state as at the first admission, in coma and shock, jaundiced, distended with ascitic fluid, and vomiting blood.

Second Admission: The physical signs were much the same as on the first entry, although he was not so deeply jaundiced, nor

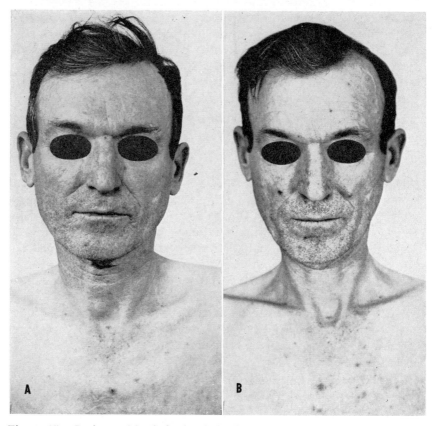

Figure 15.   Patient with cirrhosis of the liver.   *Left.*   Several small vascular spiders, one to the right of the sternum in the second intercostal space, one near the medial end of the left clavicle and small atypical lesions scattered over the face and chest.   The lesion at the Angle of Louis is a small pustule which has been traumatized.   *Right.* Picture of the same patient taken ten months later showing two large elevated pulsating spiders above each nasolabial crease, and three news spiders on the forehead.   Lesions on the chest, somewhat out of focus, are larger than they were ten months before.

were the hemorrhage and coma as severe.   There were no new spiders, but he had lost no more since discharge.   With the same treatment he responded so rapidly that he felt well enough to sign-out after ten days.

Interval: During the next three months the patient left town, but his symptoms became so aggravated that he went to another hospital.   Here the same findings were reported, and in addition his liver was observed by means of a peritoneoscope, which disclosed the diagnostic picture of hepatic cirrhosis, the liver being very small. When he returned to Cincinnati he was forced to stay in bed, except for visits to the out-patient clinic, where he was given mercurial diuretics and his abdomen was tapped.   It became impossible to treat him in this manner and he was admitted to the hospital again on November 12, 1939, complaining only of great weakness and an enormously swollen belly.

Third Admission: There had been a general decline in weight, a fact which became clear when the ascitic fluid was removed.   The two pictures (Figure 15) indicate this and show several new vascular spiders on the face.   The ones on the cheeks pulsated vigorously. By x-ray studies the presence of esophageal varices was substantiated.   After two weeks of supportive treatment the patient was allowed to go home.   His condition was becoming worse, but the main problem was ascites rather than jaundice.

Interval: Because his other hepatic functions were not deteriorating as rapidly as the portal obstruction was developing, it was decided as a counsel of desperation to perform an omentopexy.   For this the patient was admitted early in January, 1940, a year after his first visit to the hospital and seven years after the appearance of signs of beginning cirrhosis.   He had mild jaundice and advanced ascites.

Last Admission: Even with painstaking preoperative care, a liberal use of vitamins, and a high carbohydrate and protein diet, the patient could not be brought into good condition.   The omentopexy was performed and he recovered from the first effects of the operation but died in coma, with moderate jaundice, a few days later.   There were no measurable changes in his spiders.

Autopsy: The autopsy provided a second confirmation of the diagnosis of cirrhosis.   The liver weighed 1375 grams and its irregular surface was studded with fine nodules.   The spleen was fibrous and weighed 310 grams.   Esophageal varices were demonstrated.

TABLE III

LABORATORY DATA AND SPIDERS

Case 1.

Date	Icterus Index	Blood Urea Nitrogen	CO_2 Combining Power	Pro- thrombin Time	Choles- terol	Crea- tinine	30 Min. Brom- Sulphalein Retention	A/G Ratio	Van Den Bergh Indirect	Van Den Bergh Direct	Spiders
1-4-39	25	31	54	20	170	1.1	10%	2.9/3.5	+	+	16 spiders. None pulsating. Largest 3 cm. in diameter. Many faded within 6 weeks
8-5-39	15	47									No change in spiders since discharge
11-12-39	8	17					15%	2.8/3.3			Several new spiders, 2 pulsat- ing (25 in all)
1-12-40	16	21	55					1.7/4.2	+	+	No change in spiders

Comment: This man was observed during the last year of his life while remissions and relapses in his disease were occurring. Table III gives evidence that the advent of new spiders was not characterized by any striking change in the results of laboratory tests. No observations were made throughout a phase when spiders were increasing in size and number. Hemorrhage from the nose may have resulted from trauma to an angiomatous vessel in the nose, although this point was not established. This man went through an episode of severe bleeding later and observation at this time revealed only very sparse small spiders. The changes following transfusion make it reasonably certain, however, that he had larger lesions not evident during the critical period of his entry into the hospital.

Blanching and disappearance of the lesions are dependent on the changes in the cutaneous blood vessels associated with exsanguinating shock. Many of the spiders, although present, are invisible or difficult to see until the circulation is in a more nearly natural state. It is unlikely that very large spiders, several centimeters in diameter, could have developed in as short a time as twenty-four hours, although some do grow very rapidly and may reach that size in as short a period as ten days. In this patient, and in others whose spiders were watched before and during large hemorrhages, the lesions disappeared or became so faint as to escape detection unless the site had been marked. When the lesions regressed they left only a spot of atrophic or nearly normal skin, with or without pigmentation, as a mark of their former existence. Photographs made at two stages of the disease reveal some of the changes in the spiders.

2.   The Vascular Spider in Pregnancy

REVIEW

Blaschko (526) recorded the development of large numbers of "angiomas" during pregnancy in an eighteen year old girl. It is not possible to say whether they were spiders or something else. So far as I have been able to determine, the first observation of spiders appearing during pregnancy was recorded by Corbett in the *British Journal of Dermatology,* in 1914. He stated that he had seen spider angiomas appear in the skin during pregnancy and disappear entirely after it was over. This note has remained in oblivion since its interment.

Fibroma molluscum gravidarum carefully studied and illustrated by Brickner in 1906 and 1913 is possibly a related phenomenon. Although this lesion is distinct from the cutaneous arterial spider, there is much similarity between it and an unusual form of spider not described in medical writings, which I have encountered in two pregnant women who had typical spiders also. It was characterized by prominent elevation, a warty or gristly texture, and a core consisting of a coiled central artery with vivid pulsation. The alternate fading and flushing could be seen beautifully by depressing the surface with a glass slide. In both instances, the atypical lesion appeared and disappeared simultaneously with those of the usual variety. Unfortunately, I was not able to persuade either patient to part with her strange stigma and can only speculate about its structure. Never having seen the eruptive *fibroma molluscum gravidarum*, it is not possible to say whether the lesion described above belongs in this category or is something entirely different.

I have observed a pronounced erythematous change in and around pigmented moles during pregnancy in women simultaneously marked with typical vascular spiders. In one pulsations could be felt. This erythema and the associated vascular spiders faded simultaneously postpartum. This phenomenon is somewhat like the changes around pigmented nevi which Goldman has observed after use of ACTH or steroid hormones. A similar increase in the size of vascular lesions was described by Carleton and her associates in a patient with Maffucci's syndrome during pregnancy. It was uncertain whether increased blood volume or actual growth of vessels was responsible.

Ward has written of "multiple pigmented warts" in pregnancy, but neither he nor Brickner made any mention of pulsation. It is improbable, however, that it was specifically sought. Brickner's second article contains speculation about the possible relation of the lesions to glands of internal secretion.

The next note on cutaneous spiders in pregnancy was published by Zeisler who considered syphilis as a possible causative agent. A more detailed description by Konrad in 1925 called attention to the appearance of telangiectases on the face, neck and arms during the second month of pregnancy. This is the first emphasis on the distribution so characteristic of the acquired cutaneous spider in pregnancy as well as in disease of the liver. The abrupt fading or vanishing of these marks in the postpartum period was observed. In the next year a similar finding was reported in a woman who had a pituitary tumor (16), and the possibility was considered that an endocrine disorder might be responsible for the skin lesion. Two examples of spiders in pregnancy were encountered by Urbach who described the vascular lesions in detail. They vanished shortly after the end of pregnancy.

The first indication of a possible familial tendency was pointed out by Gougerot and Meyer who observed the appearance of typical spider-like angiomata during the fifth month of pregnancy in four consecutive gestations, in a woman whose sisters had also acquired spiders during pregnancy. Because of the history of syphilis in the family, they believed the lesions to be stigmata of hereditary syphilis. Distribution on the neck, arms and hands was noted. There was no mucosal lesion and no tendency to bleed.

In another report (644) spiders were not seen during the first and second pregnancies but appeared in the third month of the next pregnancy on the neck, chest and arms. The paper included a description of spiders of several varieties and sizes, with the larger ones typical in shape, having an elevated central boss and a peripheral anemic halo. The authors believed the distribution to be related to the cutaneous nerves arising from the brachial plexus.

In Madden's report on generalized angiomatosis, two cases of vascular spiders acquired during pregnancy were included. One patient was a thirty year old white woman whose spiders appeared during the third month of pregnancy and then increased in number up to the seventh month. Two months after pregnancy they had all gone. The other patient acquired them during the fifth month of pregnancy. Mitchell has referred to similar cases. Davis has contributed a learned discussion of subcutaneous hemangioendotheliomas associated with pregnancy in which he discussed the rare malignant variety and included a number of excellent photographs of typical vascular spiders. He collected a series of eleven cases during a two year period from various antenatal clinics. The description of a type characterized by "pigmented warty growth projecting under the superficial layers of the skin" classes it as one of the pigmented warts discussed by Brickner. A possible relationship to this type of lesion to the much commoner vascular spider of pregnancy has been discussed. Smith has observed spiders occurring during the last month of pregnancy in a twenty six year old woman. During her third pregnancy they appeared again on the back and upper chest during the fifth month. Some idea of the difficulty of tracking down medical reports of vascular spiders can be seen in the title of Smith's note—"The Treatment of Hereditary Telangiectasia" (791).

Special kinds of bleeding with coagulation defects are well known in pregnancy. It is possible that the vascular changes of pregnancy, producing angiomatous changes in a polyp, caused the fatal hemorrhage in a pregnant woman described by Polayes and Nevins.

Forman described a woman who acquired spiders early in the second month of each of eleven pregnancies, all of which ended disastrously with delivery of a stillborn fetus before term. The spiders faded rapidly within a week after labor. He believed that an endocrine disturbance was responsible. In addition, he observed the coming and going of spiders in phase with the waxing and waning of symptoms in a patient with peptic ulcer.

Vignes, Hanoun and Vial have reviewed the European literature on spiders in women during pregnancy and have recorded their familiarity with this innocuous phenomenon.

The study of capillaries in pregnancy with the dissecting microscope, or other microscopic technique has revealed typical changes in pregnancy. Melbard and others have shown that about two-thirds of pregnant women develop enlargement, almost varicose, dilatation of capillaries of the skin, a figure not unlike the proportion of women who get spiders and palmar erythema.

Walsh and Becker in their monograph on erythema palmare and naevus-araneus-like telangiectases gave full description of six patients who got spiders during pregnancy. In four, palmar erythema also was present. In some patients spiders existed before pregnancy. Those in whom they appeared during pregnancy observed their advent anywhere from the third to seventh month. Spiders tended to parallel the palmar erythema in the time of onset and fading, but there were some exceptions. These authors discussed the number, size, configuration and distribution of the vascular spider, and for the first time arterial pulsation was looked for and found in the spider of pregnancy. Their investigation included inspection with a capillary microscope and histologic study. A low-power view of one of their biopsy specimens gives an excellent idea of the two types of vessels encountered, the thick coiled stem artery in the subcutis branching directly into "veins" of comparable size. This they termed an arteriovenous anastomosis, but did not point out that it differs from the true arteriovenous anastomosis in having a multitude of "veins" branching from a central artery, and in the continuation of these "veins" into a capillary bed before the blood is conveyed away in true veins. They did not find any evidence of hereditary tendency except in patients with palmar erythema, nor did they see any indication that the spiders had followed the often evoked "minor trauma" such as mosquito bites, pinpricks, and the like. There was no incrimination of syphilis or disease of the liver. They believed the most probable cause to be some endocrine disturbance. Newman believed the cause to be an increase in blood volume plus the effects of progesterone.

In my monograph on the arterial spider based on observations up to 1942, I had notes of forty one women who had acquired vascular spiders during pregnancy. In many instances spiders were observed to appear between the second and third month of pregnancy. Usually they disappeared at the time of delivery or shortly thereafter. There was no indication that hepatic disease was responsible for vascular spiders in the women observed.

The neglect of the vascular spider by obstetricians is surprising since this lesion is enough of a cosmetic nuisance in pregnancy to attract attention. Little systemic investigation of it has been recorded, however. Some of the forty one were seen casually, but enough were studied with care to form a general idea of their prevalence and of their striking changes during and after gestation.

Most women first notice spiders between the second and fifth month of pregnancy. This agrees with the data cited above. One very striking exception to this rule was observed by the wife of a colleague whose interest in spiders was both personal and general. She observed vascular spiders on her face and arms about the middle of the first pregnancy. These faded soon after the child was born and were entirely gone two weeks postpartum. In a second pregnancy, for which the date of conception was certain, a spider on her face suddenly reappeared ten days after the date of conception, and three days before the menstrual period was due. From this she made the diagnosis of pregnancy, which later was amply confirmed. This lesion enlarged slowly throughout gestation, and others appeared later. It was lost to view by the third day after delivery although it could still be felt, but no trace remained on the sixth day. This spider did not reappear in a third pregnancy, although many new ones were seen.

Often spiders are thought to be pimples or acne lesions, and many women traumatize them, occasionally causing a severe hemorrhage, to their surprise. Often they are covered with face powder. Rarely they are feared as a manifestation of some malignant disease, or dreaded under the mistaken notion that they are a token of syphilis.

The habit of the vascular spider in pregnant women is to enlarge slowly until term. New ones may appear at any time during the second and third trimesters, and those already present tend to increase slowly in size. There is an abrupt decrease in size and number at, or a few days before, the time of delivery and during the ensuing ten days or two weeks. The smaller ones disappear without leaving a trace, and the larger ones either diminish in size or vanish during the period of uterine involution. These residual spiders often undergo a gradual decrease in size and number. At length the skin becomes clear. In some women they may persist up to ten years after the last child is born.

I have noticed a few instances in which vascular spiders occurred in the infants of mothers who had acquired similar lesions during pregnancy. This has occurred in children of either sex. It does not necessarily follow that one of the parents will be found to have spiders when they are present in a child. There may be an hereditary factor.

The morphology and physiology of spiders in pregnancy do not differ from those of the other types discussed. The location, pulsation, color, shape, size, and warmth are substantially the same.

When vascular spiders were observed to appear during pregnancy, I supposed that some toxemia or hepatic disorder was imminent, or smoldering; but no untoward episode marred the course of an uneventful pregnancy. The lesions vanished or faded during the early postpartum stage. Therefore I suspected that the advent and disappearance of spiders bore a relation to the endocrine tides whose normal ebb and flow are altered so spectacularly during and after gestation. The time relationship suggested placing the blame on estrogenic substances or at least related steroid hormones, for the estrogens are at a higher level in the blood during the period of pregnancy when the spider is likely to blossom forth.

Nothing in the persons studied here has indicated a relationship of these spiders to hepatic disorders, malnutrition, alcoholism, or any of the toxemias of pregnancy. Only one of the forty one women had ever had jaundice. In several cases the women were certain that spiders had antedated pregnancy, even though they had enlarged or become more numerous during its course; and there is no reason to doubt this observation.

SPECIAL STUDY

The following section is based on a series of studies undertaken directly after World War II at Cincinnati to find out the actual incidence of vascular spiders and palmar erythema in pregnant women, to assay liver function and to describe the natural history of the events under observation. With complete cooperation from the physicians and nurses of the Obstetrical Service of the Cincinnati General Hospital, I examined every patient seen on every visit to the prenatal clinic and also during hospitalization for delivery, and again at the visit six weeks after discharge following the 4 to 10 days of hospitalization for delivery. I had great help from Drs. Dexter, Cogswell, and Embick in these studies (69). In an effort to reduce subjectivity I made all the actual examinations. Beginning in October 1946 every woman who visited the clinic was examined at each visit. A detailed record was kept of the findings. Since it was not feasible to examine each person completely every time, the observations were confined to the hands, lower and upper arms, face, neck, and upper chest. The conditions of lighting were kept constant. An artificial blue light was used and all patients were examined while standing or sitting before the light. The presence or absence of vascular spiders was recorded. If they were present, we recorded their location and number. Palmar erythema was noted as either the diffuse or the sharply localized form. A notation was made of the depth of color of the skin in both white and negro patients. A great many photographs were taken. Sometimes a series of photographs was made throughout pregnancy, in the hospital shortly after delivery, and again at the final post-partum visit. In patients who had either type of vascular change in the skin, an effort was made to ascertain the time

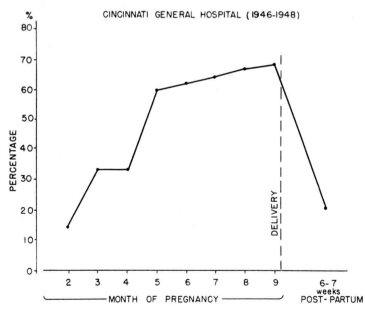

Figure 16.   Percentage of white women with vascular spiders during and after pregnancy.

of its appearance. But this information was not very reliable except when we had examined patients before lesions appeared. Some patients were aware that vascular spiders and palmar erythema antedated pregnancy. Others had never noticed either one. We collected urine over a twenty-four-hour period for hormone assay in many patients and studied liver function.

The subjects included all women examined in the prenatal clinic who were in attendance in October 1946 and all new clinic patients who came in through 23 October 1947 and were followed through July 1948. In order to make a number of correlations, we collected extensive data on age, color, parity of the mother; sex, birthweight, viability and normality of the child; lactation; season of the year; and complications of pregnancy such as toxemia, hypertension, or eclampsia. The date of the last mentrual period was recorded in order to learn the duration of pregnancy at the time of the first visit if lesions were already apparent. The date of the delivery was recorded. In the final analysis, the time of appearance of vascular changes was based on recalculation from the date of delivery in all pregnancies which went to term. A total of one thousand two hundred forty three women were observed. Of these four hundred eighty four were white and seven hundred fifty nine were negro women.

Vascular spiders were found in three hundred twenty one or 66.6 per cent of the four hundred eighty four white women observed

TABLE IV

DISTRIBUTION OF SPIDERS IN WHITE AND NEGRO WOMEN

Area	White (529 Lesions) Percent	Negro (105 Lesions) Percent
Face	11	12
Neck and anterior chest	14	5
Arm, upper anterior	7	5
Arm, upper posterior	8	3
Arm, lower anterior	14	9
Arm, lower posterior	21	17
Palm	7	20
Dorsum of hand	18	29
Others	(knee 1 case)	

and in eighty seven or 11.3 per cent of the seven hundred fifty nine
negro women. Since patients came in at varying stages of pregnancy
for their first clinic visit, figures on incidence of spiders throughout
pregnancy are not derived from large numbers seen during the
second and third months of pregnancy, while those for the last
months were high. In Figures 16 and 17 are recorded the percentage of all women seen in any month of pregnancy who had vascular
spiders at the time. Fourteen per cent of the white women under
observation had vascular spiders by the second month of pregnancy.
For the next three months there was a general tendency for the
proportion having spiders to increase rapidly. Following this, there
was a slow but steady increase in positive cases up to the time of
delivery. By the ninth calendar month of pregnancy, 66 per cent of
all white women under observation had vascular spiders. Control
figures which are, of course, not in any sense absolutely comparable,
indicate that about 15 per cent of women (in the same category)
have vascular spiders without reference to age, pregnancy, or the
number of pregnancies in the past. Nine other women had vascular
spiders which they knew had existed before the first pregnancy.
Findings in negro women are different chiefly in a much lower
incidence of vascular spiders. In Figure 17 we find that no spiders
were observed before the fourth month by which time they had
appeared in 8 per cent of all subjects seen during the fourth month.
The incidence rose thereafter until a peak was reached by the ninth
month when 11.3 per cent were found to have spiders.

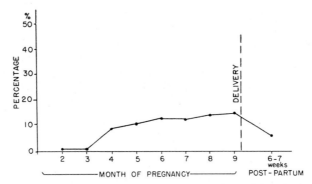

Figure 17.   Percentage of negro women with vascular spiders during and after
pregnancy.

This notable discrepancy between incidence in white and negro women highlights an aspect of the study in which we correlated the depth of skin pigmentation with the finding of vascular spiders among both white and negro women. An estimate of degree of pigmentation of the skin was made on each person and recorded as light, medium, and dark. White women with red hair were recorded in a separate category. This was checked at each clinic visit without access to previous estimate of pigment by the observer. While this is at best only a semiquantitative evaluation there was surprising consistency in the routine observations by each member of the study group, and good consistency between different observers. Thus subjectivity was not a great source of error, though it may be in various clinical studies (57). In Figure 18 we have charted the percentage of women with different, depths of skin pigment in whom we observed vascular spiders. There was a similar trend among negro women whose depth of skin pigment was recorded as light, medium, or dark.

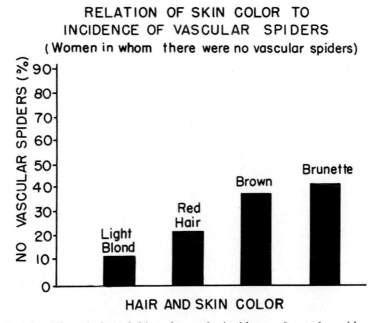

Figure 18. The relation of skin color to the incidence of vascular spiders, also giving the percentage of all pregnant women in whom no spiders were observed.

In Figure 19 the highest incidence of vascular spiders in white and negro women during the last month of pregnancy is compared with their incidence at the regular postpartum follow-up. In white women the percentage fell from sixty nine to twenty. In negroes the corresponding change was from eleven to five per cent. Thus about three-fourths of the women who had any vascular spiders in the ninth month of pregnancy had lost them all by the seventh week after delivery. Figure 19 gives the rate at which vascular spiders and palmar erythema were lost during the last month of pregnancy and during the puerperium. Data are derived from all subjects with observations, regardless of follow-up. A few women suddenly lost

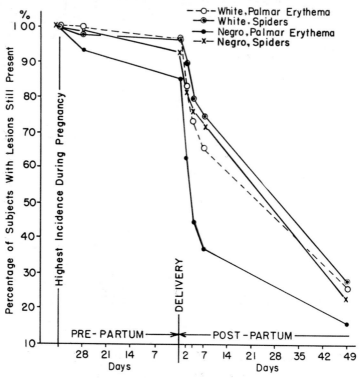

Figure 19. Rate of disappearance of palmar erythema and vascular spiders in white and negro women during the last stages of pregnancy, time of delivery, and the post-*partum* period.

vascular spiders, or they decreased in size during the month before delivery especially during the last week. Sometimes we used this herald to predict the time of the oncoming delivery. The period of most rapid loss of spiders was during the week immediately following delivery. The loss thereafter was more gradual up to the time of our final observation. In the few women whom we saw up to a year after delivery there had been a further decrease in size and number of lesions unless another pregnancy intervened. In Figure 19 the data for disappearance refer to women who had lost all vascular spiders. In those still postive at the postpartum check-up many had lost some but not all of the lesions, and in others they had decreased in size so that the quantitative aspects of the changes were even more dramatic than the figures indicate. There was a tendency for lesions which appeared late in pregnancy to fade early, and those which appeared early to disappear somewhat later. This is partly related to size of individual spiders, the larger ones usually taking longer to

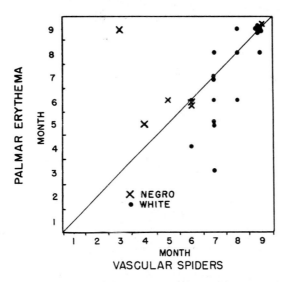

Figure 20. The relationship of the month of appearance of vascular spider and palmar erythema in white and negro women during pregnancy.

vanish completely. Without charts marking the area of each lesion, and photographic records, it was impossible to identify precisely the spot where a spider had been. At times a small freckle marked the spot, and at times the skin was slightly atrophic, but these were exceptional findings. In three instances we noted spiders after delivery which were not recorded before. We believe that this represents an earlier oversight rather than the actual development of new lesions during the puerperium.

In Table IV we have compared the location of vascular spiders in white and negro women. There are notable differences. In negroes the hand was the site of about half the spiders, whereas in white women it was the site of only a quarter of the lesions. The difference was even more striking where the palm was considered, lesions being almost three times as common in the palm of negro women as in white women. Aside from differences in pigmentation, we have no ready explanation for these contrasts.

OTHER OBSERVATIONS

Although we did not see any clinical indication of hepatic disease complicating pregnancy, we did some liver function studies in twenty six white women to see whether there was any laboratory evidence of impaired function, or any difference amongst those with vascular spiders or palmar erythema and those without such vascular changes. The icterus index, bromsulfalein retention at forty five minutes after 5 mgm. per kgm., cephalincholesterol flocculation and thymol turbidity tests were done in the third trimester of pregnancy. Those tests did not reveal any significant sign of hepatic damage; and the very minor deviations from normal were found regardless of presence or absence of vascular spiders or palmar erythema or both. There was no indication that damage to the liver comparable to that usually found in chronic cirrhosis existed in the pregnant women in this study. Nothing suggested that vascular lesion in pregnancy had been caused by hepatic malfunction, despite the observation of Ober and LeCompte of a specific form of acute hepatic disease in some pregnant women.

The vascular changes in the skin had no notable association with first, or later pregnancies, with male or female offspring, with age or youth of the mother, with lactation or its failure to occur or to continue properly. We have studied hypertension and toxemias more extensively since there is some evidence and more belief that humoral factors play a good part in their genesis. Patients having systolic blood pressure of more than 140 millimeters of mercury and diastolic blood pressure of more than 90 millimeters of mercury were classed as hypertensives. Hypertensive patients with albuminuria, edema, symptoms of headaches, or convulsions in the third trimester of pregnancy were classed as toxemias. Of one thousand one hundred forty-five patients twenty-four, or 2.1 per cent, had hypertension during pregnancy. In another ninety-nine, or 8.7 per cent, there was toxemia. These diagnoses were made by members of the obstetrical staff independently of our own studies, and the data were combined only after the records were complete. The number with hypertension was too small to have much significance, but even in this group the incidence of vascular spiders or palmar erythema, or the two in combination, was almost exactly the same

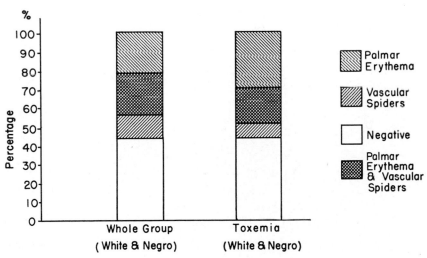

Figure 21.   Comparison of finding of vascular changes in the skin in pregnant women with and without toxemia.

as in the whole group. Since the number with toxemia was larger we have compared the incidence of vascular spiders and palmar erythema in this group with the incidence in the entire series in Figure 21. While there are slight differences the figures agree so nearly that we conclude that the changes in the skin we have observed have no essential relation to toxemia or its absence.

In the children of the women in this study there was the expected incidence of birthmarks, hemangiomas, and spiders but they had no relation to spiders, palmar erythema or any of the factors we recorded. Many of the children of mothers who had palmar erythema and spiders were marked with no blemish. Others, whose mothers never had vascular changes, had birthmarks. Likewise we found no relation between neonatal gynecomastia and the presence or absence of spiders and palmar erythema in the mother during pregnancy.

The studies indicate that vascular spiders and palmar erythema, alone or in combination, are frequent accompaniments of normal pregnancy. Since the investigation was intensive and persistent we discovered many lesions of which the subjects were wholly unaware. Many, however, were obvious and had been noticed. In some women they were the source of embarrassment or worry.

Since vascular spiders or palmar erythema may be found in normal non-pregnant women we have been particularly interested

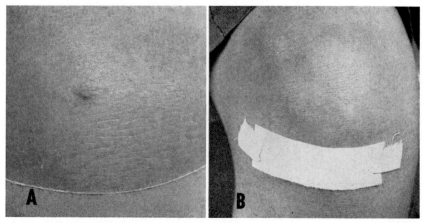

Figure 22.   *Left*. Spider on the knee of a pregnant woman.   *Right*. Disappearance after pregnancy.

in their fate after pregnancy since our control observations do not include women in a wide range of ages who have never been pregnant. Such observations as we have made indicate that a vascular spider may be found in at least 10 per cent of white women who have borne children. In a study made during a nutrition survey of American troops in various islands in the Pacific during World War II vascular spiders were seen in 14.9 per cent of the white and in none of the negro soldiers (54). Even taking off from such a base line there is a large and consistent increase in the number of spiders per woman and the number of women with spiders, from the second or third month of pregnancy until term. At this time there is a sud-

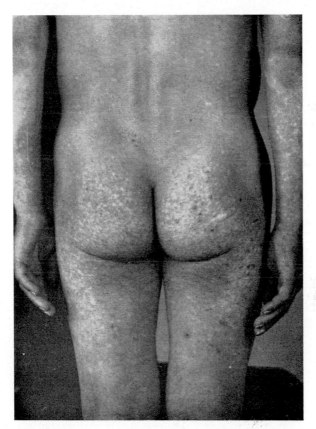

Figure 23. Speckled appearance of the skin cooled by fanning in a patient with cirrhosis of the liver. (Courtesy of Dr. Martini.)

den decrease in size of individual lesions, and a complete disappearance of many, so that by the seventh week after childbirth the number is approaching that found in control groups. Subsequently there is a further decrease which apparently continues slowly so long as another pregnancy does not occur.

These observations may be compared with those made in persons with chronic hepatic disease. Although the number of patients with hepatic disease was not as great it was ample to establish the fact that both spiders and palmar erythema often develop as complications of chronic or subacute disease of the liver. If and when the state of the liver improves these vascular changes recede just as they do following the completion of gestation, though rarely with such dramatic suddenness. Vascular spiders in well established cirrhosis are usually larger and more numerous than in pregnant women. Their similar distribution over the upper part of the body, their similar shape, palpable pulsation and intravascular pressure are strong indications of their kinship. I have not observed a woman who had known of vascular spiders during a pregnancy who later had them with chronic liver disease nor have I encountered a woman with cirrhosis who became pregnant, though some with ascites had suspected pregnancy. Martini's studies indicate that the

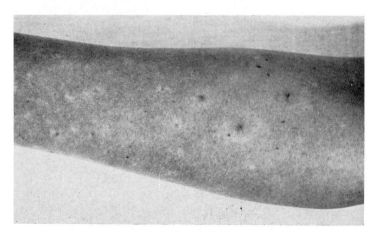

Figure 24.   The speckled mottling of the skin demonstrating small and medium-sized spiders developing in the pale regions and the progression of the anemic halo peripherally as the spider enlarges.   (Courtesy of Dr. Martini.)

microscopic details of structure of the spiders in cirrhosis, pregnancy and normals are identical. Clinical evidence suggests no fundamental difference between those which appear in pregnancy and those which appear in cirrhosis.

Our studies established a frequency of spiders and palmar erythema as banal accompaniments of normal pregnancy which surprised us. We have advanced the hypothesis that these phenomena may be caused by hormones, and have implicated the estrogenic substances in particular. The facts we have recorded should be known to obstetricians, if only for the occasional comfort they bring to women whose worry about such blemishes may add its needless burden to the trials of pregnancy.

GINGIVAL LESIONS IN PREGNANCY

Many diseases affect the gums, though much of the information about gingival lesions in dental journals is unknown to physicians. In our mutually excluding specializations, this information does

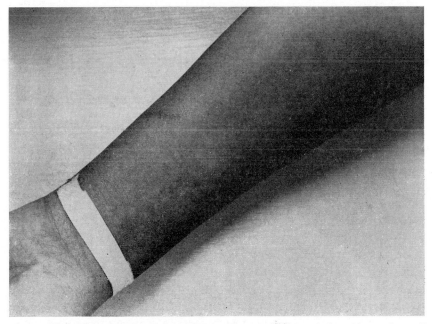

Figure 25.   Photograph of the skin showing speckling of the skin and small spiders in pregnancy.

not appear in any of the currently popular texts of medicine such as Cecil, Harrison, or Christian, nee Osler. Nevertheless gingivitis gravidarum or pregnancy gingivitis is well recognized by dentists, and by any physician so curious as to examine the mouth of pregnant woman. In most women the change is one of simple hyperplasia, the piling up of tissue sometimes spongy, sometimes firm. Because of its exposed location, bleeding from mild injury is usual and subsequent inflammation is the rule. We did not make a systematic study of the gums in pregnant women. Many were examined in the course of looking for mucosal spiders. While mild changes in the gums were common, extensive lesions were rare. We did not have enough data to see whether there was a correlation with the spiders. It is the general impression that hypertrophy of the gums in pregnancy has an endocrine basis.

Hyperplastic redundancy of the gums may occur as a complication of Dilantin therapy used in the treatment of convulsive disorders. In superficial appearance it resembles the gingival reaction of pregnancy. If there is a common pathogenic basis, it remains for the future to disclose.

3. The Vascular Spider in Normal Persons

The emergence of the vascular spider as an entity separate from other small dilatations of the vessels in the skin of normal persons cannot be assigned to any specific time or author. Von Grafe coined the term telangiectasis in 1807, but did not remark on spider-shaped lesions. There is a large and fantastic literature on the subject of birthmarks, or mother's marks, sometimes called "envies" because it was held that they resulted from some jealous passion of the mother during pregnancy. Others believed they were an indication of the noisome influence of a malevolent witch. This has been discussed, and William Harvey's role in vetoing a witch hunt has been mentioned. Most of the records contain little about the exact appearance of the lesion but are devoted to speculation concerning the hypothetical forces alleged to have caused them. They are irrelevant here. A discussion of dermal vascular markings is found in the works of John Bell, although he was not above echoing prevalent superstitions about them. Watson, writing in 1839, suggested that telangiectasis might be analogous in some ways to the post-traumatic arteriovenous fistula.

Besnier and Doyon, in a footnote to their translation of Kaposi's text described *télangiectases pontués stellaires,* but did not discuss clinical relationships. Marshall reported an infant who was born with many lesions, some evidently vascular spiders. Many disappeared as the child grew older.

Jonathan Hutchinson, in his *Archives of Surgery,* reported a typical example of the vascular spider or *nevus araneus* in a healthy subject, and gave a scholarly description of its clinical features. He stated that such a lesion, dignified by the title of *Nevus Aranarius,* was well known to the older English surgeons, but no reference was given and it has not been possible to track it down. He also remarked that spiders pulsated, blanched with pressure, filled instantaneously upon release, did not occur in very young children but were found frequently after the age of five years. He had seen more in children than adults; and more in girls and women than in men, which he attributed to vanity. He found the tip of the nose to be a favorite location. He recommended cautery for their removal.

Fitzwilliams noted the centrifugal flow. He also found that pressure caused the spider to fade. When the pressure was released the color reappeared at the center and spread rapidly to the periphery. He believed that there was some peculiar relation to cutaneous nerves because he had seen the aggregation of spiders along the distribution of cutaneous nerves.

Sequiera reported multiple telangiectasia in older persons without apparent disease. These lesions were similar to those described by Broq in patients with repeated attacks of hepatic colic. Sibley was impressed with the symmetrical distribution of spiders in a thirty five year old woman who consulted him. After a time the lesions faded and ultimately disappeared. He made no note of a connection with hepatic disease or pregnancy.

Becker has given an excellent summary and review of the clinical aspects of generalized telangiectasia, classifying lesions as congenital or acquired, although he admits that there is some overlapping of the two varieties. He did not discuss the vascular spider separately but included some examples and case reports.

Williams and Snell have commented on the spider in normal persons.

These few scattered references indicate that the vascular spider when occurring in normal persons has been recognized as an insignificant stigma. No reason has been demonstrated for its sporadic occurrence; and no considerable attention has been given it. It is important because the common association of a similar lesion with hepatic disease and pregnancy has given rise to a widespread belief that it is pathognomonic of some trouble in the liver, latent or obvious (249).

A. Observations

Up to the time when I found vascular spiders in normal children as well as in normal men and women, the notion had been entertained that the connotation of hepatic disease, past, present or future, was inevitable. With the gradual accumulation of details about a large number of persons with no history or contemporary indication of such trouble, I became convinced that the vascular spider was not invariably a harbinger or omen of disordered function of the liver. This was strengthened by observation of healthy and longevous families with several members who had been affected for many years.

I have records of more than one thousand persons with spiders in whom clinical hepatic disease, pregnancy, past or present, and malnutrition could be excluded. No tests were done to exclude latent vitamin deficiency disease, hepatic disease, or secret alcoholic addiction. The subjects were regarded as normal.

The number of lesions in a single subject was small. The average was slightly over three, and the largest number in any normal person was nine. Most often there was but a single spider. This is in sharp contradistinction to hepatic disease, where they may be myriad, or in pregnancy, where they may be plentiful.

The radicles in many of the vascular spiders in normal persons were fewer and smaller than those of spiders in hepatic disease or pregnancy. Often the lesion appeared as a red area about the punctum, with no legs. In a few instances anomalous forms occurred in addition to the more typical ones. Pulsation occurred in most of the lesions. The pressure needed to obliterate them was the same as that for the other lesions studied (see Section 1). In some persons with spiders other parts of the skin were examined with a high-power hand lens. Many had widespread changes in the cutaneous vessels. Others had none. Distribution followed the general pattern noted in Figure 4. The face and neck were most frequently marked with spiders.

The age at onset was variable. Numerous lesions were noted first at the age of puberty, but whether this was the true epoch of origin or merely denotes a developing self-consciousness is undetermined. They were frequent in young children. Some were birthmarks.

Inexplicable changes in size, even complete disappearance with subsequent recrudescence, have been noticed. The natural history may include a slow waxing and waning, months or years being necessary to complete a definite cycle. I have not discerned any rhythm of change.

B. Spiders Seen In Previously Normal Persons With Vitamin Deficiency

The vascular spider was not described as a stigma of any vitaman deficiency disease until the 1940's. No reference to it as such appears in the medical writings on pellagra. There are a few remarks on telangiectases though spiders may have been included under this classification. Majocchi observed telangiectasis in alcoholic pellagrins in 1899; and certainly cirrhosis and pellagra may have followed addiction to alcohol. Marie mentioned a pellagrous woman "covered with telangiectases," without further comment. Fearnsides wrote a paper entitled "Telangiectases in children in association with wasting and protracted diarrhea." Some of the children had complicating deficiency diseases, but there was no evidence of hepatic disorder. One may surmise that some of the lesions described were indeed vascular spiders since Fearnsides commented on the same phenomenon in adults with cirrhosis. Alessandrini and Scala described a woman with pellagra who had "venous ectasis on the nose and cheeks." They did not elaborate further. These brief notes, buried in discussions of other topics, constitute the record of telangiectasia in vitamin-deficiency diseases. That they have been noted casually may be significant. Such comment had faded from contemporary medical literature on the subject until recently.

I must take the blame for having caused, inadvertently, the belief that spiders were signs of B-complex vitamin deficiency. When I was working in the Nutrition Clinic in Birmingham, Alabama, I designed a form for keeping records, since none was at hand. In it I included a space for spiders, palmar erythema and a few other lesions I wanted data about, looking for a non-pregnant, non-cirrhotic control group. Visitors borrowed the forms, used them in nutrition surveys and the spider as casual interloper became imbedded in several reports. This curious event indicates the decline of clinical expertise in nutrition.

There was no difference between the vascular spider of normal persons and that encountered among the ill nourished folk seen in the Nutrition Clinic in Birmingham, Alabama, during 1940-41-42. I found spiders in association with angular stomatitis, conjunctival and corneal vascularizations, glossitis and peripheral neuritis. Occasionally they increased in size or number during an exacerbation of the deficiency syndrome. Usually, there was no parallelism. In two subjects spiders disappeared at the time when the symptoms of the vitamin deficiency grew worse. Some new spiders appeared during or after successful revival of health following restoration of specific vitamins and other factors lacking in the diet. By far the greatest number of patients showed no change in the spiders throughout the three seasons during which they were under observation, regardless of clinical course, nutritional status, or treatment.

A familial tendency to vascular spiders was strongly marked in the one hundred and twenty Birmingham subjects perhaps because most of the families were available for examination. Spiders were found in parents or siblings of 58 per cent of those whose families were examined. They had been *observed* by the patients in only 13 per cent so that a negative history is to be looked upon with suspicion, unless verified. Typical spiders were found in approximately 10 per cent of all the malnourished patients examined. The incidence in "normal" persons is about the same.

Vascular spiders in patients with nutritional deficiency were fewer per person than in patients with chronic disease of the liver. Ordinarily they were small, having only a few visible branches and a small erythematous macule. Few could be felt to pulsate although occasionally pulsation was very forceful. The pressure needed to obliterate them, as determined by means of the capsule technique, was the same as that recorded for spiders in hepatic disease. More spiders occurred on the hands and arms and fewer over the trunk than in persons with hepatic disease or pregnancy.

Biskind and Biskind showed that estrogens were not inactivated, destroyed, or excreted adequately in animals deprived of an ample supply of B-complex vitamins, though the metabolism of androgens was not much compromised. There is an imbalance in the estrogen-androgen ratio. There was no evidence that spiders seen in the malnourished persons in the early 1940's were related in any way to specific effects of deficiency disease or endocrine anomaly discovered on clinical examination. The entire experience indicates that spiders were the same as in normal persons.

4. The Vascular Spider in Miscellaneous Conditions

REVIEW AND OBSERVATIONS

Notes concerning the occurrence of typical cutaneous vascular spiders have appeared sporadically in medical reports of all kinds of diseases. In many patients spiders may have been merely coincidental, but it is impossible to eliminate a common cause when the pathogenesis is unknown.

Spiders are said to occur in *xeroderma pigmentosa*. Osler recorded instances in which spiders together with the more common mat-like telangiectasia occurred in x-ray scars. He also mentioned their occurrence in *scleroderma*. It is possible that Milbradt was describing the same lesion, although the diagnosis of the condition he was discussing is obscure. Spiders have been noted in *rheumatic fever*, although Keil, in his survey of the rheumatic eyrthemas, did not separate them from nonspecific telangiectasis. I have seen vascular spiders in rheumatic fever only in victims of chronic valvular disease complicated by cardiac cirrhosis. These spiders may be presumed to have the same cause as in other forms of hepatic cirrhosis. The one exception was in a young man. Several small red nodules appeared during an exacerbation of rheumatism. Although originally they were believed to be rheumatic nodules, they later developed the characteristic star-shape of vascular spiders; and after several months they disappeared. This is the only time I have seen spiders develop in such circumstances.

Vascular spiders are very uncommon in Graves' disease. Hyde presented an extensive review and reported many cutaneous vascular disturbances, among which was at least one perfectly typical vascular spider. This article attracted some attention among dermatologists, who still refer to it, but it escaped the notice of authors of systematic treatises on the thyroid gland. Only three cases have been observed among the fairly numerous examples of thyrotoxicosis I have encountered in the past twenty years. One patient knew that the spiders had appeared many months after signs of severe over-activity of the thyroid had been observed. Following iodine therapy and sub-total thyroidectomy, the metabolism returned to a normal level, and after several months the spiders vanished. Unfortunately we did not test hepatic function. McCreary has told me of a patient who got a large crop of spiders during the development of thyrotoxicosis. They disappeared during therapy with an antithyroid drug.

Radschow and Brodecher reported a large outcropping of spiders the day after bilateral stellate ganglion resection in a patient with cirrhosis and scleroderma.

Mosny and Malloizel reported an outbreak of telangiectases in a man with lead poisoning. Their sketches are somewhat suggestive of telangiectasis eruptiva mascularis perstans.

Holt described the outcropping of spiders in two patients treated for Parkinson's disease with trihoxyphenidyl. One with heart failure developed "literally hundreds of such angiomas on the face alone." They went away within three weeks after administration of the drug was stopped.

I have observed spiders appearing twice in women while getting ACTH, and in one man getting cortisone. They all had severe rheumatoid arthritis. Solem has reported detailed studies of spiders appearing in a young woman getting ACTH for rheumatism. Certainly these are unusual events. Whether they are purely chance events, cause and effect, or an indirect effect is not clear. It is possible that thinning of the epidermis, as Castor and Baker described in experimental animals, may be responsible. In this connection the observations of Goldman and Richfield are of interest. They observed the increase in size of established junction nevi and the appearance of new ones during protracted therapy with ACTH alone or with cortisone. Vascular changes were not described.

If we can trust our patients' recollection or observational capacities about the onset of spiders, in a few instances verified ourselves, these notes of curious cases should be added. I have heard of spiders appearing suddenly in the following circumstances: 1. At the time of onset of severe diabetes; 2. Six weeks after an episode of heat hyperpyrexia; 3. Two months after the termination of a normal pregnancy without liver disease or subsequent pregnancy; 4. After a severe sunburn; and 5. During an exacerbation of ulcerative colitis. These patients had careful clinical and laboratory studies which failed to reveal any evidence of disease of the liver or pregnancy. Except for the ones actually under observation, those with thyrotoxicosis, one with ulcerative colitis, one at the onset of diabetes, there was always a question of whether the history portrays discovery of long established spiders at a time of intensive examination of the patient by himself, or whether they did in fact appear suddenly.

5. Spiders and Related Vascular Changes in the Mucous Membranes

During the first part of this study I did not search for vascular spiders except in the skin. It is not possible to estimate their frequency in inaccessible regions, since the mucosal spider fades after death in the same manner as its dermal congener (46). Unless a careful endoscopic examination is made, one cannot state that spiders were not present simply because they were not seen post mortem. I have seen the mouth affected, the nose, the rectum, the cunjunctiva and the stomach. In appearance, the vessels were irregular, rarely having the characteristics of a well defined central hub with radiating spokes. Pulsation was not evident upon the somewhat uncertain palpation of the lesions in the buccal mucosa, soft palate, hard palate or gums. No lesions occurred upon or under the tongue, although a different form of telangiectasis, the caviar lesion, occurs under the tongue (59), while the dorsum often is spotted with the characteristic lesion of Osler's disease (Chapter III, Section 1). The coming and going of the mucosal spider paralleled the coming and going of the dermal type.

Mucosal spiders were seen chiefly in patients with a large number of spiders in the skin. No mucosal spider was detected in patients with hepatic disease without spiders in the skin. I have seen only one lesion bleed but suspected it in others. In most cases of grave hematemesis, the presence of esophageal varices was demonstrated after convalescence or at post mortem examination. It is not inferred that severe or even fatal hemorrhage may not occur from small bleeding arterial spiders of the mucosae, but it is rarely possible to establish such a cause.

Tortuous coils of redundant aneurysmal vessels in the conjunctiva have occurred at times, one of which is pictured in Figure 10. This change was seen to reach macroscopic proportions within a week. The shape is strikingly different from that of the spider.

The important fact has been established that macroscopic vascular changes comparable to those of the spider in the skin occur in mucous membranes. No information exists, nor have we obtained any, about the histology of mucosal lesions. Their relationship to hemorrhage is still to be defined. In my experience they are uncommon. Probably they are not important as a cause of bleeding from the alimentary canal.

6. Palmar Erythema in Liver Disease

An older Miss Muffet
Decided to rough it
And lived upon whiskey and gin.
Red hands and a spider
Developed outside her
Such are the wages of sin.   W.B.B.

One of the lessons learned during early observations of vascular spiders was the extreme difficulty of seeing lesions with the mind's eye as well as seeing them mechanically. In several case notes of patients with cirrhosis of the liver and arterial spiders I recorded and described accurately the classical clinical features of palmar erythema. I even made several charts of the color pattern in palmar erythema in case records. But I did not see the erythema reflectively until I read the paper of Walsh and Becker.

A. DESCRIPTION OF THE LESION

The color of the palms in healthy people varies considerably, not only from one person to another but in a given person from time to time. Depth of color varies more than does the design of color distribution. If a normal person lets his hand hang down for a few minutes the palm becomes speckled with pale islands surrounded by areas of erythema. Sometimes there is a little cyanosis. The design of red, white and blue, though fairly constant from month to month, undergoes slow phases of variation, indicating that the cutaneous blood vessels undergo slight changes in their structure and location.

Two forms of palmar erythema are recognized clinically. One is a very marked exaggeration of the normal mottling (Figure 29).

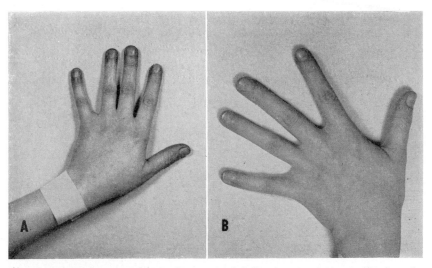

Figure 26. Palmar erythema during and following pregnancy affecting the knuckles and particularly the terminal phalanges and the root of the nail, with vivid color of the fingertip.

The hand, even though not dependent, shows conspicuous redness. This may affect not only the palm but to some extent the dorsum of hand especially the fingers and the base of the nails. In the other and more common form of palmar erythema, the disorder commences in the heel of the hand, the hypothenar eminence, which may be the only portion involved (Figure 27). There is a very sharp line of demarcation between the red portion and adjacent uninvolved areas. As time passes, the red spot on the palm enlarges toward the base of the little finger while the thenar eminence reddens. The margins in this area are less distinct than elsewhere. Frequently there may be one, two or three very prominent red spots on the palm between the regions where the fingers join the hands, but not directly under the palmar callouses (Figure 27). Finally the palmar surface of the distal phalanx of the thumb and all four fingers gets involved. When the red color is extreme the redness goes around to encompass the base of the nail. Under such circumstances *clubbing of the fingers* and digital erythema occur. This has been noted in cirrhosis (50, 53) and not only or even chiefly in "Hanot's cirrhosis." Since the digital erythema indicates an increase in blood

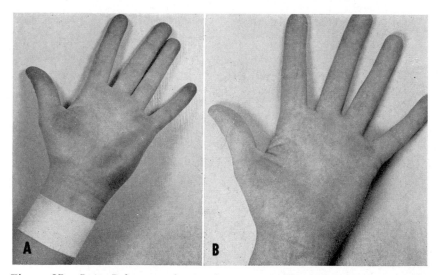

Figure 27. *Left.* Palmar erythema of pregnancy illustrating the intense discoloration of the hypothenar area as well as the discoloration of the terminal portion of the digits. *Right.* Fading of the lesions after delivery.

flow made manifest by increased skin temperature and cutaneous pulsation as well as by redness, the criteria of Mendlowitz for clubbing are fulfilled. It may be strongly suspected that the clubbing of fingers in hepatic disease results from the same forces which give rise to vascular spiders and palmar erythema. Reasons for the irregular occurrence of clubbing, spiders and red palms remain obscure.

Though studies of glomus bodies do not tell their exact anatomical distribution in the palms, the distribution of the palmar redness suggests a chronic state of vasodilatation involving primarily glomus bodies and direct arteriovenous shunts. The red portion of the palm is warmer than the adjacent pale or uninvolved portions. In many instances "capillary" pulsations may be seen. The red spots along the portion of the palm near where the fingers join it exactly overlie defects where the fascial aponeurosis is absent or much attenuated (Figure 28). Anastomoses from the deeper arteries coming to the surface of the palm are most abundant in such regions.

Information on the comparative histology of the skin, the nerves and blood vessels of various parts of the palm and sole is scanty. It is well known that those regions are more vascular than the neighboring portion of the skin on the arms and legs. But the intimate details of the vascular architecture of different areas of the arms and sole has not been mapped. The presence in the palms and soles of large numbers of direct arteriovenous shunts is significant. Since the increased redness is associated with an increase in surface temperature and "capillary" pulsation the blood flow must be increased. Circulation time and arterial blood pressure do not differ from normal. Histologic studies of a few specimens of skin indicate that the overlying skin is normal though there is a distinct increase in the number and size of the palmar capillaries in red areas compared with those in unaffected areas. As Chalmers pointed out long ago, no cutaneous nerve supplies the exact areas involved and likewise the large anastomosing arterial arcades are not limited to the strict confines of the red regions nor do the white areas seem to have a reduced blood supply.

The relationship of palmar erythema to the arterial spider is a fascinating one which was first emphasized by Walsh and Becker. Redness of the palms in liver disease seems to be remembered as a tradition by many clinicians but I have found no early written record of it. A great many physicians including Doctors Longcope and Hamman at the Johns Hopkins Hospital, Soma Weiss and Christian in Boston, Blankenhorn and Schiff in Cincinnati, could not point out ot me any published reference to this topic in earlier medical writings. Almost simultaneously Perera, Ratnoff and Patek, and I

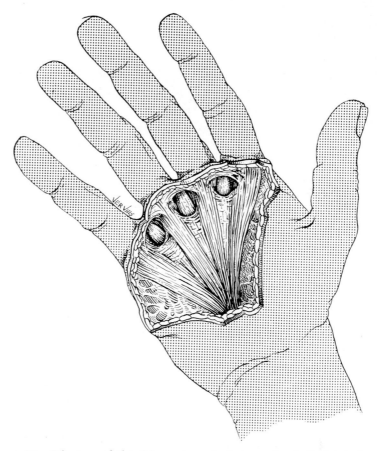

Figure 28. Diagram of the thin spots and absence of palmar fascia in areas exactly underlying portions of the hands where redness is most intense in palmar erythema.

published papers on the occurrence of palmar erythema or "liver palms" in patients with chronic disease of the liver. After these papers appeared many physicians told me that they had known it all the time, but I believe this to be an example of the *devant vu,* the belief that something happening for the first time had happened before.

The occurrence of "liver palms" in pregnant women, many of whom had vascular spiders, was pointed out first by Walsh and Becker. Lofgren also commented on them in pregnancy. He presented evidence that the cause might be estrogenic substances, or the general alteration in hormones associated with gestation. Palmar erythema as a complication of pulmonary tuberculosis has been noted by Trosler who believed it to be caused by toxins. The parallel clinical variations in intensity exhibited by vascular spiders and by redness of the palms suggest a common cause, at least for lesions associated with hepatic disease, pulmonary disease, and pregnancy.

B. HISTORY

In surveying medical writings, one encounters difficulty in deciding whether to include certain obscure conditions of the palms and soles among authentic cases of palmar erythema. Reports during the last quarter of the 19th century were often vague about details and it is difficult to make a diagnosis from the description. Into the category of doubt must fall the erythrokeratosis or erythema keratosis of the soles and palms and related disorders. Palmar erythema as a distinct entity seems to have been described first in an all too brief note by Chalmers written in 1899, although until I resurrected it, this short paper had not been noticed by subsequent writers. Chalmers was impressed by a remarkable palmar redness symmetrically disposed, most pronounced in the palmar pad of the hyperthenar eminence. He described the condition in Europeans who were residing in the Gold Coast of West Africa. There were no symptoms and the condition was entirely innocuous although apparently it was common among the patients he studied. He suggested nothing concerning the nature of the stigma. Bizarre erythema of the palms and fingers with or without cyanosis has been noted in a number of conditions.   Osler (50) noted it in a patient with a fractured skull but it is not known whether it had existed before the fracture or not. A somewhat similar condition may be observed in instances of the painful shoulder and hand syndrome following myocardial infarction. But here the disorder seems clearly to be a vasoneurosis and different from the ordinary variety of palmar erythema. Rheumatoid arthritis is known to be associated with palmar erythema which is indistinguishable from the kind associated with liver disease and pregnancy. I have never been able to correlate this with any disordered function of the liver, low serum albumin, or other alterations in the electrophoretic pattern of serum proteins in rheumatoid arthritis. It is much more common in women than in men. I have never been able to get certain evidence that it had developed after the arthritis began though many patients think it did. I have seen it grow more intense as the disease progressed.

In 1914, there was an interesting discussion of a patient presented at a meeting of the British Dermatological Association. The diagnosis was thought to be erythromelalgia but in the absence of pain this is wrong by definition. Parkes Weber compared the palms with those noted in 1901 during an outbreak of arsenic poisoning where the term "arsenical beer drinkers hands" had been in vogue. It seems to have been painless. Since palmar erythema usually produces no symptoms there is no difficulty in distinguishing it from acrondynia or erythromelalgia which by name and by definition are painful.

The next report, the one usually considered to be the original, was made by Lane in 1929. He observed two men who had had red palms for as long as they could remember. Other members of the family had identical discoloration of the hands. Lane named the condition *erythema palmare hereditarium*. He was the first to observe hereditary and familial features. From the comments at the presentation of his paper and the discussion of several subsequent reports it is clear that many physicians have had a vague familiarity with similar cases but had given them no careful consideration. After Lane's paper sporadic reports and notes appeared. In a review of the subject, I listed these in detail (50). Ambler observed it in liver disease. Mierowsky was the first to observe similar erythema of the soles in a patient who had the palmar change. From the description given by Parkhurst it does not seem likely that isolated plantar erythema with sweating and occasionally with eczema is the same but this must be settled by further study. Slight pain in the hand has been recorded only by Gottron. I have seen two patients who developed palmar erythema rather acutely in whom the process was distinctly painful. There was a sensation of pins and needles with a feeling of fullness and the description by the patient that the hands felt as if they were about to burst. Bloeman noted clubbing of the fingers in a patient who had had palmar erythema over a period of twenty-seven years. Schmidt-laBaume's patient had dermatographism. The patient had noticed that his palms were especially red after drinking alcohol. Aguilera Maruri found the condition in a man with syphilis and tuberculosis. It gradually disappeared under antisyphilitic therapy after it had been present for at least three years. Feldman seems to have been the first to point out the association of palmar erythema with pregnancy. Walsh and Becker presented a large series of cases and cited many of the antecedent reports. The thing that excited their attention was the association of palmar erythema and vascular spiders in pregnant women. This association had not been reported before. Their detailed study included observation of the skin with the capillary microscopy and histologic studies of the vascular spider. Their paper should be consulted by those who wish details of this interesting disorder.

The acroerythrosis associated with pulmonary tuberculosis, described by Banyai and Hirsh, seems to be significantly different from that recorded by Trostler who described changes which are like the "liver palms" of cirrhosis of the liver. Banyai's patients had erythema which was diffuse and homogeneous in appearance. It was painless and not associated with edema, desquamation, or ulceration, or with hyperhidrosis. Some asymmetry occurred in the color of the hands or fingers. The discoloration was not thought to be the same thing as the palmar erythema of liver disease. Some years ago Johnston and Hecht observed palmar erythema, calling attention to the frequency of low serum albumin. I have observed dozens of patients with low albumin but no palmar erythema. I cannot find a casual relationship. Here it is very important to have data on controls. At most if there is a significant connection it is with some common underlying disturbance rather than that palmar erythema causes hypoalbuminemia or hypoalbuminemia causes palmar erythema. Hibbs has called attention to mottled erythematous skin in patients with dry beriberi and said "the soles of the feet and palms of the hands were often fiery red and excellent pictures of so-called palmar erythema."

Observers have called attention to classical palmar erythema in disseminated lupus erythematosus. Baehr, Klemperer, and Schifrin noted erythema of the ends of the fingers and around the nail beds, the thenar and hypothenar eminences and occasionally on the ends of the toes and the ball of the foot. The high proportion of women of childbearing age in collected cases of lupus erythematosus is another bit of testimony suggesting some relationship of estrogens to palmar erythema. Palmar erythema in pregnancy has been described at length by Lofgren. He used estrogenic materials to induce palmar erythema in nonpregnant women who had had palmar erythema during pregnancy but had lost it. He suggested a possible relationship of the lesions to high levels of estrogens.

My experience has been that palmar erythema is a less reliable sign of severe or chronic liver disease than is the advent, or enlargement of vascular spiders. It may increase while spiders are increasing in number and in size, and it usually fades when spiders are on the wane.

7. Palmar Erythema in Pregnancy

Palmar erythema in pregnancy seems to have been reported first by Feldman in 1939. He made a brief comment about it in a woman in whom palmar redness appeared during the second, third, and fourth pregnancies and disappeared as soon as each pregnancy ended. He speculated about a possible relationship to increased blood volume and the hormone progesterone. The classical observations on palmar erythema and pregnancy were made by Walsh and Becker. I have suggested that vascular spiders and palmar erythema observed in pregnancy and chronic hepatic disease might be caused by estrogenic hormones, and I reported a few studies which indicated that such changes in blood vessels in the skin might be induced by administering estrogens to susceptible persons (47-50). In the first paper devoted exclusively to the subject of erythema of the palms and pregnancy, Lofgren gave the details of three patients he had investigated. He reproduced excellent photographs of the return to normal by the fourth postpartum month in a woman with palmar erythema of pregnancy. Independently he made the suggestion that estrogenic substances might be responsible for the reddening of the hands. To test his notion he administered estradiol benzoate to one of the women four and one-half months after delivery. There was a definite increase in the palmar redness but it did not reach the intensity which occurred with pregnancy.

A. SPECIAL STUDIES

We searched for palmar erythema at the same time we were studying spiders. In pregnant women palmar erythema was ob-

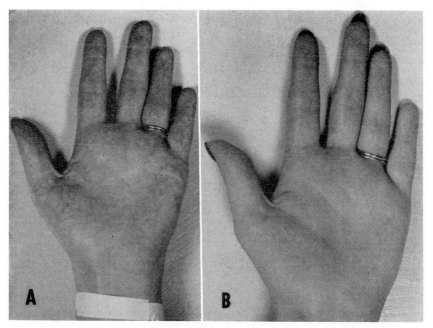

Figure 29.   *Left.* Diffuse palmar erythema occurring in pregnancy. *Right.* Fading of the discoloration at the end of pregnancy.

served in a total of three hundred, or 62.5 per cent of the white women and two hundred and sixty-three, or 35 per cent of the negro women. Figure 30 gives the incidence throughout pregnancy and by the time of the postpartum visit six weeks after discharge. The trend of appearance time of palmar erythema was considerably different from that for vascular spiders. While only 14 per cent of the white women seen in the second month of pregnancy had vascular spiders, palmar erythema was present in 33 per cent at that time. From the second through the ninth month there was a gradual rise. The dip in the curve from the third to the fourth month does not mean that some women lost their palmar erythema during this time but that it happened to be less common in the women making their first clinic visit during the fourth month. By the time of the regular postpartum visit palmar erythema had faded in all but 9 per cent of the women. This compares with 20 per cent who retained

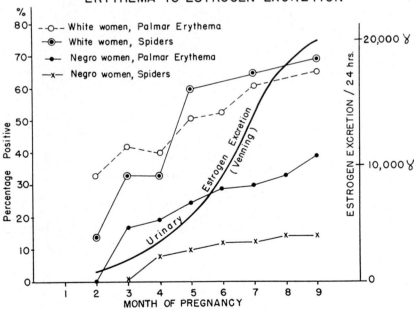

Figure 30. The relationship of the presence of spiders and palmar erythema at various stages of pregnancy to the urinary excretion of estrogens.

one or more vascular spiders at this time. Three white women had palmar erythema before the onset of the first pregnancy and in two of them other members of their family had red palms also.

In Figure 30 the curve for incidence of palmar erythema in negro women is given. This may be compared with a similar curve for vascular spiders in Figure 17. While none was found in the second month, palmar erythema had appeared in 17 per cent by the third month, and there was a slow but steady rise to a peak of 39 per cent by the ninth month. This had fallen to 4 per cent by the

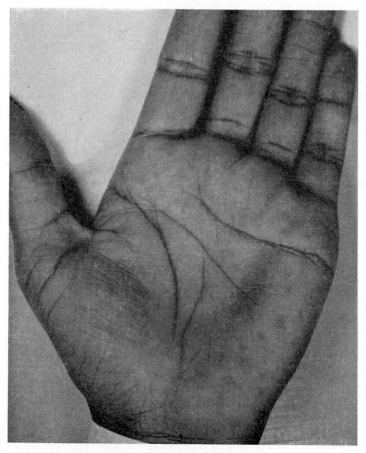

Figure 31.   Palmar erythema in the negro with irregular islands of intense redness and small anemic halos.

postpartum follow-up. Palmar erythema was almost three times as common as vascular spiders in negro women while there was only a slight difference in the incidence of vascular spiders and palmar erythema in white women. The most probable cause is the variation in skin pigment which is much less deep in the palms than in other areas of skin of Negroes.

In Figure 32 the time of appearance has been compared with the time of fading of palmar erythema. There is an indication that the lesion appearing late fades early and lesions occurring early disappear late. The longer they last during pregnancy the longer they remain afterwards, perhaps because they are larger. In 10 per cent the lesions disappeared before or during the last week of pregnancy, a larger proportion than in the case of vascular spiders. Palmar erythema tended to fade more rapidly in negro than in white women (Figure 19). The change in the vessels in the palm is more labile and has a large functional element. The distribution and intensity of the redness vary from time to time. There is spontaneous variation in the combinations of mottled erythema, cyanosis, and pallor in many instances. There is a more abrupt onset, and fading is complete in more women at the time of follow-up.

TIME OF DISAPPEARANCE OF PALMAR ERYTHEMA IN 114 WOMEN WITH KNOWN MONTH OF APPEARANCE(Percentage)

TIME OF DISAPPEARANCE	3	4	5	6	7	8	9	TOTAL
STILL PRESENT				1		1	1	3%
7 WEEKS POST-PARTUM	1	2	1	1	3	2	7	17%
1-7 DAYS POST-PARTUM		2	3	8	6	8	15	42%
24 HOURS AFTER DELIVERY			1	3	5	5	14	28%
LAST WEEK OF PREGNANCY				2	3	4	1	10%

MONTH OF ONSET DURING PREGNANCY

Figure 32.   The relationship of the time of disappearance of palmar erythema to the time of onset in pregnant women.

We have found no explanation for the fact that palmar erythema or vascular spiders may occur alone, or together. Palmar erythema was observed in 67 per cent of the white women who had vascular spiders. Vascular spiders were observed in 71 per cent of the white women who exhibited palmar erythema. Thus if either type of vascular change was found the other was about twice as likely to be present as to be absent. This suggests but does not prove that there may be a common cause. In Figure 20 we have plotted the known month of appearance of vascular spiders and of palmar erythema. There is a tendency for them to occur at about the same time but there are notable exceptions. Further data are needed to determine whether the observed tendency for palmar erythema to

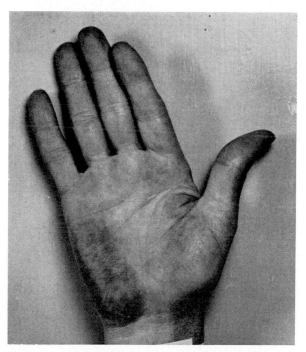

Figure 33. Palmar erythema of the kind commonly called "liver palms" revealing the regions of most intense discoloration on the hypothenar area with less intense color on the palmar surface of the terminal digits of the thumb and fingers, and the roughly circular areas between the points where the fingers join the hand. They are between and not below the palmar calluses. See also Figure 28.

appear before spiders in negro women and the reverse in white women, is characteristic. Their parallel increase in intensity throughout gestation, and then the simultaneous rapid decrease or disappearance further support the idea that spiders and palmar erythema have common etiologic mechanisms. One may suggest that the sites affected, i. e., palms or other parts of the body, are determined by inherent properties of the vessels to react to the stimulus which provokes the change. This may be a genetic peculiarity though there is no proof that this is the case. In the few women observed in two or more pregnancies we have found a tendency for either or both types of lesions to recur. There have been exceptions. Thus the supposition that there is only one mechanism at work in pregnancy which evokes vascular spiders or palmar erythema or both is far from established though the natural history of the phenomena points in this direction.

8. Plantar Erythema

George Pernet first described plantar erythema under the title "symmetrical lividities of the soles of the feet." Plantar erythema occurred in one of his patients with scleroderma. In another lad who was normal it was apparently an independent affection. He did not mention any association with palmar erythema. A striking feature of the color change in the skin was the remarkable symmetry and the clear separation of the red part of the skin from the adjacent uninvolved skin. It was confined strictly to the soles of the feet, being most prominent on the heels, next most prominent was the area under the ball of the foot, and finally it occurred also on the toes.

On the feet the redness appears on the plantar surface involving the pads, the toes, the ball of the foot and less intensely along the lateral half of the plantar pad. Usually it involves most of the thick skin over the heel. Studies by Wetzel and Zotterman indicate that by actual counts of capillary loops, the palms and soles contain vessels arrayed more densely than in other areas of the skin. This may account for the distribution of the erythema. Herzman gives the following descending order of richness of arterial blood supply to the skin—fingerpads, ear lobes, toe pads, palms, forehead, face, dorsum of fingers, hands, feet, forearms, knees and shins.

I have observed plantar erythema only in persons who had palmar erythema. In no case was the redness of the foot greater than that of the hand; usually it was much less pronounced. I have observed it most often in persons with cirrhosis of the liver, rarely in pregnancy, and in only one person who had hereditary palmar erythema as the major change in the skin.

9.   Some Speculations on Mechanism

Years ago when I suggested the hypothesis that spiders and palmar erythema acquired in normal pregnancy or in chronic disease of the liver resulted from an increased circulation of estrogens, I thought that it would be simple to verify or disprove the idea. My notions of the great complexity of causality were naive. Though I have studied the problem intensively off and on during the intervening time, a final answer seems always to elude me as the fast ebbing waters fled before a thirsty Tantalus. Any hypothesis which proposes to explain the mechanisms whereby vascular spiders are produced in the skin, their nature and their meaning, must account for (1) their occurrence in normal persons with no disease; (2) their appearance and enlargement in progressing parenchymal disease of the liver and their rarity in obstructive jaundice; (3) their advent during the progress of normal pregnancy with normal liver function; (4) their peculiar distribution with high concentration in the upper exposed parts of the body; (5) the significance and mechanism of the enhanced flow of arterial blood; (6) the reasons for their abrupt disappearance just before, during, or soon after the natural end of pregnancy and similar but less spectacular decline when disease of the liver improves clinically; and (7) the significance of palmar erythema which may come, go or endure in similar circumstances.

Spiders and palmar erythema may exist singly or together in persons whom we call normal. I have secured data from many sources, Army inductees, soldiers in training or in combat areas, persons attending a cancer screening clinic, patients with a miscel-

lany of diseases and well persons having a routine physical examination. I have records of more than two thousand persons without
obvious liver disease or pregnancy. The various groups show much
individual variation but among them spiders were found in 9 to 15
per cent of white persons but not in normal negroes of whom I have
had occasion to observe few. Palmar erythema was found in 3 to 5
per cent regardless of color. Only about a quarter of the persons
with spiders had palmar erythema but two-thirds of those with palmar erythema had spiders. Spiders are fewer and smaller in "normal" persons than in cirrhotics or pregnant women. There may be
only one or a few. If there are more than five, other conditions
should be suspected. On the other hand, palmar erythema may be
very intense in normal persons. In children, whom I have observed
less systematically, my impression is that spiders are more common.
I know that they may fade away after a few years, or in early adult
life. Or a new one or several may appear, enlarge and then vanish.
A few persons not pregnant and not cirrhotic may have crops which
come and go under the influence of I know not what ecological
forces, internal or external.

Are there any common denominators of cirrhosis and normal
pregnancy? When this question first forced itself on my attention,
I supposed that pregnant women with vascular marks must have
a disturbance of liver function. Observing the smooth course of
pregnancy, childbirth and the normality of offspring made me
doubt this. Later on, tests disclosed no aberration in hepatic function and no connection with the toxemias of pregnancy. Up to this
time spiders and palmar erythema were segregated away from each
other; unknown to obstetricians or beyond the notice of those integrated at the level of the mechanical problems of the pelvis;
known to dermatologists in normal persons, or pregnancy, or cirrhosis but not in all three; and known to internists as curious stig-
mas of cirrhosis. This fragmentation of clinical medicine required
a view of the forest and recognition that the trees, though in different places, might be of the same species.

Thus a search for a common factor began. My initial hunch
that there was a deficiency of B-complex vitamins, which might induce vascular changes in skin and mucous membrane, soon proved

sterile. Then, I observed the endocrine changes which may attend cirrhosis, read about other observations and got the idea of a possible estrogenic effect. One of the early observations attracting my attention to endocrine dyscrasias in hepatic disease was the advent of profuse but irregular uterine bleeding in a fifty-three year old woman with cirrhosis. She had had the menopause nine years earlier. The bleeding occurred at the same time that a new crop of spiders appeared. The uterus had no gross lesion to account for the bleeding. While the patient was under observation several weeks later, bleeding recurred, along with a new crop of spiders. coma, increase in ascites, and worsening of liver function as revealed by laboratory tests. Prothrombin deficiency was not found nor did vitamin K therapy help. Subsequent studies have revealed no connection between vitamin K and spiders (46). Since I saw this patient, many others have been observed and questioned for disturbed endocrine function.

Cirrhosis before the menopause may be associated with an irregular increase in bleeding or intermenstrual hemorrhage. As the disease advances amenorrhea may develop. Still later this may be punctuated by profuse bleeding. Such disorders are well known to gynecologists and students of liver disease.

Impotence is common in men as cirrhosis worsens. It may bring a cirrhotic patient to the doctor. While inquiry into this problem is treacherous, as critics of Kinsey have observed, some reliable patients observe that libido and potency may fail as the disease advances and return as the disease improves. Similar changes may occur in other diseases, perhaps from nonendocrine mechanisms, but testicular atrophy, gynecomastia, prostatic changes and more rarely the development of pectoral, axillary and sometimes pubic alopecia reveal an endocrine disorder.

French observers long ago called attention to situations in cirrhosis which were thought to indicate polyglandular dyscrasias. Paisseau and Oumansky described cirrhosis with hypotrichosis, changed distribution of body fat and retarded sexual development. This picture was elaborated by others (496) who reported complete hairlessness and reduced thyroid and ovarian activity. Comparable disorders have been described in patients with the cirrhosis of hemachromatosis with atrophy of thyroid, pancreas, adrenals, and testes, prostatic hypertrophy, low basal metabolism and heart failure (10),

Gynecomastia has many recognized causes, and others not understood. Karsner made a comprehensive review of the subject up to 1946. Much has been written on the endocrine aspects since that time. My concern is with the relations of the endocrine abnormalities and the liver. Silvestini first described gynecomastia in cirrhosis and Paula made an early detailed study of it in 1930. Corda added testicular atrophy to the combination which in Europe came to be called the Silvestini-Corda syndrome. Detailed studies of estrogen excretion in cirrhosis with gynecomastia by Edmondson, Glass and Soll indicated that a high level of total or free estrogen was the probable cause.

During and after World War II many studies of prisoners of war revealed a form of gynecomastia, sometimes associated with orchitis, which occurred in starved men who suddenly were given large amounts of good food. Various studies indicated that if the liver was abnormal, a good diet might revive activity of pituitary, adrenal and gonad faster than the liver could resume its function in maintaining the metabolic balance between androgen and estrogen. After a time with estrogens circulating at a high level, gynecomastia might appear. Kark and his colleagues have suggested that it might be an effect of the positive nitrogen balance and remasculinization, presumably through the agency of male sex hormone. Testosterone may produce gynecomastia.

Perhaps the best evidence for a direct relationship of estrogens to the feminizing sequels of cirrhosis is in Klatskin's obervation of gynecomastia developing in men with severe serum hepatitis when the estrogen level was high, and receding as the levels returned to normal as the disease improved. This emphasizes the great importance of making endocrine assays and clinical observations before and during the acute stage of liver disease rather than in the chronic inactive stage. Here lesions may remain after the cause has disappeared. In early pregnancy and progressing cirrhosis such studies are notably sparse.

Biskind and Biskind have suggested that a deficiency of B-complex vitamins may be the mechanism by which malnutrition and disease of the liver cause endocrine disturbances. They believe that the relation between estrogen and androgen may be as important as the degree of absolute rise in estrogens.

Gynecomastia occurring in paraplegia is another variety which has not been explained satisfactorily.

In addition to the well known feminizing effects of estrogens it is important here to recall the effects of estrogens and androgens on blood vessels. The role of estrogens has been expounded in great and elegant detail by Barthelemez and Markee for the spiral arteries and other vascular changes of the endometrium and myometrium.

Reynolds has discussed spiral arteries in ovaries and kidneys and has suggested that such a structure may be able to reduce or increase pressures abruptly and to some extent help in control of temperatures. Edwards, Hamilton, Duntley and Hubert demonstrated that male sex hormone has a profound effect on the color and vasculature of men. Eunuchs have a notably pale skin. This is restored to its normal pink color by testosterone. Castrates have less hemoglobin than normal in the skin and much of it is in the reduced state. Thus the cutaneous vascular bed is smaller and has less blood flowing through it. Areas with a large amount of venous blood had dilated veins with an increased amount of reduced hemoglobin. Male hormone restored these aberrations to normal. The observations were extended by Reynolds, Hamilton, di Palma, Hubert and Foster. They found that the vascular bed of eunuchs was more labile than that of normal men, and that the low threshhold of response was restored to normal by testosterone and somewhat less by progesterone. Estrogens increased the excitability of blood vessels for a short period in all subjects. Testosterone increased the finger volume of normal men. In men with testicular deficiency more than in normal men testosterone, progesterone and desoxycorticosterone increased the threshhold of cutaneous vessels to oxygen lack. Still further studies were reported by Edwards and Duntley in normal and ovariectomized women. Just as in men, removal of the gonads did not reverse or destroy the basic peculiarities which distinguish the skin of men and women but did reduce them. This indicates a fundamental genetic difference. Unlike the response in many animals, the effects of hormones were not confined to one area, but involve the entire skin. After the ovaries were removed the cutaneous blood flow became reduced and sluggish but there was no dilatation of venous networks such as were noticed in men. Estrogens or progesterone given singly increased cutaneous blood flow and the proportion of oxyhemoglobin in the blood. Given together they diminished the hemoglobin and more of it was in the reduced form. In the first part of the normal menstrual cycle the skin resembled that in ovariectomized subjects but by mid-cycle and afterwards vascularity increased greatly, reaching an acme in the premenstrual period.

Other hormones can produce vascular changes in the skin. Ebert and his colleagues have shown that adrenocortical steroids have an important role in maintaining normal vascular tone and alter the reactivity of small vessels to many different inflammatory stimuli. Cortisone increased vascular tone in the intact animal without modifying the response to histamine. In man cortisone does not modify the response to histamine.

A direct effect of adrenocortical steroids on the skin has been reported by Castor and Baker who found that prolonged percutaneous application made the epidermis thinner, reduced the size of sebaceous glands and arrested the growth of hair. Collagen fibers lost substance and the thickness of the dermis was reduced. Howes has observed some increased vascularity of experimental granulations in rabbits ears when open wounds are dressed with stilbestrol ointments.

I have made a number of trials of potent estrogenic hormones, both locally or systemically in a number of cirrhotics in remission. In a few normal persons the trials have been negative. I have never been able to cause a spider to appear by extended percutaneous application of estrogens in oil, by implanting pellets or by repeated local injections. On the other hand, the parenteral or oral administration has been followed by the development or the reappearance of new spiders or of palmar erythema in just over a third of the persons in whom it was tried. There was no clinical suggestion of worsening of the disease or deterioration of liver function tests.

I am much troubled by the negative findings, which must be explained. The positive results are consistent with the hypothesis that estrogenic hormones may be a major factor in provoking spiders and palmar erythema in chronic disease of the liver and in normal pregnancy. My belief that I would be able to demonstrate a close relationship between levels of urinary excretion of estrogens and the frequency of spiders in cirrhosis was tested in collaboration with Doctors Mirsky and Broh-Kahn in Cincinnati, and Schedl in Iowa. We found the level of excretion of estrogens in twenty-four hours too inconsistent to allow us to predict that a person would have spiders. If, however, the test was repeated at intervals throughout a long illness, a rising level of estrogen excretion was associated with the appearance or enlargement of spiders or palmar erythema or both as the disease worsened. If the trend was to improvement, vascular lesions diminished or disappeared along with the lowering of estrogen levels and clinical improvement. Nothing tells us whether this parallelism represents cause and effect, simultaneous effects of some other casual process or an accidental circumstance.

The excretion of 17-ketosteroids was low throughout fluctuations in the clinical course of cirrhosis until late in the period of improvement. Many years ago I had suggested that a possible common factor to normal pregnancy and chronic liver disease might be a high level of circulating estrogenic hormones (47, 48, 49) or related endocrine substances, perhaps of adrenal origin in the men at any rate. The fact that no significant abnormality of hepatic function was detected in pregnant women with palmar erythema and vascular spiders as compared those who did not have them reveals that disturbed liver function in pregnancy is not responsible for their occurrence.

As collateral testimony that estrogenic hormones may produce an effect on the vessels of the skin qualitatively similar to the well-documented effect on vessels of the uterus, we have superimposed Venning's curve of estrogen excretion throughout pregnancy upon figures for the incidence of vascular spiders and palmar erythema in white and negro women during pregnancy (Figure 30). Although the forms of the curves do not agree with precision there is similarity. Evidence from tests in the critical early months is not adequate. Crucial data from individual patients very early in pregnancy are wanting. There is no established finding which invalidates the hypothesis that humoral agents with estrogenic function give rise to vascular changes in the skin during the course of normal pregnancy and during the active stage of chronic liver disease.

If estrogenic substances and related steroid hormones are indeed a major factor in causing spiders to appear, the estrogens are not necessarily of ovarian origin since lesions occur in men and women equally and in boys and girls before puberty and in women after the menopause.

Unpublished studies done with my associates, Franklin and Schedl, of fifty normal persons and fifty-eight persons having various hepatobiliary diseases revealed that the urinary ketosteroid level in hepatitis was low in the acute stage and returned to normal as the patient convalesced. On the other hand, levels of estrogen were high during the acute state and returned to normal or subnormal levels as the patient convalesced. In cirrhotics, the 17-ketosteroid level often was much depressed and showed little tendency to return to normal. In benign or malignant extrahepatic obstruction of bile ducts, the 17-ketosteroid excretion usually was depressed. In general the 11-oxyketosteroid excretion was elevated and in randomly selected subjects the eosinophile response to ACTH was normal. These findings might be interpreted as indicating a nonspecific reaction to the stimulus of the disease rather than a particular humoral effect, at least as far as the 17-ketosteroids are concerned. These observations gave us no grounds for determining whether or not the depressed 17-ketosteroid level represented a reduced manufacture of precursors or altered metabolic pathways.

A. Relaxin and Antistiffness Factor

In 1926, Hishaw demonstrated that the separation of the pubic bones in guinea pigs was under the control of a specific substance later called relaxin. The same process occurs in varying degrees in many mammals. There has been much controversy about its nature and its relationship to estrogen and progesterone which have similar properties of inducing pelvic relaxation.

The identification of the antistiffness factor as stigmasterol by Rosenkrantz, Milhorat, Farber, and Milman puts it in a very different category from relaxin. Numerous studies from Hishaw's laboratory and elsewhere have revealed that relaxin is a compartively low molecular weight protein. It has been prepared in adequate purity for clinical testing. It seems to reduce uterine activity and thus may be of use in treating prematurity. Preliminary tests with this compound in persons with a variety of orthopedic conditions have not been followed by the appearance of spiders or palmar erythema but the subject has not been explored systematically. I know of no clinical studies where vascular changes in the skin were sought in persons getting stigmasterol.

B. Arguments Against Estrogens in the Causation of Spiders

No one should be so pleased with his own hypothesis that he fails to see a case against it and there is certainly one which can be made out against estrogens being responsible for the occurrence of spiders and palmar erythema in cirrhosis of the liver and in pregnant women. In the first place the humoral mechanism cannot explain localization. This phenomenon is recognized in such things as gynecomastia which may be unilateral or quite asymmetrical even when induced by steroid hormones. Pellagra, the unilateral variety, is an example of local and regional forces collaborating with a humoral process. Certainly in pellagra, syphilis, the acute exanthems, lupus erythematosus and many other diseases, characteristic lesions of the skin are evoked by humoral forces. Biochemical or infectious agents cooperate with local factors which determine the location and extent, and no doubt, the course of the alterations in the skin. However little the term *locus minoris resistentiae* offers as an exact explanation it expresses a well known phenomenon. Thus while the peculiar localization of spiders and palmar erythema provides no testimony to support a humoral mechanism it is consistent with one.

The abrupt, almost precipitous appearance, and sometimes the sudden disappearance of spiders is unusual for a humoral agency although menstruation may commence abruptly. We might assume that an algebraic factor of time and some X force might suddenly produce an effective result after a given threshhold had been exceeded. As for the disappearance of spiders the thrombotic obliteration of actual spasm of the artery might account for it. In most instances the coming and going is relatively slow and not a dramatic entrance or exit.

The major argument against a humoral mechanism is the fact that a patient may be developing a spider or one may be growing larger while another is vanishing. Chance thrombotic occlusion might explain the loss of one while another is appearing under increased humeral forces, but this is speculative. In any event we must assume there are very strong regional forces operating to explain the curious distribution. Clark and Clark have noticed the puzzling simultaneous appearance and disappearance of arteriovenous shunts in adjacent areas of the rabbit ear as though some kind of homeokinetic see-saw were operating.

Persistent failure to find spiders in persons who have received large doses of estrogenic substances for a long time, although not been searched for systematically, suggests that the hypothesis may be in error though it is plausible that some alteration in liver function must obtain, or actual disease of the liver occur, or the time-dose summation was inadequate in such patients. In short the observations are on much firmer ground than the hypothesis; and this is good.

II

VASCULAR LESIONS CAUSED BY HUMORAL MECHANISMS

1. The Dermovascular Aspects of the Syndrome of Metastatic Carcinoid

Serotonin, isolated and identified ninety years after its biologic effect was discovered, has emerged as a fascinating natural humor of the body. Its myriad, miscellaneous and mystifying functions are the pleasure and confusion of the pharmacologist, the fascination and mystery of the internist and surgeon, the hope and bewilderment of psychiarist and psychologist and a will-o'-the-wisp of the hematologist. Even dermatologists are in on the fun. Ninety years ago Ludwig demonstrated that defibrinated blood contained a vasoconstrictor substance which had not been demonstrable in the same blood before clotting. This was a paradox. Most of the attention to the clotting mechanism traditionally focused on what had been removed from blood in the process of clotting. Here something was added. Rapport, Green and Page, seeking this mysterious vasoconstrictor, identified it in 1948 and since that time its structural formula has been elucidated and it has been synthesized. Thus eighty years elapsed between the discovery of a biological principle recognized and known only by what it did and the final identification and synthesis of the active compound serotonin, 5-hydroxytryptamine, a derivative of tryptophane. This is enteramine which Erasmer had been working with for many years, having discovered it in extracts from various portions of the gut. Hematologists have demonstrated that platelets contained much serotonin, which, however, apparently is picked up and carried around as cargo. Though it aids in clot retraction it is not necessary for effective hemostasis. It has been thought that serotonin may accumulate in areas of the body in concentration sufficient to cause regional vasoconstriction. The potentially harmful effect of serotonin on blood vessels and the heart has been demonstrated by elucidation of the syndrome of metastatic carcinoid and hyperserotoninemia,

The central nervous system contains large amounts of serotonin. Both the central and peripheral effects of serotonin are blocked by lysurgic acid diethylamide which produces effects resembling those of temporary schizophrenia. It has been suggested that the action of reserpine may result from its ability to cause cells in the brain to release serotonin, for when it is free outside of the cells monoamine oxidase destroys it. I have had under observation three patients with the carcinoid syndrome, two of whom were described in association with Olch and Weinberg and one with Funk.

Case Report

Our patient, a man with a harrowing tale of many vicissitudes, was observed first when he was fifty-seven years of age. About nine years before we saw him he had hemorrhoids and intermittent diarrhea. Two years later he had an automobile accident in which he was shaken up but not badly hurt. He dated his major trouble from this episode. His main complaint was the irregular coming and going of an indescribable kind of nervousness. The diarrhea he had had earlier recurred frequently but in no regular association with the erratically eddying waves of anxiety. In his work as a railroad telegrapher he probably sent peculiar and interesting messages because he became easily excited and flustered whenever he addressed himself to the simplest problem. He would feel a sensation of warmth in the neck and face together with lightheadedness. It was hard to concentrate. In any unpleasant situation he tended to get cramping abdominal pains. When embarrassed he would get severe abdominal cramps. Three and one-half years before admission x-rays revealed "spastic colitis and diverticulitis" which did not responded to special diet, antispasmodics, antibiotics and other preparations. During the seven years before admission he had lost forty pounds but only eight pounds during the eight months immediately prior to admission. There had been no respiratory distress, palpitation, bronchial spasm, or symptoms suggesting heart disease. He was under observation from 22 March 1955 to the time of his death on 11 July 1956 and had a total of four hospital admissions.

On examination he was quick in movement and in speech. He had obviously lost weight. His hair was grey and silky. His skin was warm and of fine texture with tiny telangiectases over the torso, head, neck and upper extremities. The complexion was fair and persistently ruddy. Playing in variegated pattern on this florid hue was a transient waxing and waning of the erythema in blotchy patches around the face and neck (Figures 34 and 35). It grew more spectacular as time went on. He had a fine tremor of the tongue and outstretched fingers, a somewhat labile blood pressure, and inconstant lid lag. The heart was without murmurs and was not enlarged. The liver was somewhat enlarged as was the prostate gland. Psychiatrists evaluated his several problems and said he had "chronic brain syndrome without psychosis but demonstrating neurotic reaction" and he was given chlorpromazine, 200 mg. a day, without any improvement. On subsequent examinations it was found that his liver had descended to the region below the umbilicus and was irregular and tender. Pressure on the liver caused a

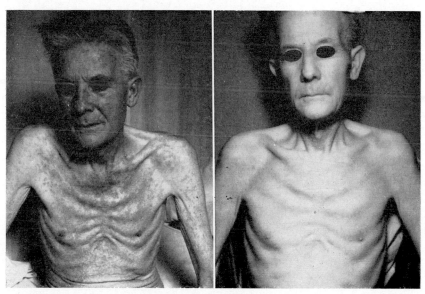

Figure 34 (left). Carcinoid. Black and white photograph of a patient with the syndrome of metastatic carcinoid showing the speckled erythema and his unhappy expression during intense flushing.

Figure 35 (right). Carcinoid. Infrared photograph taken during the same phenomenon. The mottled cutaneous pattern of flushing, pallor and cyanosis is not seen. There is an angiomatous lesion on the anterior aspect of the right shoulder.

violent fit of flushing. There were still no abnormalities of the heart or lungs. After negative upper GI series, on two occasions a barium enema revealed obstruction in the mid portion of the descending colon. On 20 March 1956 he had an operation which revealed in the lumen of the upper ileum a nodule 5 mm. in diameter which had extended through the wall of the bowel, invaded the mesenteric lymph nodes and completely encircled the celiac axis (Figure 36). There were extensive metastases in the liver. Whenever the tumor mass about the root of the mesentery was manipulated, systolic blood pressure fell to about 50 mm. of mercury. No obstruction was found in the colon, spasm having vanished with anesthesia. Biopsy of the metastatic nodule in the liver revealed a characteristic malignant carcinoid. During the next few months he continued to have loud and painful hyperactive peristalsis, paralleling in severity the quantity of food he ate. He continued to have a low-grade fever. His weight had risen twenty pounds during the time as he was developing peripheral edema. A soft, systolic murmur was now heard along the left sternal border.

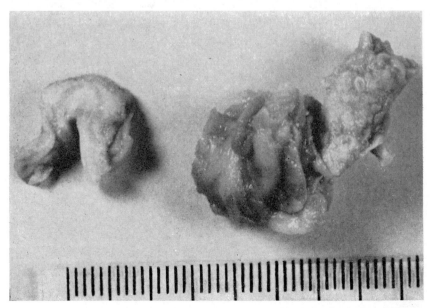

Figure 36. Carcinoid. Autopsy specimens of the primary tumor of the ileum on the left, and the metastatic lesion involving the ileum and celiac axis, on the right. The ruler is marked in centimeters.

Bronchial wheezes occurred at times. Abdominal pain, vomiting, increasing edema, and psychotic behavior were the major problems. He had auditory and visual hallucinations of a paranoid nature. Later he became disoriented, developed ascites and edema in all portions of the body, bilateral pleural friction rubs, an apical systolic murmur, and a similar murmur over the aortic and tricuspid valve areas. His hemoglobin was reduced to 9.7 grams. There were no gallops, shocks or thrills and no diastolic murmurs. The liver became increasingly knobby as it expanded in size. The color changes in the skin became more and more conspicuous; the brighter redder hues predominated over the upper part of the body, and the darker, bluer hues over the lower part. He developed numerous dark, flat angiomas from which the blood could be compressed fairly readily. They were most numerous on the front of

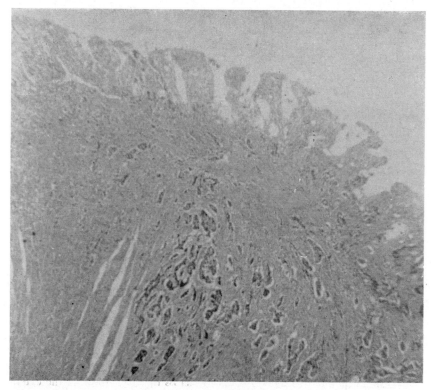

Figure 37.   Carcinoid. The microscopic section of the primary tumor in the ileum.

the chest and on the dorsal aspect of the upper arms. In diameter they ranged from specks just visible to 3 mm. The structure of the lesion is revealed in Figure 42. In addition, there were numerous networks of fine telangiectatic vessels widely disseminated over the skin. During his declining days the disorientation continued, the ascites and peripheral edema accumulated, the superior rectus muscle of the left eye became paralyzed and a friction rub was heard over the liver. He died quietly on 11 July 1956.

At autopsy the principal abnormalities were: a small, discrete yellow-gray tumor in the wall of the proximal ileum (Figure 36); gross metastases to the regional lymph nodes and the liver; moderate hypertrophy of the right ventricle; thickening without stenosis of the tricuspid and pulmonic valves which were rubbery to the touch, shimmering with increased highlights, and somewhat succulent. A similar but less extensive valve disorder was found in the mitral and to a lesser degree the aortic valve. There was no septal opening between the atria or the ventricles. The coronary arteries were almost occluded by sclerotic plaques but there was no infarct. Ascites, bilateral hydrothorax, acute esophageal and duodenal ulcers, testicular atrophy, acute passive congestion of the right lung

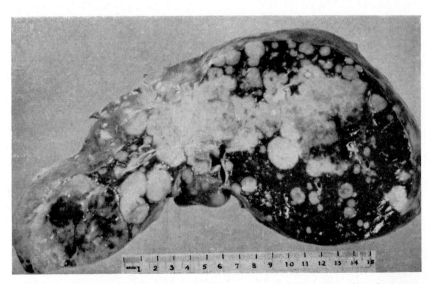

Figure 38. Carcinoid. Transverse section across the liver, showing the extensive coalescing and isolated nodules of metastatic carcinoid which had replaced much of the liver.

and aortic sclerosis completed the findings.   Microscopically the tumor nodules had the characteristic structure of carcinoid tumor (Figures 38 and 39).   There was very intense fibrosis of the adhesions which developed at the site of the abdominal operation far out of proportion to the local tumor growth.   Sections of the tricuspid and pulmonary valves disclosed a cartilage-like proliferation of connective tissue (Figure 40).   There was no calcification.   I have fixed some of the features of this dramatic clinical cinema in mind by this limerick:

> *This man was addicted to moanin'*
> *Confusion, edema and groanin',*
> *Intestinal rushes,*
> *Great tri-colored blushes,*
> *And died of too much serotonin.*   W.B.B.

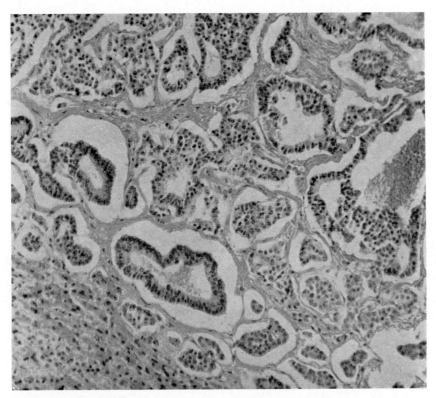

Figure. 39.   Carcinoid.   Metastatic nodule compressing the liver cells.

A. SPECIAL STUDIES

Two serotonin antagonists were used without any obvious effect. BOL 148, two tablets five times a day, were given for four days, and on another occasion 25 mg. of 1-Benzyl 2-Methyl 5-Methoxy tryptamine HCl, was given for two weeks. Urinary excretion of 5-hydroxyindolacetic acid ranged from 195 to 921 mg. in twenty-four hours but there was no particular relationship of this fluctuation to any form of therapy. There was no abnormality in blood coagulation. Platelet deficient plasma from the patient produced no improvement in the defective prothrombin consumption of the patient with severe thrombocytopenia. Serum from the patient caused no more improvement than a normal control did in correcting defective prothrombin consumption from the same patient.

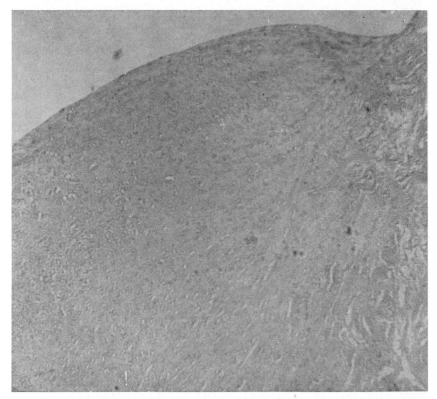

Figure 40.   Carcinoid. The pulmonic valve lesion with fibroblasts and amorphous ground substance.

There was a slight but not significant increase in the speed of clot retraction.

The Undefriend test for 5-hydroxyindolacetic acid in the urine is simple and apparently reasonably specific though a banana diet may cause false positives. In many hundreds of tests we have found none strongly positive except in patients with metastatic carcinoid and the test has been negative in two persons with carcinoid of the bowel without metastasis. This suggests that the liver or the lung inactivates, sequesters or destroys serotonin.

B. Special Features

In this syndrome angiomas arise in the skin. They are unlike spiders, cherry angiomas or venous stars but have some resemblance

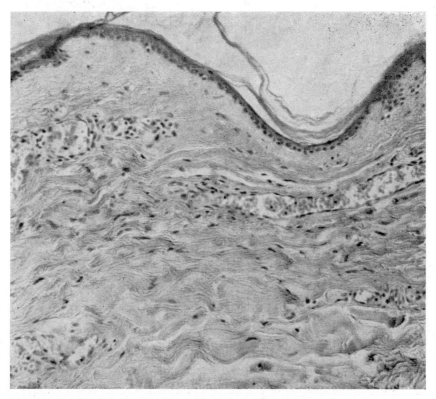

Figure 41. Carcinoid. Angiomatous lesion consisting of dilated vessels with very thin walls near the surface of the skin.

to venous lakes, though smaller and having a completely different distribution. The histopathology suggests angiomatous and telangiectatic changes, proliferative and degenerative (Figure 41). The analogy with spiders, and the liver's role in excreting, inactivating or destroying estrogens is in keeping with the fact that the carcinoid tumor must have metastasized to the liver to produce the syndrome. In addition to the personal cases under observation, I have seen several others and have never seen a lesion characteristic of pellagra. If pellagra does indeed occur in patients with metastatic carcinoid, I would ascribe it to the loss of vitamins from the hypermotile diarrhea. There is no evidence that nicotinic acid metabolism is affected but tryptophane metabolism is seriously impaired. The avid carcinoid tumor has a high metabolic priority for tryptophane with which to build serotonin. It is possible that, with the intake of nicotinic acid at a critically low level, the diversion of trypto-

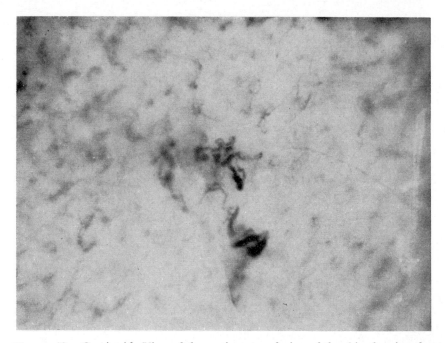

Figure 42.   Carcinoid. View of the angiomatous lesion of the skin showing the irregularly disposed, tortuous, dilated and bulbous vessels.   They are many times the diameter of normal capillary loops.   (Courtesy of Captain Davis.)

phane from its possible conversion into nicotinic acid might give rise to clinical pellagra.

Flushing, with the curious triple reaction may be caused by a vasoconstrictor agent by: (1) release of histamine; (2) stimulation of peripheral vasomotor nerves; (3) local reactions aiming at restoring a steady state, or (4) something else. We do not know whether the regional effector mechanism or local factors are important but tissue reactivity has some bearing on the matter since the most intense flushing occurs repeatedly in precisely the same place. Release of serotonin by massage of the liver triggers the effect with precision approaching that of a circulation time test. The bizarre mingling of erythema, cyanosis and pallor are not explained as uniform effects of a vasoconstrictor so that local reactions and homeokinetic mechanisms may play a part.

Bronchial spasm, which may be induced in experimental animals, probably accounts for the difficulty in breathing. Hypermotility of the gut and plentiful watery diarrhea molest the victims of the syndrome. Clifton and his colleagues have demonstrated a sharp contraction of the bowel in normal persons after intravenous infusion of serotonin, a reaction not shared by persons with cirrhosis of the liver or sprue. This is of interest in conjunction with the occurrence of spiders in chronic disease of the liver and is in keeping with an altered responsiveness of the vascular bed of the skin in cirrhosis.

The acquired valvulitis, particularly on the right side of the heart, seems to be caused by repeated injury to the valves produced by the intermittent but frequent surges of high concentrations of serotonin which reaches the right side of the heart where the endocardium may undergo invisibly the same vascular torment which plagues the skin. Spasm and reactive hyperemia in a structure whose mission leaves little repose give rise to inflammation, fibrotic reaction with an abundance of amorphous ground substance and final scarring with stenosis. Since there was no opening between the right and left sides of the heart in our patient, the fact that some damage is done to the valves on the left side suggests that the lungs were not quite able to remove all the serotonin which came to them in such abundant quantities.

Clotting is active and retraction is excellent but apparently there is nothing supernormal about clotting in people with hyperserotoninemia. It is possible that intravascular clotting may be connected with the development of angiomas.

Fibrosis of a very dense variety may be related to the general increase in collagen, fibrinoid and hyaline material seen in the several lesions.

2. Epidemic Dropsy

From time to time in the land of India there have been remarkable outbreaks of a plague called epidemic dropsy. Even from the very earliest description of it, it could be separated from beriberi to which it had some resemblance. It was recognized as a distinct entity. My attention was called to this phenomenon some years ago by Dr. Farrell. In company with many physicians from Calcutta and elsewhere he had observed an outbreak in India during the winter of 1934-35. He had been much impressed by the eruptive angiomatosis associated with this disorder. Some of the published clinical descriptions are not complete. It is not always clear that the histopathologic studies were made from classical lesions. This eruptive angiomatosis may affect blood vessels throughout the body as well as in the skin. There is a weakness and dilatation of capillaries together with destructive and proliferative changes in which both telangiectasia and angiomatosis join hands. In the skin this acute vascular anarchy may give rise to erythematous areas which dot the skin with spots and red lumps. When they are large, they tend to be somewhat elevated. Because of the weakness of the vascular wall, hemorrhage may occur in the lesions. Purpura may dominate the clinical findings. There is no description known to me of their fate if the patient recovers.

Careful studies by Lal and his associates indicate that this is an intoxication. Epidemiological studies demonstrated a relationship to mustard in the diet. Further studies showed that it was mustard contaminated by the seeds of *argemone mexicana*. A great many efforts to reproduce the disorder in animals have been only partly successful and the precise compound responsible for changes has not been identified. Nonetheless there is strong evidence that it is a toxic material, which, eaten in fairly large amounts, causes vascular changes. There is no indication that any other process is intermediate. The effect produced has some analogies with the toxic exanthems, ergot poisoning, lathyrism, and some of the rickettsial diseases. It would be be of much interest if the toxicology were worked out with modern methods for here is an example of an eruptive angiomatosis at least partially understood. It might throw light on neoplasia as well as vascular lesions of various kinds.

3. The Skin Lesions in Pellagra

A high degree of symmetry is usual in lesions caused by humoral mechanisms. The cutaneous lesion of pellagra is characteristically symmetrical, has a very sharp line of demarcation from the adjacent apparently uninvolved skin. Histopathologic studies reveal that similar processes are going on in the clinically unaffected skin even without a lesion. Any portion of the skin may be affected. It is typical for mucous membranes to be involved—notoriously any part of the alimentary canal and sometimes the vagina in women.

Before any lesion occurs the skin may be mottled. The true skin lesion in pellagra begins as a diffuse erythema which looks just like any mild burn. There is redness, increased heat, some edema of the skin, increased sensitivity, and spontaneous burning, though itching is rare. Pellagrous dermatitis may occur in exposed portions of the face, the neck, the arms and hands, the legs and feet, or in the moist regions beneath the breasts, in the pudendal or perianal region or other places where exposure to sunlight has not occurred. After the erythema has continued for some days, usually at a fairly steady degree of high intensity, the color begins to diminish and slight pigmentation appears. If the reaction is very violent, blisters and blebs may occur and secondary infection may confuse the picture. Where it is relatively mild, the erythema fades, and desquamation of skin may occur in fine scaly flakes or more commonly in pieces several centimeters long. Occasionally almost a complete cast of the superficial skin may be thrown off, though it is relatively uncommon for the lesion to encircle a limb. During the stage of erythema when there is some edema, the superficial aspect of the skin may appear parchment-like. Pressure with a pencil or the finger may squeeze blood from a very wide area since the skin may take on some of the characteristics of a hard translucent shell.

As the erythema fades pigmentation with melanin appears and spreads as did the original erythema from the center to the periphery or along the arm or leg in advancing bands. The new skin is soft, may be heavily pigmented and is likely to display a prominent mottled pattern. It is a mistake to consider pellagra as a skin disease only. This was the source of much of the almost interminable historic confusion about the nature of pellagra. Some aspects of pellagra are vascular and concern the skin.

A great deal of work has been done on reasons for the localization of skin lesions in pellagra. This theme has been a recurring motif in medical polemics. The skin lesions in pellagra and the reasons for their localization illustrate the principles of interaction between internal and external stimuli as they produce their effects in causing a disease, determining the localization of lesions, the progress of symptoms, the course and in many instances the outcome of illness. Another reason for much confusion in understanding skin lesions was the fixed idea that pellagra was a skin disease. The emphasis was on static rather than dynamic aspects of the unfolding natural history. Some years ago I had occasion to observe approximately seven hundred persons with the many symptoms and various lesions of pellagra and other B-complex deficiency disease. I made a detailed study of factors affecting localization. Asymmetric lesions which appeared spontaneously gave me the clue. I was able to induce unilateral lesions in undernourished persons who were going into the phase of relapse of pellagra.

If the diet has been deficient in nicotinic acid, perhaps low in tryptophane, and ordinarily but not necessarily high in corn, and perhaps containing toxic materials such as naturally occurring antimetabolites, or other unknown factors, people get pellagra. Why do skin lesions appear and what determines their localization? Pellagra long ago was called *the disease of the sun*. Exposure to sunlight was recognized as likely to produce more serious damage in a pellagrin than in a normal person. The supposed dependence on the sun even led to the belief that a photosensitizing process operated. This notion was abetted by the confusion about urinary pigments in pellagra which were at one time supposed to be porphyrins. While porphyrin may be excreted, usually the levels are not very high. No one has shown a relationship between an increased excretion of porphyrin or of the indolacetic acid pigments and the suscepti bility to, the extent, or the course of skin lesions.

One of the problems in the study of skin lesions, particularly those concerned with blood vessels is the fact that we have no way of separating for physiologic measurements the relatively small basal flow and the conspicuous increases in flow which occur in certain diseases and in states requiring a rapid loss of heat. Among the important neglected observations in pellagra, is the fact that skin lesions in different parts of the body may be at different stages at the same time in one patient. There may be an early erythema in one place, peeling and desquamation in another, and advancing pigmentation in a third. This indicates that though humoral mechanisms, the disturbances in respiratory function and the dynamics of enzyme action, are essential in producing the trouble, local factors are very important. Not only location but time of development of lesions and the speed of their progress and other elements in dynamic natural history have eluded physicians who were either not interested or did not have the time to busy themselves with such details. The analogy with vascular spiders, though not close, should be emphasized since in an occasional patient new spiders are appearing and old ones are disappearing at the same time. This also implies that very important regional forces operate. Furthermore, since Martini and others have expressed the conviction that localization is conditioned by exposure to light, wind, and air, the analogy with pellagra may be permitted but not stretched too far.

In an effort to study factors in localization, I found thirty-two instances of unilateral or conspicuously asymmetrical skin lesions out of eight hundred and eighty-nine cases. In patients who were bedfast, leaning on one elbow when they ate might cause localization on this elbow. In persons up and around, unilateral lesions developed on the side of severe varicosities. Unilateral lesions occurred in scars. In one instance the pellagraderm appeared in the non-paralyzed hand of a patient with hemiplegia. In the majority of instances it was possible to demonstrate irritation, injury, or disturbance in blood flow to account for the unusual localization of the lesion (Figure 43).

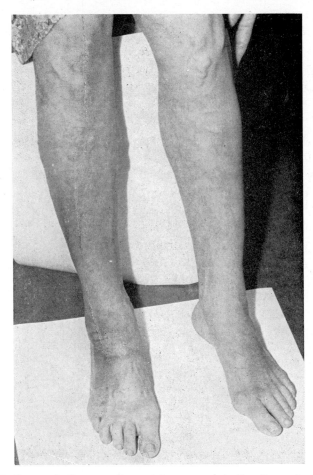

Figure 43. Pellagra. Pellagrous dermatitis asymmetrically disposed over the dorsum of the foot in a patient with an asymmetrical arrangement of varicose veins. The silhouette of the veins on the right leg is displayed. There were no comparable veins on the left leg and foot where no lesion developed on the dorsum. At the time this photograph was taken the patient had bilateral dermatitis on the back of the hands and arms, glossitis, diarrhea, and mild mental disturbance.

On the basis of these observations, efforts were made to increase the metabolism in particular regions of the skin by using heat from an ordinary electric pad while the cutaneous circulation was impeded by sandbags weighing three and one-half pounds. In several susceptible pellagrins who were so treated during the one or two weeks before a spontaneous outbreak of pellagra, unilateral lesions appeared in the area where the heat and ischemia had been employed, while none occurred in the opposite side which had not had such treatment. Symmetrical lesions appeared elsewhere at the same time. Since the experiment in no way involved the sun, photosensitivity was not responsible.

By far the most fertile cause of localization of lesions in the skin pellagra is exposure to the sun. Not only does this frequently give rise to an acute pellagrous skin lesion but relatively minor degrees of exposure may be followed by a severe clinical illness. Even when there has been no recent exposure to sun, it is common for lesions to appear in areas which have been intensely exposed in the past suggesting that the altered state of circulation and other changes may continue and thus provide sites for localization at a subsequent period.

Pellagra, fortunately now very rare with us, is a good example of a systemic disease produced by a specific deficiency operating at the humoral level. Local lesions produced by enzymic disturbance are situated where the skin has been damaged recently or long ago by nonspecific agents, of which sunlight is the traditional villain, the most important but not an essential culprit.

4. Diabetic Angiopathy

There will be room for no more than a note about the angiopathies in diabetes to which innumerable workers have made contributions. They are not cutaneous but I put them here for interest. Current investigations suggest that vascular changes in diabetes are intimately and essentially related to the whole complex process of diabetes and are not a sequel to just a part of the metabolic disturbance. One group of observers sees these disorders as potentially preventable complications; another views them as concomitants, as part of Calvinistic doom fore-ordained when the disease begins or before. The vascular syndromes of long standing diabetes are characterized by the equal risk of men and women. Most striking is the ophthalmological picture of the retina with venous anomalies, vascular proliferations, exudates, hemorrhages, blood spots, and pigmented lesions of the macula. Generally the retinal veins are overfilled. They are enlarged, tortuous and sometimes beaded. Minute globular aneurysms occur in the retinal capillaries, particularly on the venous side, beginning singly or in small numbers within or near the macula. They are the earliest unequivocal retinal sign of diabetes.

Exudates in diabetic retinopathy present many unsolved problems. They have a tendency to coalesce and form large waxy patches. Rounded solid hyaline masses may be seen in sections of the retina. Phlebosclerosis of the retinal veins may occur as well as infiltration around nerve fibers. Ultimately hemorrhages, exudates, and opacification of the lens may develop. Unfortunately there is no detailed study of individual subjects with a description or photographs of the retina from the earliest stages to the final appearance of severe damage, and ultimately autopsy examination.

The small, round, sanguinolent spot seen with the ophthalmoscope has been recognized for more than a half century as pathognomic of diabetes. Ballantyne demonstrated that retinal lesions are true microaneurysms. They are very numerous in histological sections of the retina of persons whose diabetes has lasted a long time. Changes in the veins of the retina appear as dark irregular areas of congestion suggesting actual beading of the veins. Proliferations of blood vessels occur in protracted diabetes. Fine new blood vessels work their way into the vitreous, followed later by formation of a rather scanty connective tissue which may obscure and later destroy vision. Diabetic proliferative retinopathy can be distinguished by ophthalmoscopic examination from other similar proliferations as long as the vitreous is not opaque. In contradistinction to the retinopathy of hypertension which is located more on the arterial side of the capillaries, the diabetic angiopathy is primarily venular.

Ditzel and others have observed the vessels of the bulbar conjunctiva. In a study of young and old, diabetic and normal, it was possible to define the vascular changes attendant upon aging, separate them from those peculiar to diabetes and evaluate the effects of aging and diabetes taken together. In brief, the arteries and veins in youth had a ratio of 1:2 to 1:3. The flow of blood was smooth and perivascular edema was absent. With aging irregularities developed in the terminal arterioles and the venules, large and small. As age advanced hyaline infiltration occurred in the vessels. Erythrocytes aggregated in clumps and clusters within the lumen of the vessels. Flow became sluggish in capillaries and venules. In addition to these changes diabetics had capillary and venular alterations, exudates and plugging of arterioles with aggregates of red cells. The older a diabetic at the onset of the disease, the more his vessels showed lesions characteristic of aging. The younger he was at onset the more exclusively "diabetic" were the lesions. Diabetic capillary changes which were reversible were varying degrees of venular distention and arteriolar narrowing. The permanent changes consisted of elongation of venules and the venous limb of the capillaries with evidence of degeneration.

It is essential that the characteristic diagnostic features of diabetic angiopathic be recognized and that we understand those elements which serve to differentiate them from other lesions superficially similar and sometimes mistaken for them. We still are far from understanding the relationship of vascular changes to the metabolic disturbances in diabetes to degree of control and to the passage of time. Fortunately, the only one we may hope to control, namely the adequacy of metabolic regulation, appears to have the most influence on angiopathies.

5.   Cushing's Syndrome

The opium of forgetfulness is spread widely with a random distribution. It is well that we forget much of the nonsense and confusion of past generations. What we remember, however, is dependent upon the strange fortuity of recollection and other subtle forces. Few people who first describe or understand a disease achieve eponymic immortality. Goldstein has reported several strange quirks of fate in the survival of a name attached to signs, syndrome, or symptom complex while the originator usually is forgotten. A pressure campaign by friends and admirers is more likely to achieve results than actual priority. Such certainly is the case with Cushing's syndrome since it was already well recognized in the 1920's and Cushing's paper on the subject was not published until 1932. Bauer had addressed himself to this interesting problem. Perhaps even more remarkable in the case of Cushing's disease is the fact that what we call Cushing's syndrome was thought by him to have its symptoms produced through the intermediation of basophilic changes in the pituitary without any necessary lesion or malfunction of the adrenal. We now know that it is the other way around.

However this may be, Cushing's disease and Cushing's syndrome in classic form present several striking vasocutaneous abnormalities. The most flagrantly spectacular, the purple striations, are not primarily a vascular change. By stretching and shearing pressures, superficial layers of skin are pulled apart along lines of cleavage which leave the underlying vascular bed readily exposed. Another part of the mechanism is increased vascularity of the skin as is demonstrated when the color of the striations changes conspicuously under the influence of appropriate therapy. They undergo somewhat the same alterations as the red striations of pregnancy after the termination of pregnancy. While Cushing's disease is active, however, the vascular bed of the striations has a purple hue. This fades leaving merely the silver striation after the disease is brought in hand therapeutically. The florid appearance of the face with a vivid red color is produced partially by telangiectases and partially by dilatation of the subpapillary venous plexus and its increased content of oxyhemoglobin.

Another aspect of the vascular change in the skin is the increased fragility of blood vessels. This accounts for the easy bruising. It is not rare for petechial hemorrhages, purpuric spots, and larger ecchymoses to occur in a region sometimes already marked by telangiectases. I have seen typical spiders in two patients with Cushing's syndrome.

There are many published photographs illustrating the cruel metamorphosis which occurs during the evolution of Cushing's disease or syndrome. What may have been a fine looking, normal man, woman, or child, becomes disfigured, developing a type of obesity which tends to spare the limbs, a buffalo hump, great jowls, a look of florid plethora, hirsutism, telangiectasis, the purple slash marks of striation and lesions which superficially resemble acne. Similar but less advanced changes may occur with the use of various steroid hormones. I have not seen actual striations develop in such people though some of the other vascular changes in the skin do occur.

III

CONGENITAL AND HEREDITARY LESIONS AND BIRTHMARKS

1. Hereditary Hemorrhagic Telangiectasia: Osler's Disease

Osler's disease or hereditary hemorrhagic telangiectasia has an interesting history. One wonders whether the disease is new, still arising here and there from some chromosomal mischance, an easily triggered mutation, or whether the syndrome has emerged from hiding before our eyes, as we slowly learn to observe and reflect. It was the first "bleeding disease" for which the mechanism was understood reasonably well. In 1865, Babington wrote a brief note on "hereditary epistaxis." His letter in the *Lancet* was a response to Sutton's report on some curious cases of increasing nosebleeds. Babington described epistaxis in five generations of a family. This was perhaps the first true hereditary hemorrhagic telangiectasia although he failed to comment on a diagnostic skin lesion. Legg in 1876 described "a case of hemophilia complicated by multiple nevi" which was almost certainly another example. Chiari described a probable case in 1887. Rendu gave a brief discussion of the clinical features and called the disease pseudohemophilia. Chaufford and Kopp reported early examples. Churton reported a probable case with epistaxis, hemoptysis and multiple pulmonary aneurysms. The disease was not really fixed as an entity, however, until Osler established its true character in a series of classic reports (628-630). He finally brought it out of the mysterious cluster of diseases characterized by hemorrhage; recognized that the clotting mechanism was normal; and that bleeding resulted from inadequate vessels. Parkes Weber elaborated upon the description and emphasized the clear-cut differences between hemorrhagic telangiectasia and hemophilia. He noted specially the absence of sex-linked transmission and the tendency for nose bleeds to occur before telangiectases were

132

hemorrhage, and the recurrence of often repeated hemorrhage at the time telltale telangiectases become prominent, usually in the third decade. Skin lesions may occur in young children but apparently are not well known or often searched for. Ehrenborg and his associates have recently discussed this problem and reported a five year old boy who had nosebleeds from birth, hematemesis and melena at three and later had to have a partial gastrectomy. Classical lesions were found on the skin and telangiectatic capillaries with recent hemorrhage in the stomach as seen through the gastroscope and in the surgical specimen. I have under observation a child of seven with fine networks of telangiectases in the face but not the typical lesions her father has.

In my original observations, I stated that the lesions do not go away spontaneously and that unless a profound anemia causes them to fade they can always be found (53). Subsequent observations indicate that this is only half true. It is true in the sense that I have always been able to find lesions, once they make their first appearance. Careful study, repeated inspection and pictures taken over a period of ten years in individual patients reveal three states or processes. First, some lesions have persisted without any alteration over this span of time. Second, some lesions have disappeared completely over periods ranging from six to thirty-six months. They left no trace to be detected by the most searching inspection in a hunt guided by photographs of the skin or mucous membranes. Even 20-power magnification disclosed no old footprint to tell where a lesion had been. One assumes that thrombotic obliteration occurred. Third, new lesions have appeared, have grown in size, and in some instances have also disappeared. They may reach full size within three months though my records do not tell exactly how rapidly. The lesions which came and then vanished usually were small.

E. Gross Morphology

It is possible to differentiate the telangiectatic lesion of Osler's disease, the classic pinhead angioma, from spiders and other vascular spots by its clinical characteristics alone. In Osler's disease the typical lesion is punctiform. It is a spot. Usually it is not elevated. Sometimes it is even depressed. The margins connecting it with the normal skin are sharp. A single vessel may be connected with a punctum, or there may be several branching vessels so the lesion assumes the appearance of the arterial spider. But in such cases there are other spots or papules, sharply isolated, with no vessels attached (Figs. 44 and 45). Furthermore, the central red area of the

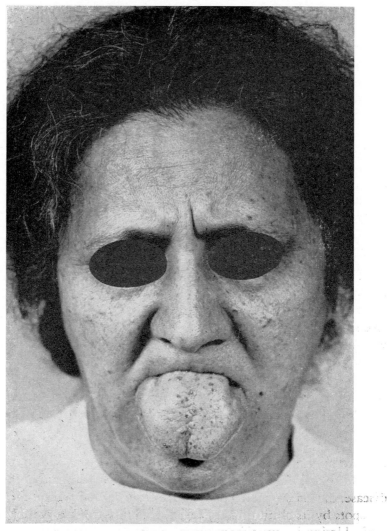

Figure 44.   Osler's disease. Angiomas of the tongue and face in a woman with characteristic hereditary hemorrhagic telangiectasia.

telangiectatic lesion of Osler's disease is very much larger than is the body of the spider in relation to the spider's much more numerous effluent vessels. The very thin skin over the lesion may flake off in fine silvery scales. At times there may be a ring of white dry scales around the lesion, especially the lesion on the fingers.

In patients with Osler's disease I have never failed to find perfectly characteristic lesions elsewhere in the body when there was some trouble in identifying a particular lesion as a spider or a telangiectatic mark of Osler's disease. Solid, somewhat cyanotic, nodular forms occur (Fig. 46). They may be elevated. Probably when the spider-like lesion occurs in Osler's disease the vascular weakness involves one of Renaut's terminal arteries in the skin. Its arteriolar

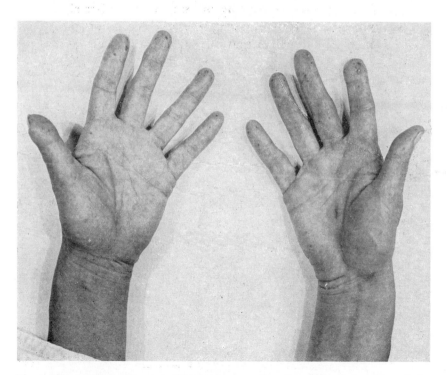

Figure 45. Osler's disease. The punctate telangiectases of the skin of the palm of the hand, most prominent on the distal phalanges. The lesion on the right index finger has a soft scale over it where bleeding and healing occurred in the past.

ramifications accentuate the normally invisible vascular structure to the point of visibility.

Pressure on the vascular spider produces complete blanching. When pressure is released the centrifugal blood flow fills the larger branches and a bright red color immediately suffuses the region rendered pale by compression. Pressure on the lesion of Osler's disease may cause complete fading. Frequently, however, it is not complete because volvulus and strangulation of some of the loops occur in the telangiectatic mass of coiled vessels.

Studies with transparent pressure capsules connected to mercury manometers disclose that the pressure required to blanch the lesion in Osler's disease is of the same order as that required to obliterate the arterial spider, 60 to 100 mm. Hg. Although frequently pulsation may be seen by pressing with a glass slide, palpable pulsation is rare. The average size of the lesion in Osler's disease is much smaller than that of the arterial spider. Skin tem-

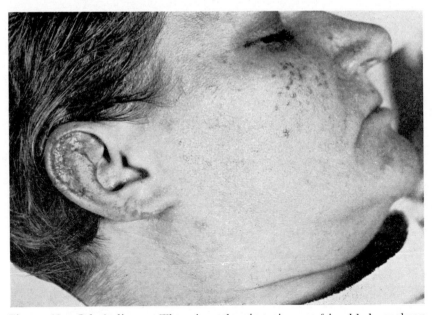

Figure 46.   Osler's disease. There is a telangiectatic mat of jumbled vessels on the right ear, and the slightly elevated, nodular telangiectases on the cheek. Lesions such as the ones on the cheek ordinarily do not fade with pressure and rarely pulsate.

perature over Osler's disease lesions is not higher than that over adjacent uninvolved skin, except in large pulsating lesions.

F. DISTRIBUTION

In Osler's disease the mucous membranes are affected almost always. The disordered vascular structure may exist in any part of the body. Lesions have been described in most vessels except the aorta and the great veins. The lesion, with thin weak walls leading to ubiquitous bleeding, presents almost infinite variety. At the very early stages and in an occasional patient having only a few lesions the mucous membranes of the mouth and nasopharynx may disclose no lesion. I have watched one man in his twenties from the time I found but one lesion on the lip till now eight years later he has scores. With the disease known in the family it was possible to make the diagnosis from one typical spot. They may appear in any part of the skin though more occur in the upper part of the body than in the lower portions. Mucosal telangiectases are almost always visible in Kiesselbach's area on the nasal septum and on the tip and dorsum of the tongue and rarely beneath it. They may occur at the opening of the eustachian tubes. I have observed them in conjunctiva, esophagus and bronchial tubes, stomach, intestine, vaginal and rectal mucosa. In the skin they are notable for their frequency on the palmar surface of the fingers and the hands, the fingernails (Fig. 47), the lips, the ears including rarely the tympanic membrane, the face, the lower portions of the arms, the toes, with the trunk and abdomen being less often affected. The toes and soles may be marked also. Their disposition on the palmar surface and their occurrence in the nail bed, lips, and ears and fingertips, following the distribution of glomus bodies, suggests that the glomus body, with its intricate vascular arrangements, may be especially liable to suffer the vascular weakness of Osler's disease.

Hemorrhages from or into the stomach, bowel, lung, meninges, brain, retina, sclera, kidney, bladder, liver and mesenteric vessels attest the universal range of weakened vessels involving the remote inner reaches of solid organs and tubular structures as well as mucous and cutaneous surfaces.

Martini has adduced strong evidence that there may be a specific form of cirrhosis of the liver associated with Osler's disease.

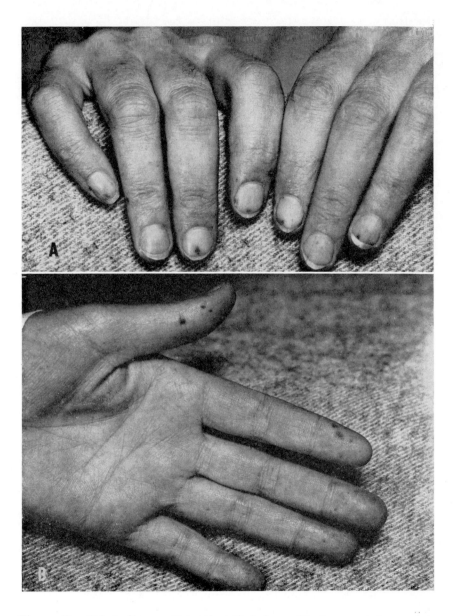

Figure 47.   Osler's disease. Telangiectatic lesions with characteristic punctate areas on the palmar surface of the fingers and the typical diffuse, sometimes linear spots under the nails.   These ordinarily do not have very sharply defined margins.

I had been somewhat reluctant to accept Fitzhugh's conclusions and those of a number of others, marshalled by Martini to support his contention. This was based on the fact that not more than 2 per cent of all the people with Osler's disease had been reported to have cirrhosis of the liver. This seemed scarcely more than a chance occurrence since we know of no immunity conferred by either disease against the other. I have not seen the two together. Remembering our long failure to associate arteriovenous aneurysm and Osler's disease I do not deny Martini's idea of a specific kind of vascular anomaly in the liver in Osler's disease. Martini describes the following characteristics. The liver is enlarged and has porcelain-like thickening of the serosa with shallow indentations of the surface. Retractions are produced by connective tissue septa which traverse the liver and communicate with the thickened capsule. The connective tissue is frequently arranged in an intracinar fashion with epithelial sprouts similar to those of gallduct proliferation (Fig. 48). In these connective tissue strands are enlarged cavities lined with endothelium, frequently filled with blood, very

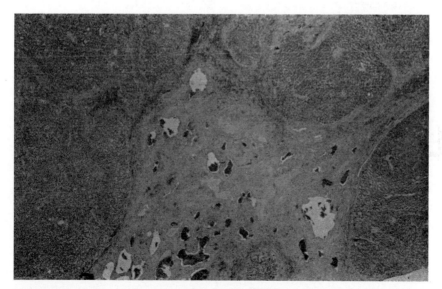

Figure 48.   Osler's disease.   Cirrhosis, fibrosis and numerous irregular blood lakes and channels occupying one of the fibrous tissue septa.   (Courtesy of Dr. Martini.)

similar to those found in the skin. They do not appear similar to any normal liver cavities. Collections of lymphocytes, histocytes, and plasmocytes infiltrate into the connective tissues. Telangiectatic lesions in the liver without cirrhosis, have been reported by Snyder and Doan, Schuster and others. We may have here a form of vascular anarchy leading to serious disease of the liver. Whether this is to be explained on the basis of inadequate blood flow or a more subtle effect of distortion upon the normal functions of the liver cannot be answered on the basis of evidence we have now.

G. PULMONARY ARTERIOVENOUS ANEURYSMS

It is not possible to say who made the first clear-cut connection between acquired pulmonary arteriovenous aneurysm and hereditary hemorrhagic telangiectasia. There are a great many scattered references to telangiectases noted in people with pulmonary arteriovenous aneurysm. Many of the reports of surgical cases do not mention the skin. There seems to have been no thoughtful connection until Goldman's papers on the topic. Since that time, there have been many case reports. By 1950, it was possible for Giampalmo who reviewed the topic to add fifty-seven new cases to those reported up to that time.

The rich and complex vascular arrangements of the lung, even in normal persons, include little arteriovenous shunts, particularly along the intralobular zones. They are favorable sites for dysplastic vascular lesions. But why they should give rise to signs and symptoms for the first time in early adult life and not before, is a mystery. The appearance of pulmonary arteriovenous fistula comes in the same post adolescent period when vascular lesions in the skin and bleeding become established or are noticed.

The history of arteriovenous fistula of the lung is well illustrated in the following case report.

Case Report

A twenty-seven-year-old man was admitted to University Hospitals because he had had convulsions. The morning of admission he had a seizure which started with drawing of the head to the left. This was followed by convulsive movements of the arms. There was loss of consciousness during the convulsion, followed by confusion for thirty minutes. The patient complained of headaches in the post-convulsive period. Later in the day there were two other convulsions, with rolling of the eyes upward and convulsive movements of the upper extremities for five to ten minutes. There was no aura, no biting of the tongue and no incontinence.

Past medical history revealed that the patient had never been as active or as strong as his siblings. In recent years he had become cyanotic. At the age of seventeen he was confined to bed with swollen knees for two weeks. At that time bluish lesions were found on his lips and clubbing of the fingernails was noted. At the age of twenty he was in an automobile accident. Though he was comatose for four days he recovered without known sequelae. Epistaxis and bleeding from the lips had occurred for many years. Ten months before admission he was seen at a nearby tuberculosis sanitorium because of a persistent cough. Although on roentgenographic examination a shadow was seen in the left hemithorax, there was no evidence of tuberculosis. Osler's disease with pulmonary arteriovenous shunt was diagnosed by Dr. David Funk, then one of our residents.

The family history revealed the father to be alive and well at the age of sixty. The patient's mother and sister and several maternal aunts and uncles had recurrent severe nosebleeds (Figure 48). Three brothers were alive and well. At the age of twenty-seven the patient's sister had died of an acute illness which began with a headache. The spinal fluid examination in her case was suggestive of a head injury or "brain tumor." She died within forty-eight hours of the first symptom.

The young man was husky and well nourished, not then acutely ill, lying quietly in bed, alert and cooperative. The pulse rate was 78 per minute. The blood pressure was 120/70 mm. Hg. The respiratory rate was 18 per minute. The body temperature was 101° F. rectally. The lips were cyanotic. Small blue raised lesions were noted on the lips and on the tongue. The neck was supple. Crusted blood was observed in the nose and in the naso-pharynx. Examination of the heart and lungs was negative except for a soft systolic murmur heard best at the right border of the chest in the fourth interspace. Clubbing of the fingernails was noted. It was my impression that he had Osler's disease, had burst a blood vessel in his brain and had an expanding hematoma.

Laboratory data: A voided specimen of urine was acid in reaction, and the specific gravity was 1.028. Chemical tests for albumin, sugar and blood were negative. The hemoglobin was 17 gm. per 100 ml., and the red blood cell count was 6.23 million per cu. mm. The white blood cell count was 13,600 per cu. mm. The differential count showed 60 per cent segmented polymorphonuclear leukocytes, 1 per cent basophils, 31 per cent lymphocytes and 8 per cent monocytes. X-ray studies of the skull were normal. X-rays of the chest showed the lung fields to be clear except for a rounded sharply circumscribed area of increased density 1.5 cm. in diameter in the left lung field in the fourth interspace anteriorly. A lumbar puncture revealed clear fluid with an initial pressure of 170 mm. of water. With compression of the jugular veins, the spinal fluid pressure rose to 220 mm., and a free rise and fall of the column were observed. The Pandy test was negative. Three polymorphonuclear leukocytes and ten erythrocytes were seen per cubic millimeter.

Second hospital day: The patient was treated with anticonvulsant drugs and had no fits.

Third hospital day: The patient had a good day and was able to read a magazine. Headache was minimal.

Fourth hospital day: The patient awakened with a severe headache. He had a fit in which his eyes deviated to the left. This episode was followed by two other fits and he then remained in a state of nearly continuous convulsions. Another lumbar puncture revealed an initial pressure of 210 mm. of water with a free rise and fall. One mm. of clear fluid was withdrawn and the Pandy test was 1 plus. Without acid there were 39 mononuclear cells and 15 red blood cells. With acid there were 43 mononuclear cells. It was noted that there was a fine nystagmus to the right and to the left. The cranial nerves were intact to examination.

Fifth hospital day: He was comfortable but his appetite was poor. Headaches continued with point of maximal intensity in the suboccipital region. He had no fits and was less drowsy.

Seventh hospital day: He began having rapidly repeated grand mal convulsions early in the morning. There were four within fifteen minutes, with clonic movements of the left arm. The convulsions were observed to be entirely on the left side. They ceased after we gave phenobarbital and 25 per cent magnesium sulfate intravenously. Following the convulsions, a left facial paralysis was noted. The left arm was weak and could not be extended into the air. The patient was drowsy but he cooperated fairly well. Weakness of the left leg appeared later in the day. Angiocardiography and ventriculography were not thought to be indicated. Later in the day Dr. Schwidde did a craniotomy. A brain abscess was found, not a hemorrhage. The pus removed at the time of operation contained anaerobic nonhemolytic streptococci, alpha hemolytic streptococci and anaerobic actinomyces.

Ninth hospital day: The color was good and the vital signs were stable. The right pupil was dilated but had a slight light reaction. He was able to move both arms on stimulation. The hemoglobin was 13 gm. per 100 ml., and the red blood cell count was 5.0 million per cu. mm. The plantar responses were extensor.

Tenth hospital day: The vital signs were normal but the patient's airway was poor except when the head was extended and the jaws elevated. The initial pressure of the spinal fluid was 160 mm. of water. The fluid was observed to be smoky with erythrocytes.

Thirteenth hospital day: The patient showed some movement of the left arm and leg. The vital signs were steady. A Levine tube was put in the stomach and gavage feedings were started.

Fifteenth hospital day: There was some pharyngeal obstruction so an oral airway was inserted, but this caused laryngospasm. A nasopharyngeal airway through the left nostril relieved the obstruction. Because of accumulation of secretions in the tracheobronchial tree, plus episternal retraction, it was believed that a tracheotomy would be beneficial. At the completion of the tracheotomy, the patient became cyanotic and respirations were slow and shallow. Oxygen was administered but the heartbeat ceased. A thoracotomy was done through the third left interspace and cardiac massage was started at a rate of twenty to twenty-five per minute. Measures to initiate spontaneous heart action were unsuccessful. The patient died.

The significant findings at autopsy were as follows: There were multiple blue non-elevated angiomatous lesions of the lips and tongue. A similar lesion was found on the tip of the right great toe. The skin of the hands and feet was ashen-gray. There was clubbing of the fingers and curling of the fingernails.

The most conspicuous finding was the multiple arteriovenous aneurysms of both lungs. They were numerous and varied in diameter from 2 mm. to 3 cm. The tracheobronchial tree contained much tenacious mucopurulent material. There was no evidence of pneumonic consolidation either grossly or microscopically, and numerous sections of the left lung were taken to study the arteriovenous fistulas. The veins and arteries were patent. A few colonies of anaerobic actinomyces were grown from the lung. The right lung was injected by Dr. Tabor.

There was mucosal erosion of the distal one-half of the esophagus but there were no telangiectases of the gastrointestinal tract. No telangiectases were found except those involving the skin and mucous membranes and the lungs. There was the operative defect resulting from draining the brain abscess.

The angiomatous lesions of the skin and lips had small dilated vascular spaces lined with endothelium. "They do not have much of a wall. What wall is seen is made up of loose fibroblastic tissue. The vascular spaces extend to the very base of the epidermis" (Figure 50).

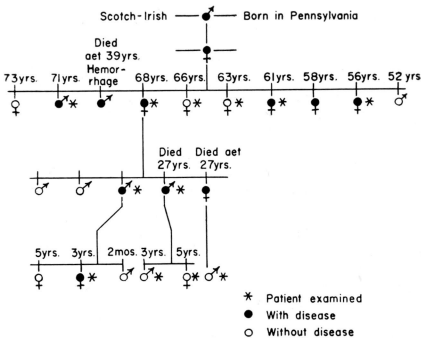

Figure 49.   Osler's disease. A kindred with three generations under observation. Presumptive evidence of the disease existed for the older ones. This kindred has been followed for four years since the diagram was made. There was definite evidence of Osler's disease in the girl when she was three years old.

The angiomatous lesion from the lip showed acute cellulitis throughout. In some instances the cellulitis was so extensive as almost to simulate an abscess.

The type of reaction found in the brain at autopsy consisted principally of infarction and hemorrhage. There was very little purulent material, nor were any sulfur granules found in the numerous sections studied.

Anaerobic nonhemolytic streptococci, alpha hemolytic streptococci and anaerobic actinomyces were cultured from the brain abscess. These organisms are commonly part of the flora of the mouth. The telangiectatic lesion from the lip showed an acute inflammatory reaction. It seems likely that the port of entry of the organisms was this telangiectatic lesion, not the lung.

Discussion

Some trend to ill health may be suspected by vague complaints in youth and a tendency to lag behind in classroom and in sports.

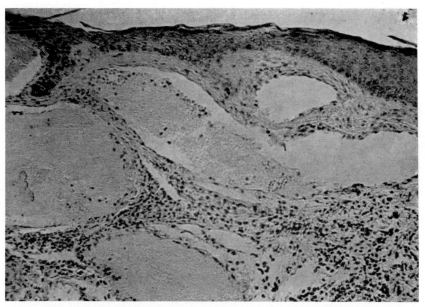

Figure 50.   Osler's disease. Angiomatous lesion of the lip with extremely large, dilated, thin-walled areas containing blood. In the lower part there is infection with cellular exudate and inflammation. The skin over the lesion is thin, in places only three or four cells thick.

Cyanosis may occur. There is no history of having been a blue baby. Then come the telltale lesions on the lips, bluish because of cyanosis. Nosebleeds and other bleeding occur in parent or siblings. Clubbing of cyanotic fingers develops and if the nails also harbor the telangiectases a finger may display clubbing, cyanosis and vascular lesions of skin and nail. Close ausculation often discloses a systolic or continuous bruit, sometimes so far away from the heart that its nature is evident immediately. Since many of the larger shunts are central, hilar bruits may be mistaken for heart murmurs or lost in the heart sounds. Clubbing and cyanosis may lead to confusion with congenital heart disease. Should such a person have an x-ray, pulmonary shadows may be noticed. The telangiectases and cyanosis provide the diagnostic clue, unless intercurrent hemorrhage disguises the clinical pattern for a time. Ordinarily polycythemia wins out over anemia, but a seesaw contest may present a fluctuating series of clinical states.

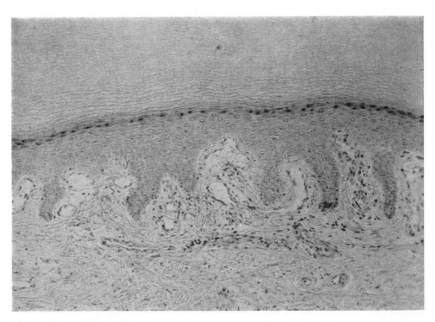

Figure 51.   Osler's disease. Lesion from the skin of the finger showing the distortion of the papillae by small dilated vessels wandering about amongst them. In none of these and many other sections have I been able to identify the sphincter structure described by Nödl.

The pulmonary shunt may be single. Usually several exist but one large one dominates. It makes the loudest murmurs, shunts the most blood and produces the largest x-ray shadow.

I have found no record of pulmonary A-V fistulae in children with Osler's disease. This does not mean that they do not occur. A review of the x-ray films of the chest of many patients with Osler's disease which were made in Cincinnati from the middle 1930's up to 1942 did not reveal any pulmonary shunts. One was discovered in 1946 and two since then (213). It is not possible to say what the frequency of the pulmonary shunts is among persons with skin lesions diagnostic of Osler's disease. I have seen two out of one hundred and fifty. Since, it may take some time to develop, however, these figures have little meaning, and a much higher frequency is probable.

The dynamic state of pulmonary arteriovenous fistulae is illustrated by the fact that when lobectomy or pneumonectomy brings respite and corrects the cyanosis, polycythemia and dyspnea, after months or years new shunts are apt to grow in the remaining lung tissue. We do not know that this would not have happened anyhow without an operation. It is plausible that increased blood flow and ventilatory action of the remaining lung favored this development.

Figure 50 shows the complexity of the actual lesion. Injection studies by Dr. Rodman Tabor with plastic materials of different colors demonstrated that an aneurysm may have two arterial supplies, from bronchial as well as pulmonary arteries, and the pulmonary venous drainage. Dynamic studies of the forces favoring the development of a shunt we do not have. The problem of A-V shunts in the low pressure pulmonary system is interesting in comparison with the high pressure systemic A-V shunts, but comparable studies are not available. There is increasing evidence that pulmonary shunts may exist, actual or potential, in normal persons. Their negligible dynamic effect leaves them unrecognized; though in pregnancy and in some cases of cirrhosis of the liver they may have some significance, enlarging under the influence of unknown stimuli.

H. Other Lesions

Aneurysms of systemic arteries have been discovered in victims of Osler's disease. Shuster has reported an interesting example of aneurysm of the splenic artery. A search of medical reports of miscellaneous aneurysms not syphilitic or arteriosclerotic might reveal others. More important would be the study of patients with such aneurysms for stigmata of Osler's disease. Systemic attention seems the hardest task for most physicians. It is rarely tried. Much more detailed study is needed for information adequate for useful generalization.

A patient with full blown telangiectasia, an aunt of the patient E. R., had a remarkable aneurysm of the hepatic artery and its branches. Excessive bleeding from the bowel and a thrill and continuous murmur above and a little to the right of the naval, led me to make a preoperative diagnosis of an arteriovenous shunt in the portal circulation, a condition I could not find described in medical writings. At operation Dr. Ehrenhaft found an aneurysm of the artery arising from the superior mesenteric artery. An aneurysmal extension formed a complete arterial circle. A thrill in this arterial-artery aneurysm was eliminated by occluding temporarily the main feeding artery. The dynamic arrangement suggested the mechanism of a midget arterial cyclotron with blood accelerated in a curious circular arterial structure causing thrill and murmur. Through and through suture reduced but did not eliminate these remarkable signs. No true arteriovenous aneurysm was found. There has been no known bleeding from the bowel since the operation.

I. Histopathology

In addition to Hanes' detailed observation on the histopathology of the telangiectases of Osler's disease, Beek and others have contributed studies. Fingerland and Janousek reported their observations of the enormous dilated papillary capillaries, some of which had liquid blood but others had old organized clots. The papillae over the larger bulbous capillaries were narrow and there was pronounced hyperkeratosis. Between capillaries and epidermis was a layer containing new capillaries and macrophages with blood pigments indicating an organized extravasation. Subintimal hyalinization was common and might be so large as to fill the greater portion of the telangiectasis. The precapillaries of the reticular layer had proliferation of the adventitia leading to encroachment upon the lumen.

Though the lesions of Osler's disease may affect very large or very small vessels the process seems to be much the same (Figure 51). It is a failure of muscle and connective tissue to develop properly in the wall of the vessel. The small vessels may be nothing but a layer of endothelial cells with little else except meager connective tissue. Elastic tissue may be attenuated but may be normal. Thus contraction is impossible and bleeding is inevitable from minor leaks and trivial trauma. Davis, using a special device for shearing off the keratin layer of the skin with very little trauma, has demonstrated a decrease in the number of capillary loops. Coiled distended vessels constitute the telangiectasis. They reach the size of one to several millimeters. In addition there are remarkable little circular vascular channels which may become telangiectases.

Martini, Nödl, Staubesand and their colleagues have made serial sections of the lesions in the skin and have come to the conclusion that there is a specific vascular anomaly in which there is a double spiral pattern of a vessel with irregularly placed thick muscle elements and a well formed sphincter. Accompanying veins of very small size have well developed valves. It is suggested that the sphincter mechanism may lead to the development of cavernous convoluted angiomas in the abortive attempt at functional adaptation of a deranged circulation. It is possible that the deforming sphincter and related changes are the same as the alterations discussed by Fingerland and Janousek.

The fact that bleeding in Osler's disease is usually a surface phenomenon indicates that trauma and irritation are accessory causes. Atrophy of the skin overlying the lesion tends to reduce the mechanical protection ordinarily afforded.

J. PHYSIOLOGY

Lewis found that the capillaries and small blood vessels do not react to stimuli which affect normal tissues. Macfarlane observed "sharply localized abnormalities of the capillaries. Those forming the lesions do not contract after injury and it is from these that persistent bleeding occurs. * * * Temporary pressure is an effective measure because a firm blood clot which is capable of maintaining hemostasis forms during its application." Though there is some variation in reports of the histopathology especially as regards elastic tissue there is no question that people with Osler's disease bleed, and bleed because the tissue composing blood vessels is deficient in structure and function. Contraction is inadequate and the blood with a normal clotting mechanism cannot get a firm footing and seal the leak. Most detailed studies of clotting stress: (1) coagulation; (2) structure; or (3) contractility. The fact that mankind has not disappeared long ago is because an integrated system of repairing minor disaster in the small vessels of the body combines proper function of vessel, structure of vessel and the co-agulability of the fluid blood.

K. TREATMENT

The emergency treatment of Osler's disease is to stop bleeding with pressure, packs, thrombin or fibrin sponges and other mechanical devices if the site is known. Cautery of vessels in the nose may give temporary relief but healing occurs with unsupported vessels in the soft mucosa so that hemorrhage recurs at least as often as when conservative methods of packing are used. As in any acute bleeding the problem of when and how much to transfuse is hard to solve. Tolerable degrees of shock may reduce bleeding, but the exact time for transfusion has to be determined by clinical judgment. Since the cause of bleeding is the vascular fault which renders active vasoconstriction ineffectual, nothing is to be gained by treatment directed at coagulation disorders. Studies by Macfarlane with the capillary microscope disclosed the failure of small vessels to contract enough to grasp a clot.

For the anemic patient, and anemia may be severe without obvious external bleeding, the specific treatment is iron, employed as long as anemia persists.

The introduction by Koch and colleagues of estrogens in therapy was hailed as a hopeful advance. The dose of ethinyl estradiol used, 0.25 mg. a day, is about ten times the amount used to control menopausal symptoms. It is curious that estrogens should be helpful since bleeding becomes a problem of importance after adolescence and in the time of full flood of sex hormones. Evaluation of this form of treatment in a disorder with such clinical variability is extremely difficult. Stefanini and Damashek found the treatment to be of no value. Harrison studied four patients intensively using larger doses and taking biopsies of the inferior turbinates before and after therapy. The normal columnar epithelium had become squamous and this change may have protected the fragile vessels. He thought treatment very effective and was still giving it when he wrote his report. Walker described a patient who seemed to become refractory to treatment after an initial response. My own observations indicate that though it seems to be helpful in some patients for periods up to six months or a year it really does no good. Either because the patient becomes lax in taking the drug, or because it has no effect, bleeding remains a problem still. The undesirable feminization of men is a nuisance. Some of the women I have treated, having passed the menopause, did not like the reactivated menstrual bleeding. They preferred to take no estrogens and bleed from the nose. Perhaps some of the newer steroid hormones will provide a really satisfactory palliation.

L. PREVENTION

Since the trait for Osler's disease is transmitted as a mendelian dominant anyone with the disease may expect to transmit it to about half of the children. Signs of the disease rarely may appear late so it may be transmitted before a parent knows that he or she has it. With the high risk of propagating the strain, and the chronic disability of recurring crises, prevention is our only satisfactory method of dealing with the problem today. Since there is no impairment of fertility the number of victims must increase, with all their private woe and public burden. This lesson is brought clearly before us in the family story depicted by Wintrobe where a genealogical ladder or tree was not enough for a many-wived Mormon patriarch with the trait—a wheel with spokes going in all directions was needed to encompass the increasing number of afflicted descendents. Bird and his colleagues have a pedigree which they depict as an oval, shaped like a football stadium with many tiers.

M. Inferences and Speculations

The notion that there is a dynamism in the structure and architectural fabric of small blood vessels, a homeokinesis rather than a homeostasis, is emphasized by these observations on the changes which occur in the visible telangiectases of Osler's disease. We think of the circulation to the skin, if we consider it at all, as in the fixed conduits of gross anatomy and the fixed sections of histology or pathology. No doubt the larger vessels do get and keep their final pattern by the time adult life is reached. But the dynamic potential is there, as we see when an artery is closed or clots and the need downstream somehow calls forth the expanding or new growth of a series of collateral tubes large enough to sustain the tissues. The nature of collaterals arising to drain venous blood when a large vein is blocked, a mechanism completely different, gains the same end, even when the upper or lower vena cava is occluded. Here pressure, dilatation and compensatory expansion of veins accommodate the venous return in a new pattern which can be observed easily since so much is superficial. So the potential for vascular new growth can be evoked to restore inadequate supply and carry off blood in new vessels when the drainage system goes bad. This is in addition to the better known new vessel growth of granulation tissue, callus formation and wound healing.

Sir Thomas Lewis, to whom I go frequently for his luminous observations and thoughts on the skin and its vessels, emphasized the constancy of the pattern of vascular designs. For instance, the mottling of the palm in red and white speckles which can be seen easily after holding the hand dependent for a few moments is relatively constant. Lewis noted no changes over a period of months. I have mapped my hand pattern at irregular intervals for seventeen years and during that time selected areas of it have undergone at least four complete changes. A slow shift ultimately reversed the red and white areas. There has been very little change near the palmar creases. The point I wish to make is that there is significant variability superimposed on a pattern of regularity. Though the theme is constant it is subject to variations. One can imagine the spreading network of small vessels subject to change as a slow motion film of undulating coral fronds which move in slow and scarcely perceptible tides on the quiet ocean floor.

Platt has observed differences in retinal vascular patterns of identical twins, although he saw no dynamic shift in configuration. This is further testimony of potential for variability in vessels.

Observations in the rabbit ear using various kinds of chambers in which small vessels can be studied and photographed over long periods of time indicate considerable variability from time to time. A remarkable influence of environmental temperature has been found (163). There may be an extensive proliferation of arteriovenous shunts during hot weather. These shut down and then disappear when the temperature becomes cool. The physical state of the small vessels and capillaries throughout the body is one of dynamic equilibrium. The numerous though often minute changes probably can be explained by forces no more esoteric but no less subtle than the tissues' requirement for blood supply and drainage. Just as Schoenheimer has recast our thinking in terms of a dynamic equilibrium of the chemical constituents of cells and tissues of the body, so it would appear that the micro-structure of blood vessels experiences continual rearrangement, reformation, obliteration— in everyday wear and tear, in healing and repair. Forces which give rise to the eruption of arterial spiders and the characteristic change which occurs whenever new vascular tissue develops in Osler's disease must extend and reorder our thoughts about such homeo-kinetic phenomena.

2.   Congenital Dysplastic Angiopathies of the Skin and Underlying Tissue

One rapidly gets lost in a sea of eponyms which designate the various bizarre vascular syndromes characterized by angiomatous lesions of the skin, with underlying vascular anomalies of the brain, extremities, or other tissues. These are developmental anomalies in which the skin change often resembles an ordinary birthmark. It would be well to discard the eponyms once for all and call them congenital dysplastic angiopathies. They are all examples of the same kind of trouble. They have some points of similarity with

Maffucci's syndrome on the one hand and hereditary hemorrhagic telangiectasia on the other, though there is no difficulty in distinguishing one from another in typical examples.

In 1860, Schirmer observed epilepsy in a patient with cutaneous telangiectas's of the face and head but he did not speculate on any connection between a lesion of the skin and a companion one of the brain.

In 1879, Sturge reported "A case of partial epilepsy apparently due to a lesion of one of the vasomotor centers of the brain." He told of a six year old girl who had a congenital vascular nevus on the right side of the head and face, and both sides of the trunk, extending down to the third or fourth dorsal vertebra posteriorly and down to the second costal cartilage on the front of the chest. The nasal and oral mucosa and the eye on the right were affected. The nevus did not cross the midline at eye level but on the chin and below it was bilateral. The right eye was enlarged. The choroidal and retinal vessels were involved. After the age of six months, the patient had had convulsions affecting the left side. Weakness of the left arm and leg began at about the same time. Sturge speculated that the seizures might be caused by a focal cerebral lesion similar to that found on the face. In 1886, Duzea wrote his medical thesis at Lyon on developmental troubles which are sequels to superficial angiomas. Weber in Germany had already discussed the problem and Thomas Smith in England had reported cases in the Transactions of the Clinical Society of London in 1882. The topic was ventilated by Masmejan of Montpellier in his thesis in 1888. Trelat and Monad in 1896 observed that hypertrophy of an extremity frequently was coupled with varicosities and hemangiomas though they described nothing which could be designated certainly as Maffucci's syndrome. All this makes it seem wonderfully curious that Klippel and Trenaunay should be given eponymic rememberance for the rare syndrome they described in 1900 as "nevus variqueux osteohypertrophique," a combination of angiomatous nevus and the congenital varicosities with hypertrophy consisting mainly of elongation of various parts of the skeletal system. In 1906, Cushing reported three cases of vascular nevi and neurologic involvement. In a series of papers beginning in 1918, Parkes Weber

(883, 890, 891, 892) described the problem of hemangiectatic hypertrophy of limbs. Later he discussed a patient with right-sided hemihypertrophy, right-sided congenital spastic hemiplegia and widespread cutaneous vascular nevi, chiefly of the superficial port wine type, involving the trunk only on the left side of the back but both sides anteriorly. There was bilateral involvement of the face more extensive on the left with a very deep cavernous angioma. The patient was blind on the left with optic atrophy, glaucoma and heterochromia irides. X-rays of the skull showed the left half of the brain to be more opaque than the right. This patient had had no fits. It was Parkes Weber's belief that in the hemihypertrophies the arterial component was meager but that the main lesion was a venous anomaly. At times he called them congenital varicose veins.

Kalisher's patient first reported in 1897, with an autopsy report in 1901, had a small cerebral hemisphere covered with a diffuse meningeal angioma. This was the first evidence for Sturge's suggestion. Apparently Volland in 1912 was the first to describe calcium deposits in the affected part of the cerebral cortex. This phenomenon may be analogous to the calcium deposits in the veins in Maffucci's syndrome and scleroderma. In addition to the distinguished contributions of Parkes Weber, there are excellent reviews of the ocular phakomatoses (birth spots) which have been discussed in detail by Kirby, encephalotrigeminal angiomatosus by King and Schwartz in 1954 and of the so-called Klippel-Trenaunay syndrome of congenital dystrophic angiectasis by de Reus and Vink in 1955. Parkes Weber who has a vast collection of rare diseases never brought together the skin-brain combination with the skin-extremity combination. All the descriptions available leave no doubt that the basic process may involve different parts of the body. Occasionally the same sort of inborn architectural error gets completely out of hand. The victim has widespread involvement of various viscera as well as the skin. Wood, White, and Kernohan described cavernous hemangiomas involving the brain, spinal cord, heart, skin and kidney in a woman who lived to be 87 years old so that minor degrees are compatible with longevity. Most reported examples, more-extensive and more-disastrous, are fatal at a younger age. The association of such vascular anomalies with tumors of brain and spinal cord was reported by Kinney and Fitzgerald.

Case Report

The patient is a seven-year-old boy who was seen in the Orthopedic Department first in June 1951 because of a very large mass over the entire right leg which had grown larger than the left, the foot growing nearly twice the size of the left foot. A retroperitoneal cyst was removed at the age of two months after a fit of vomiting caused his admission to the hospital. At this time a large hemangioma was noted over the outer aspect of the right knee and lower part of the thigh with very large subcutaneous veins coursing along the whole extremity. There was also a small hemangioma on the skin of the penis, the right side of the scrotum, the lateral aspect of the right hip and one over the medial portion of the crest of the ileum. The cyst removed at operation was diagnosed as a cyst of unknown origin. It was almost completely extirpated. Early in 1954 biopsies revealed congenital lymphangiectases in the right leg and right groin; but a femoral angiogram was not particularly unusual. Later there was a recurrence of the abdominal mass which was aspirated and 500 cc. of bloody fluid were removed. In the fall of 1954, the hemangioma on the right thigh was excised and a split thickness skin graft was made after excision of huge arteriorvenolymphatic beds in the popliteal space in the thigh. The specimen revealed "vascular malformation (angiectasis) involving the skin and soft tissues of the right lower extremity." Early in the spring of 1956, the patient had a transmetatarsal amputation and late in the fall of 1956 a modified Kondolean procedure was done on the right leg and the proximal portion of the right foot. The black and white and infrared photographs in Figure 52A and B reveal the extensive lymphangioma before it was removed. The considerable increase in the venous structures is revealed in the infrared photograph. The angioma of the upper portion of the right thigh and buttocks had a purplish-brown background color which faded on pressure with a glass slide but there were embedded in this region of dilated vessels small angiomas which did not fade on pressure. They were elevated slightly above the surface of the lesion and resembled punctate elevated angiomas which may be seen in the photograph of the thigh.

A. ATAXIA TELANGIECTASIA

Boder and Sedgwick have described a familial syndrome of progressive cerebellar ataxia with oculo-cutaneous telangiectasia

and proneness to pulmonary infections. The telangiectasia is a very
faint hair-like change on the bulbar conjunctiva, the butterfly area
of the face and the external part of the ears. There are peculiar eye
movements. The eyes halt midway on lateral or upward gaze though
movement can be completed if enough time is given. Rapid blinking occurs with the halting as though it were an effort to overcome

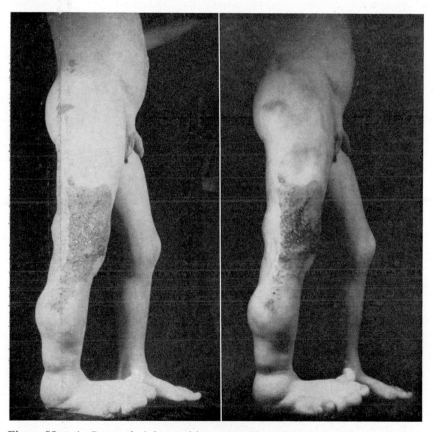

Figure 52.   *A*. Congenital dystrophic angiectasis. Black and white photograph
revealing the conspicuous distortion of the foot and lower leg, the very large
superficial angioma in which dark brown punctate angiomas are scattered upon
a background sheet colored chocolate brown to pink. In addition to the
hemangiomatous anarchy of blood vessels, some of the lesion in the right calf
was a lymphangioma.

Figure 52.   *B*. Congenital dystrophic angiectasis. Infrared photograph illustrating the increased size of the veins of the leg which has the lesion.

the interrupted movement. Coarse nystagmoid oscillations occur with return to forward gaze. The facies may be dull and mask-like, but intelligence is normal and disposition equable. There is progression of the cerebellar ataxia with ultimate deterioration and loss of voluntary movements. Because of the distribution of the vascular lesions in the cerebellum, this syndrome does not fit as one of the congenital dysplastic angiectases of the Sturge-Weber or Hippel-Lindau variety though it may be a variant of this group of troubles.

3. Angiokeratoma Corporis Diffusum Universale (Fabry's Syndrome)

Among the truly rare vascular lesions of the skin is a form of diffuse angiokeratomas scattered unevenly over the body. So far the trouble has been reserved "for men only." Fabry was the first to

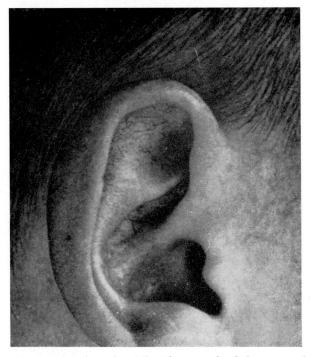

Figure 53. Ataxia telangiectasia. The photograph of the external ear revealing faint hair-like telangiectases in the ear similar to those seen in the butterfly area of the face and on the bulbar conjunctiva. (Courtesy of Dr. Elena Boder.)

study the condition systematically. Mibelli introduced the term angiokeratoma to identify little vascular aneurysms of the skin, elevated, hyperkeratotic and tending to occupy the extensor aspect of the fingers, toes and other exposed surfaces. Angiokeratoma is a lesion of childhood or early adult life. It is commoner in girls and women than in boys or men. It is preceded for some years by chilblains. In time minute scattered telangiectases develop and these become larger, more numerous, and coalesce in groups. The epidermis over them becomes horny and opaque. Similar but not exactly identical angiomas on the scrotum of elderly men, the angiokeratoma scroti (Chapter VII, Section 9), are called Fordyce lesions or the Fordyce syndrome after their early describer. They have no relation to chilblains and their owners may not have followed Osler's advice, and kept their "emotions" on ice.

Fabry's original communication, entitled purpura hemorrhagica nodularis indicates the superficial similarity of the lesion to pupura from which it is easily distinguished. This similarity has given rise to mistakes in identifying the lesion and in understanding its proper and very different significance. In recent years this rare skin lesion has come to be recognized as the surface clue to a disseminated systemic disease, obscure in nature and of unknown cause. Fessas, Wintrobe and Cartwright reported a patient whose history was a sad tale of confusion from past errors in diagnosis. These observers surveyed the medical reports, all from Europe, and described a victim of this disorder. Their studies extended the evidence that it is a bizarre systemic disease. Some of my records of patients with unusual vascular lesions of the skin suggest that there may be formes frustes of the disorder but I have not recognized a case.

A. THE SKIN LESIONS

The angiokeratomas may vary in size from those visible only with magnification to easily seen ones whose size varies from pin point specks to those about two millimeters in diameter. Their deep red color is intermediate between the purple of purpuric specks and spots and the brighter red of telangiectases. Some angiokeratomas look black. The small ones are flat, the large ones elevated slightly above the surface. The bigger ones are apt to be on the trunk, clustered around the navel, the buttocks, or scrotum. Smaller ones are found on the knees, elbows and upper arms. The skin has a speckled look reminiscent of coarse mill-ground pepper sprinkled on a white tablecloth. Because of the elevation of the larger lesions the skin feels rough and goose-pimply. Sustained pressure on the small lesions causes blanching. The larger ones cannot be obliterated. Similar lesions may be found on the mucous membranes of the mouth. Aneurysmal dilatation of conjunctival vessels occurs in rare cases. The uninvolved skin appears to be completely normal except that edema of the eyelids and of the lower legs is common. Sensitivity to cold is common but this does not seem to be connected with the mechanism operating in chilblains which may give rise to the angiokeratoma of Mibelli. The lesions have a predilection for the trunk, and in this regard resemble cherry angiomas. Distally they diminish in frequency and size. Corn-like lesions of the palms and soles may be found in addition to the vascular lesion, somewhat suggestive of the changes of chronic arsenic poisoning.

B. SYSTEMIC INVOLVEMENT

Increasing evidence points to the fact that this disease is not just skin deep. As our insight increases this is found to be true of many disorders of the "skin." Symptoms and signs point to the implication of other systems. Pains, paresthesias and arthritic complaints are common. The patients have trouble accommodating themselves to changes in temperature. The Raynaud phenomenon is common. The legs may swell. In the third and fourth decade, weakness, headaches, dyspnea and urinary complaints occur in varying combinations. Hypertension, enlargement of the heart, and electrocardiographic signs of myocardial disease occur. Eventually cardiac and renal failure may develop. A feature common to all autopsy and biopsy material has been a widespread abnormality of the smooth muscle cells of blood vessels. The media is wider than normal and its smooth muscle is vacuolated by a material birefringent under polarized light. Curious deformities of the nuclei may occur. Vascular lesions are most serious in the kidneys. Foam cells and vacuolation with lipoid material may be present in many tissues. The angiokeratomas in the skin are vascular spaces, irregular in size and shape, lying in the papillae. They contain blood or small thrombi. A single cell layer of endothelium and the sometimes hyperkeratotic skin comprise the surface.

The urine commonly contains albumin, but this is of small degree, a trace to one plus. Large foam cells resembling macrophages with clusters of lipoid globules are found in the sediment, and similar cells have been found in preparations of bone marrow (264). There is no evidence of a disturbance of fat, phospholipid or protein metabolism though such possibilities are not excluded.

C. CLINICAL COURSE

Red spots in the skin appear in childhood or adolescence. They increase in number as time goes on. The older, large ones are dark. We do not know whether old lesions disappear. Later indications of cardiac, renal or other systemic disease appear. Ultimately such disorders may lead to death.

D. SPECULATION

There are certain features which suggest that this may be a metabolic disease of the storage variety where a substance is made too readily or eliminated too poorly and, piling up, has to be deposited or stored somewhere. Some concepts of atherosclerosis hold that such mechanisms may operate to produce the serious complications of much "degenerative" arterial disease. Or some subtle damage may occur which attracts such strange deposits. Whatever the cause, the angiokeratoma of Fabry is the cutaneous signal of an all-pervasive disease of smooth muscle. It may be caused by some genetic accident in which a chromosome is injured or ruined. Reported instances have been confined to males. This, with its occasional familial trend, suggests that it may be transmitted through women to their sons as is classical hemophilia. Such are our uncertain notions. Familiarity with the syndrome will no doubt discover other cases and perhaps with more attention our understanding may explain what are now darkly held riddles.

4. Hemangiomas and Dyschondroplasia (Maffucci's Syndrome)

"If you have the good fortune to command a large clinic,
remember that one of your chief duties is the tabulation
and analysis of carefully recorded experience."   —Osler

Maffucci, in 1881, described the association of hemangiomas and dyschondroplasia, though I have seen a copy of his original paper only recently. Indeed, apparently no one else who has written about it in contemporary time has found a copy. Alice Carleton with Elkington, Greenfield and Robb-Smith, resurrected Maffucci from his ancient oblivion and restored to him the dignity of eponymic fame in their classic account of the syndrome he seems to have identified and described first. I missed the report by Carleton and associates until I read about it in Parkes Weber's book on "Rare Disease" but since then have not only studied their original and all other available reports but have been on the lookout for patients with such a bizarre and horrible disease. This alert has been rewarded by finding four examples which provide the basis for the following comments.

Maffucci's syndrome is an inborn disorganization in which there are defects in cartilage and bone formation, dyschondroplasia, and vascular hamartomas. It is a morphological anomaly characterized by mesodermal dysplasia. In such disorders characterized by two distinct abnormalities it is important to determine whether one is conditioned by the other or whether they are both produced by a common mechanism, usually a genetic one. For instance, in Wilson's disease it was thought formerly that the lenticular degeneration was secondary to the lesion of the liver. Now it is believed that both are caused in a way still quite mysterious, by a disorder in copper metabolism and transport. The cerebral agenesis of the Sturge-Weber syndrome, since it exists only in the region of the vascular anomaly, is undoubtedly a result of the anomalous vessels doing an inadequate job and starving part of the brain which then atrophies. In Maffucci's syndrome, all the evidence indicates that the vascular anarchy may exist in regions where the cartilage is not disturbed. Either lesion may occur separately and where they affect the same area either one may dominate. Therefore, they must be independent manifestations of the disease presumably accounted for by the topographical architecture of chromosomes which has somehow gone wrong. Ollier's disease, a dyschondroplasia, is an irregular bending and dwarfing of a limb, usually one-sided or quite asymmetrical. Ossification of the cartilage does not take place normally at the end of the growing bones. The dyschondroplasia of Ollier's disease is the same as that in Maffucci's syndrome. In both conditions, as the bone extends in length, islands of nonossifying cartilage persist in the metaphysis. The long bones of the arms, legs, hands and feet are commonly involved. Here and in the phalanges grotesque deformities may be produced by multiple enchondromas. X-rays shows thinning of the corticalis with area of pale mottling in the metaphysis, sometimes expansion of metaphysis and speckling of the epiphysis. Exostoses arising near the epiphysis may point in any direction in an irregular fashion. Of the forty-one reported patients, fourteen have been women. The small number scarcely lets us generalize about sex incidence. In a classical case, the child is normal at birth or no gross abnormalities are noted. There is no strong evidence for a family tendency. During early life one or more nodules begin to appear, usually on a finger or toe. Soft bluish tumors, frequently with dilated venous satellites or with phlebectasia, may be found connected with the nodules or else where. The affection is grossly asymmetrical. It may even be unilateral. Pathologic fractures are common and such fractures heal very slowly or may fail to unite. Fractures may recur repeatedly at the same site. Skewing and warping of the body may result from differences in growth of the two sides. The long bones are likely to have a club-like expansion at the ends, with cartilaginous tumors near the epiphyseal line. Curvature of the long bones produces gross deformity. Sometimes the long bones may have very short shafts or they may be of normal length. During the time of growth, because of the unequal expansion and irregular development, deformities become more obvious and grotesque. Unless operations trim off the expanding cauliflower-like excrescences, all normal elements of the hand or foot may be lost (Figure 59). The original structure may be unidentifiable. Sometimes a terminal phalanx or a protruding nail may give a clue regarding the tissue from which the growth arose. Any bone in the body may be affected but the major lesions are found distally in the extremities, in long bones, in ribs, scapula, pelvis, and vertebra, and rarely in the bones of the skull, wrist, or ankle. At the completion of growth in the mid-twenties, the process may become stationary unless pathologic fractures or accidents give rise to further disfiguring deformity. Many victims of the disease die of malignant neoplasms, particularly sarcomas of carti-lage or blood vessel. Perhaps mild examples of this disorder are more common than is suggested from the poverty of reports. In any event, I found in one hospital two certain examples and a probable additional one seen during a period of several months and another

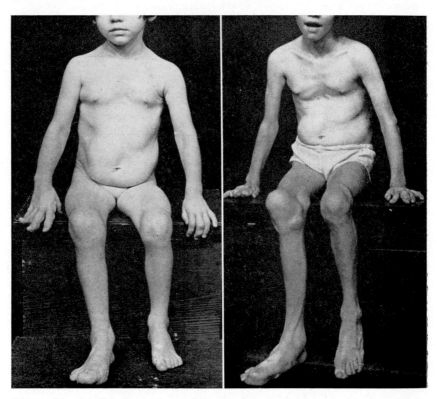

Figure 54.   Maffucci's syndrome. On the left the patient at the age of three already has anomalies of the finger, the right leg, and a lump on the right side of the abdomen.

Figure 55.   Maffucci's syndrome. Development of the disease and the patient. By the end of the sixth year there is funnel breast deformity, early scoliosis, and progress of the lesions involving both feet and both hands.

patient, hearing of my interest, makes a total of four, almost a corner on the clinical market.

The details of this disease are illustrated most graphically by the case report and in Figures 54 to 60.

Case Report

A girl now 21 years old has been attending one or another service of the University Hospitals for eighteen years. She was born October 28, 1937. Her parents were normal, the mother twenty-one, the father twenty-eight at the time of her birth. There was no consanguinity. The father's brother had died at the age of two with some congenital deformity of the spine which had prevented him from sitting up. An older brother and younger sister have always been normal. Gestation and birth of the patient were normal. She was breast-fed for thirteen months. Not until she was eight months old did her mother notice that the right hand was larger than the left. A little later the right leg and foot were noticed to be abnormally large. There was a slight limp. At the age of two years large veins were noted on the lateral aspect of the thigh and knees. When she was thirty-three months old the left middle finger had become larger than the others. When first examined at the University Hospitals she was thirty-four months old. Her general appearance is best observed in the photographs. She was somewhat thin, with irregular enlargement of the right hand, leg, and foot and middle finger of the left hand. Behind the right ear was a still-draining sinus from a mastoidectomy. The right side of the face was slightly larger than the left. Cervical lymph nodes were enlarged. The abdomen revealed "soft fatty masses in the right upper quadrant of the abdominal wall and the lower left ribs anteriorly." The right leg was larger than the left. Range of movement was normal except for the right hip, where it was limited. There was grating of the right knee on moving. The right foot was large, the great toe bulbous, with large creases in the plantar surface, which was thick, wrinkled, and tender. The index, middle, and ring fingers of the right hand were gnarled, enlarged, and knobby, with limitation of movement. A diagnosis of hemihypertrophy was made.

During the next seven years there were twenty admissions, mostly in an effort to correct and palliate the progressively distorting growth of bones of the extremities. A series of photographs illustrates better than words the cruel progress of the deformities and the modest results of repeated operations. In spite of her plight the girl has managed to make some adjustments and has kept up in school.

The following list outlines her hospital admissions and the progress of the disease for the period of observation.

March 24, 1943: X-rays showed the enlarged bones to be osteoporotic. The great toe of the right foot was amputated, and epi-

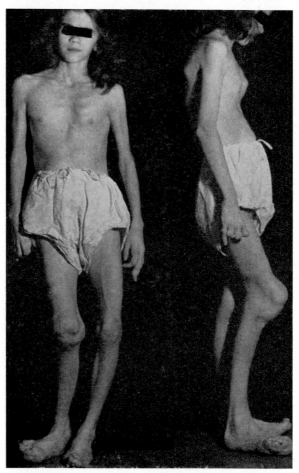

Figure 56. Maffucci's syndrome. The patient at the age of eleven years illustrating the warping and bowing of both legs in the same direction, the progressive enlargement of the veins of the lower legs without venous obstruction, the cauliflower lesion of the foot and the progressing asymmetry.

physial arrest was established in the distal femur and proximal tibia and fibula on the right. Wound healing and convalescence were normal.

October 18, 1943: Admitted for several courses of x-ray therapy to the affected areas. The second, third, and fourth fingers of the

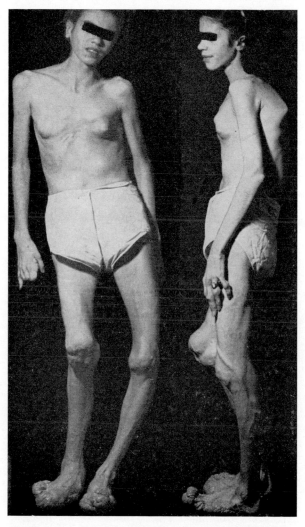

Figure 57.   Maffucci's syndrome. The status at the age of fifteen, revealing the progressive warping of the skeleton and deformities in the legs, hands, knees, and trunk.

right hand were amputated at the proximal interphalangeal joint. The wounds healed per primum.

January 10, 1944: Excision of redundant tissue of right foot.

August 3, 1944: Return visit.

January 3, 1945: Chronic otitis media. Amputation of left little toe. Microscopic examination showed a thick, horny layer over a thickened epidermis. The subcutaneous tissue was very thick and contained many sudoriferous glands. The bone of the phalanx was normal. Between the bone and subcutaneous tissue there was a thick layer of fibrocartilage without malignant characteristics.

April 26, 1945: Return visit. Healing complete. Shoe lift fitted.

April 25, 1946: Increasing valgus deformity of right ankle.

June 12, 1946: Return for shoe correction.

August 27, 1946: Return visit. Continued slow increase in deformities. Complete skeletal survey by x-ray revealed similar changes in bone structure in all sites of enlargement, with overgrowth of bone with hazy outlines and increased trabecular markings with a honeycombed appearance suggesting hemangioma. Treated for otitis media.

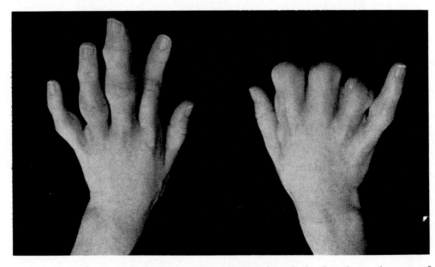

Figure 58. Maffucci's syndrome. The deformity of the hands at the age of six after portions of three fingers of the right hand had been amputated. There has been relatively little involvement of the thumb. The hands are surprisingly useful.

August 5, 1949: Shoes adjusted.

September 21, 1950: New shoes prepared.

March 31, 1952: Return visit.

August 22, 1952: Return visit.

December 18, 1952: Return visit.

May 19, 1953: Return visit. Very little change.

January 29, 1954: Return visit. No apparent change.

March 15, 1955: Return visit. Slight progression of bony deformities.

June 22, 1956: Condition static.

July 2, 1958: No change.

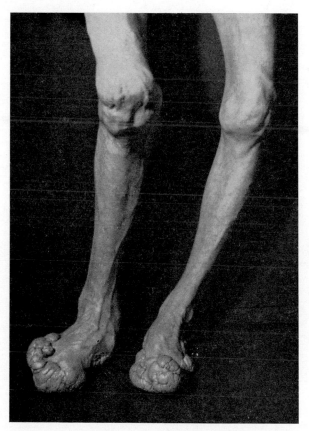

Figure 59.   Maffucci's syndrome. The deformity of the legs emphasizing the conspicuous enlargement of the veins and the proliferating red cauliflower-like deformity of the feet and toes.

Comment

The main problem posed by Maffucci's syndrome concerns the relationship between the disorders in two separate tissues. Does the vascular lesion determine the dyschondroplasia; or are the two produced by some other mechanism, probably a genetic one? Without recapitulation of all the evidence Carleton and her associates brought out, the asymmetry of the lesions of blood vessels and cartilage demonstrates that the localization of the lesions in the same place is not obligatory, any concurrence is apt to be coincidental rather than consequential. Most probably multiple effects from trouble in a single gene are responsible. Perhaps the subsequent developments in our third patient will cast some light on the matter. Patients with only dyschondroplasia (Ollier's disease) or only vascu-

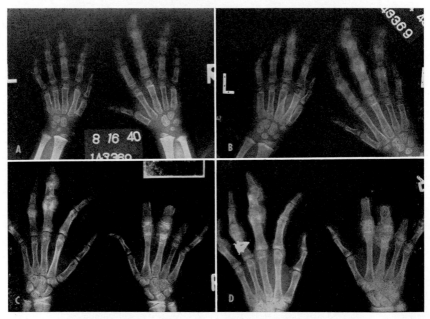

Figure 60.   Maffucci's syndrome. X-rays of the hands corresponding to the photographs in Figures 55, 56, and 57. The pathological process is well established at the age of three. The widespread occurrence of osteochondromas, overgrowth of the bones, calcification around the distal metacarpophalangeal junction of the third digit together with overgrowth of soft tissues and the progressive nature of the deformity are illustrated.

lar hamartoma should be studied for disease in the other, apparently normal, tissues. Umansky's observations suggest that only one in fifty to one hundred persons with either type of lesion might be expected to have the other also.

The experience recorded here permits the extension of generalizations already made and the suggestion of others. First, the disease may be suspected very early in life if unusual hemangiomata of the skin do not regress or disappear. In childhood, the dyschondroplastic disorder may cause various deformities and pathologic fractures. In any dysplastic anomaly, mild examples, formes frustes, are overlooked until the classic form is familiar. The occurrence of three cases in one hospital and another seen in consultation suggest that this rare disease is not so rare as the small number of case reports would suggest. The fact that a diagnosis was finally made in two of the patients after they had been observed for many years demonstrates again that we see, not what we look *at* but what we look *for*. In my own experience, finding rare diseases has resulted from being familiar with them and looking for them.

The several kind of malignant tumors to which different victims of Maffucci's syndrome have succumbed: chondrosarcoma (four), angiosarcoma (one), malignant lymphangioma (one), glioma (one), and ovarian teratoma (one)—demonstrate the very high risk of malignant neoplasm.

Observations of Inglis (428-429) on local gigantism include the suggestion that somewhat related lesions are manifestation of neurofibromatosis or von Recklinghausen's disease. Certainly in the classical examples of the Maffucci's syndrome neurofibromatosis has not been a significant or important feature of the disease.

The disorder has been reported in widely separated regions—England, Germany, Australia, and several parts of the United States. It has been reported in negroes and in those of Anglo-Saxon, Polish, and Italian stocks. With increased familiarity we may expect that it will be recognized at an earlier age, and more frequently.

Conclusion

The curious association of dyschondroplasia and hemangiomas, the devastating deformity which makes the victim a tragic carica-

turo, the high incidence of malignant neoplastic change all
challenge the geneticist, the practicing physician, and the cancer
specialist to provide a better understanding of this disorder. Maffucci's syndrome probably is commoner than the recorded cases
suggest. Any advance in our understanding depends on recognizing
the disorder. This is ample reason for calling attention to it for we
cannot eliminate a disease until we illuminate it.

5. Cirsoid Aneurysm and Arteriovenous Aneurysm

From time to time nature plays most discerning tricks. The
organization which enables so many embryos to develop with fabulous perfection escapes the template. The expected pattern fails
and we have every kind of structural deformity from headless mon-
sters to a mere extra digit or accessory breast. Among the developmental errors, congenital arteriovenous aneurysms, sometimes
called cirsoid aneurysms, may appear in various parts of the body.
When they involve the vessels of the face or scalp they may be a
troublesome nuisance (Figs. 61 and 62).

Their characteristic is active pulsation which can be suppressed
by compressing the main feeding artery. They may suggest a writh-
ing coil of worms or snakes. Brisk pulsations against sensitive
structures may cause pain; and actually erode bone or deform it by
a slow etching process with or without pain. Pulsation felt as unpleasant throbbing is common. The treatment is surgical ligation
of the main artery and large effluent veins. Mattress suture with
obliteration or rarely a complete excision may eradicate the lesion.
Unless the entire cirsoid aneurysm is removed it tends to grow back
and may require several operations.

A. CONGENITAL ARTERIOVENOUS ANEURYSM

Coursley, Ivins and Barker have reviewed the subject of congenital arteriovenous fistulas of the extremities and pointed out the
relation to congenital angiectasis of skin and underlying tissues.
They emphasize the common multiplicity, resistance to complete
extirpation and the probability of ultimate amputation. The dynamic alterations of the circulation are the same as in traumatic
arteriovenous aneurysms.

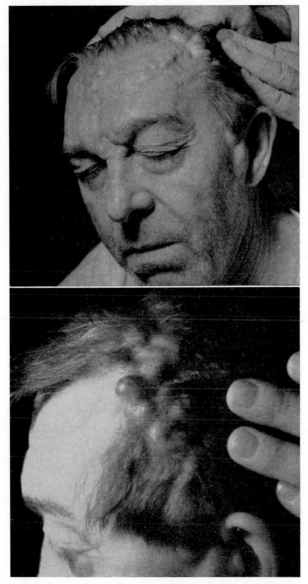

Figure 61.   Cirsoid aneurysm of the scalp.   Irregularly beaded and rumpled skin which on casual inspection suggests the hypertrophic cutis verticis gyrata.

Figure 62.   Cirsoid aneurysm.   Lateral view illustrating the obvious vascular structure of the irregular snake-like lesions.   All were compressible and pulsated freely with a loud bruit, continuous but much louder in systole.

B. TRAUMATIC ARTERIOVENOUS ANEURYSM

The havoc of World War II was not without its minor by-product of experience which advanced medical knowledge. With reference to the acquired arteriovenous aneurysm few discoveries were made. The traumatic arteriovenous aneurysm may occur when a penetrating or crushing wound lays open an artery or vein in close contact. Blood coming out of the artery under high pressure finds its way into the open venous channel. In time as healing occurs instead of obliteration of the new connection it enlarges. The coats of the vascular sac even on the venous side become thick. If an arteriovenous fistula is large it may throw such a burden on the heart that congestive failure occurs. Ultimately it may prove fatal. Arteriovenous aneurysms are a recognized cause of overgrowth of an extremity if they last long enough. They are diagnosed by the large throbbing pulsating mass which has a machinery-like continuous murmur usually louder in systole, the elevated venous pressure especially distal to the aneurysm, and an increase in cardiac output characterized by high pulse pressure, low diastolic pressure, and cardiac overactivity. A thrill is the palpable counterpart of the murmur. If one compresses either the aneurysm or the artery leading to it, there is a very prompt reflex bradycardia called Branham's sign. The circulatory state in cirsoid aneurysms, congenital arteriovenous aneurysms, acquired arteriovenous aneurysms, and the congenital dysplastic angiectases is very similar if the lesions are of comparable size. In congenital lesions of the extremities it is uncommon for a cure to be produced though there may be some improvement. Occasionally the lesions can be excised and corrected. Eventually, however, it may be necessary to amputate.

6. Blue Rubber-Bleb Nevi of the Skin and Gastrointestinal Tract

There is a characteristic variety of bluish nevus of the skin found in association with angiomas of the gastrointestinal tract which cause serious bleeding. The larger angiomas have some of the feel and look of rubber nipples, are compressible and refill fairly promptly from their rumpled compressed state. I have called them rubber-bleb nevi though they vary in size, shape and number.

This lesion has been described by surgeons but has not been empha-sized in writings of internists and gastroenterologists. In association with Dr. Robert Tidrick I have observed a child with this condition, and there are records from Surgical Pathology of others. In Albu-querque with Dr. Lyle Carr I saw another patient, a Latin Ameri-can girl, with dark brown skin who had bled from the bowel, was anemic, and had the characteristic lesions of the skin. At the same time sections of the resected specimen from another patient were inspected.

While much less common than hereditary hemorrhagic telan-giectasia, the syndrome of erectile bluish nevi of the skin and angio-matosis of the gut associated with enteric bleeding is definite. It should be known better. The disorder is referred to briefly in the comprehensive survey of Gentry, Dockerty and Clagett, but is de scribed in great detail in Shepard's beautifully illustrated mono-graph on angiomatous conditions of the gastrointestinal tract. Gascoyen, in 1860, seems to have been the first to record a case. The patient was a man of forty-four who since birth had had a vascular tumor of the parotid region which in later life grew, making swal-lowing difficult, imperiling the airway and finally causing death by suffocation. It had no bruit but it became livid and tense under excitement. Pressure reduced the size. "Numerous other nevi were scattered over various parts of the body and limbs forming tumors of greater or less size." At autopsy several nevi studded the surface of the intestine. The nevi arose in the submucous cellular tissue, projected into the cavity of the bowel but the covering mucous membrane "was still entire." There was a large heman-gioma in the liver. The vessels in the nevi appeared to be enor-mously distended "capillary veins" opening into large pouches, forming true erectile tissue. Many of the pouches were filled with pheleboliths.

McClure and Ellis in 1930 observed a 30 year old woman, anemic, dyspeptic and worried about tarry stools or bright blood which had appeared at intervals for ten years. For a long time she had had a large number of "blood tumors" over the skin. One had ruptured, bled profusely and healed with an extensive scar. "Scat-tered over the entire body but chiefly on the back, buttocks, and legs, were a large number of vascular tumors ranging in size from a pinhead to 1.5 cm. in diameter. These were reddish or purplish-red in color. Some were entirely within the skin, others were elevated, thin-walled blood sacs containing liquid blood and thrombotic masses occasionally partly calcified. A few were pedunculated. They could be partially emptied by pressure. On the right leg just above the external malleolus was a large stellate scar and a bluish discoloration where one of these tumors had been ruptured by a blow." There were more than twenty of these tumors which exceeded 0.5 cm. in diameter. Three large ones were on the sole of the right foot. At operation the liver border was seen with a large group of mulberry like tumors from 1 to 3 cm. in diameter. Gallbladder was normal. Much of the liver was replaced with cavernous hemangioma. The spleen was affected with a similar lesion being "three times normal size and the capsule entirely covered by dilated blood vessels." There was another tumor in the anterior wall of the stomach, another in the posterior wall of the duodenum, and eight widely separated single tumors in the jejunum. Some were deep in the wall. Others appeared as firm, elevated, circular, oval plaques just below the peritoneum. A few were pedunculated, intruding into the lumen of the bowel. Intussusception was beginning at the site of one tumor. The largest one half filled the lumen of the bowel a short distance from the iliocecal valve. There were none in the large bowel and no other angiomas elsewhere.

A similar case was described by Lazarus and Marks. Their patient, a fifty-eight year old man, had indigestion, belching, abdominal distention, and anemia. Nevi were found on the abdominal skin. Several operations before eventual colectomy revealed multiple small thin walled cavernous capillary angiomas of the colon.

Holman described a nine year old girl, seen first at the age of fifteen months, with a large hemangioma of the hand, another of the suprascapular region, and another of the tongue. Bleeding from the bowel was caused by an extensive hemangioma of the upper part of sigmoid. The lesion was a cavernous hemangioma, most of the vascular spaces having thick fibromuscular walls.

Heycock and Dickinson reported another patient, a six year old girl who had recurring episodes of pallor. At birth she had six toes on each foot. The spare ones were removed though the feet remained misshapen. A hemangiomatous lump appeared on the left side of the chest, and was not wholly excised even after three attempts. Another lump appeared over the spine. Because of recurrent falls in hemoglobin, an operation was performed revealing multiple red purple angiomas from 2 mm. to 1 cm. in diameter at intervals along the entire small bowel and a few in the colon. Nineteen lesions were removed. Subsequently bleeding recurred and eleven more were taken out. The report was written two months later. There was no bleeding during the interval.

Rickham reported the same general situation in a ten year old boy with an erectile tumor on the hypothenar eminence of the left hand. An abdominal operation revealed three angiomas in the small intestine, the size, shape, and color of "small blackberries." These were excised and the patient recovered.

In addition to describing a patient with congenital dysplastic angiomatosis of the trunk, right arm, and leg with overgrowth of bone and multiple angiomas of the bowel, Shepherd described and illustrated two examples of blue angiomas in the ileum and elsewhere in the gut but without the telltale lesions of the skin or other tissues which can distort the body surface.

Case Report

In March 1944, a three-month-old boy was admitted to the Pediatric Service because his mother discovered a swelling of the medial aspect of the right knee. It had been present at birth. There was no restriction of motion or pain on movement and no therapy was tried. He was next seen in the spring of 1949 with the same complaint and the soft, nontender mass which prevented full extension of the leg at the knee. Numerous solitary telangiectases on the trunk (Figure 63), the extremities, and the soles of the feet and soft, bilateral nontender masses in the parotid regions were found. An operation was done to remove the large hemangioma which extended into the knee joint. He was seen twice in 1950, having had no recurrence of the lesion. Motion at the joint was normal. In the spring of 1951 he was admitted for persistent anemia and given iron and transfusions. There had been the passage of some bloody stools. Hemangiomas were noted on sigmoidoscopic examination. X-rays of the upper and lower parts of the alimentary canal revealed no obvious abnormality. The hemoglobin, despite transfusions and the use of iron, ranged between 3.5 and 10 gm. per 100 ml. In May 1951 a resection of part of the small bowel was performed. A photograph of the gross specimen of bowel and microscopic section of an

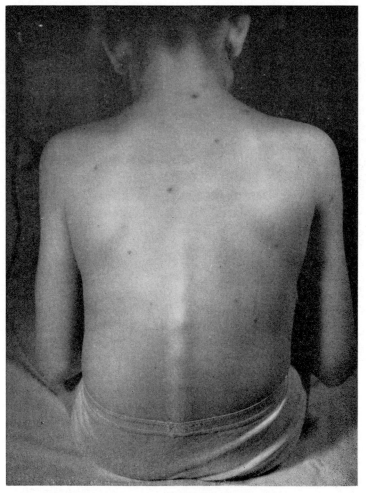

Figure 63.   Blue rubber-bleb nevus.   Many of this young boy's lesions are revealed better in this infrared photograph because many lesions do not appear at the skin surface.

angioma are in Figures 64 and 65. Though there was some occult blood in the stool after operation, the hemoglobin returned to normal but has fallen at times, usually responding to iron therapy. At intervals there is probably bleeding but there has been no gross hemorrhage. He has done well most of the time but has been given two transfusions. Once in 1956 he had a convulsion involving the left arm and leg. An electroencephalogram revealed a few focal spikes in the right temporal region. On his last visit when the photograph in Figure 63 was taken, he was asymptomatic, there were no new findings, and the hemoglobin was 11.5 gm.

In the syndrome exemplified by these few cases we have a spectrum of angiomatous lesions distributed widely throughout the body. I emphasize the fact that in a rare case angiomas of the gut can be inferred with assurance from their presence in the skin. In number, size and location, the vascular lesions may range from

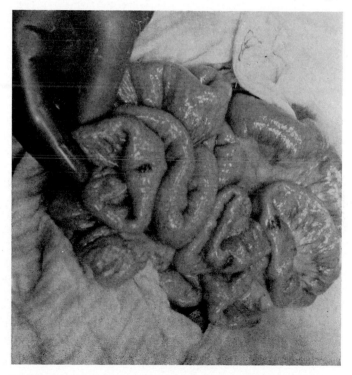

Figure 64.   Blue rubber-bleb nevus. This photograph was taken at operation. It reveals three of the many hemangiomas of the gut in the patient shown in Figure 63.

the trivial single lesion of the skin or gut to the disastrous destructive angiomatosis when the lesion is almost everywhere. The family history is negative. There is no sign of lesion in the parents or siblings of our patient.

The bluish nevi of the skin seen in this syndrome may occur in three main forms. One is the large disfiguring cavernous angioma which may replace vital structures, or growing too large size, obstruct the airway, alimentary canal, or some other important tubular structure. Another variety is the blood sac, looking like a blue rubber nipple covered with a milk white tissue of thin skin. These can be emptied of much or all of their contained blood. From the irregular mussed and rumpled state they resume their distended state by the gradual influx of blood. The third major variety of lesion is the irregular blue mark, sometimes with punctate blackish spots, merging with the adjacent normal skin in a series of color gradations through pale blue to white. Such lesions are elevated above the skin surface only if they are large. The small ones may or

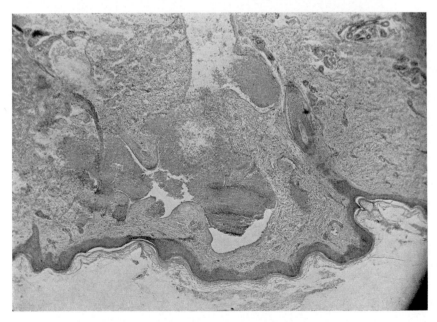

Figure 65.   Blue rubber-bleb nevus. Microscopic sections of one of the cutaneous lesions showing the enlarged and dilated vascular space in the skin. Though lesions of the skin may bleed with injury, spontaneous bleeding is rare, whereas it is characteristic of the lesions in the bowel.

may not blanch on pressure. There is rarely complete fading perhaps because of the complex tangle of coiled vascular spaces which trap blood when the structure is compressed.

7. Generalized Telangiectasia

A serious condition which appears to be an inborn dysplastic state, an inborn error of vascular structure is the universal telangiectasia. The victim may have several varieties of telangiectases of the skin and vascular weakness throughout the interior of the body. It is a kind of universal nevus, of which the nevus unius lateris is a one-sided forme fruste. Internal bleeding may be more violent and distressing than in hereditary hemorrhagic telangiectasia. In a patient we have had under observation for ten years there have been several dozen visits to the clinic or admissions to the hospital for bleeding from the alimentary canal; from the nose, cerebral hemorrhage; pulmonary hemorrhage; bleeding from the skin and mucous membranes of the mouth. This bleeding occurred "spontaneously" with little or no injury though a trivial bump might set it off. The skin has three kinds of alterations. The general color of the skin is bright red instead of the ordinary slightly red or pinkish or sometimes pale color. Almost the entire surface of the body is one telangiectatic mat. Pressure produces blanching and there is very rapid filling. The whole skin resembles a strange universal birthmark. Another characteristic is the purplish or dark red elevated angiomas which resemble but do not look exactly like cherry angiomas. They fade very little with pressure. Frequently they have an elegant anemic halo surrounding them to set them off clearly as dark purple islands with a white coral fringe in a red sea. The third lesion is the gross hemangioma which may have lymphangiomatous elements. One of these makes the upper lip of our patient stand out perpetually in a melancholy pout (Figure 66). These merely surface phenomena reflect the angiomatous and telangiectatic vascular anarchy which prevails widely within the body where there is ubiquitous and troublesome bleeding also.

In generalized telangiectasia we have a vascular lesion which is universal. Whatever the basic flaw, the capillary bed, the arterioles and venules, are deficient in muscle and elastic tissue. They

contract poorly so that the vascular element of hemostasis is wanting. Reaction to the usual mechanical or humoral stimuli is absent.
Hemorrhage is all pervasive, and life is a torment, a contest be-

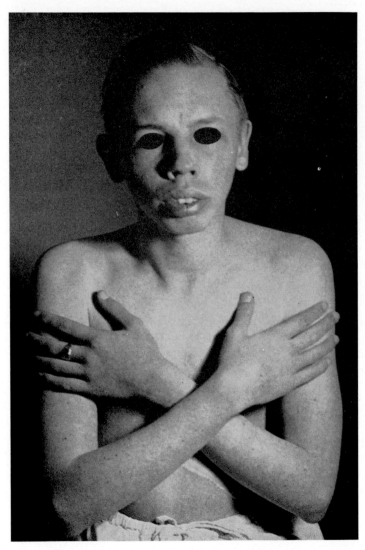

Figure 66.   Generalized telangiectasia.   The scar of the previous splenectomy
is seen.   The skin has a uniform bright color, conspicuously pinker than normal
skin.   Dark areas are angiomas.   On the forearms they are surrounded by
anemic halos.

tween bleeding and regeneration of blood, or bleeding and transfusion. The sword of Damocles is held by a narrow thread, wavering
with the threat of lethal hemorrhage into some vital organ or bleeding to death into a hollow tube, or from some mucous surface, or
the skin. No surgical therapy or local cautery is of any avail, the
fragile vessels leak blood into spongy tissue, the surface of the skin
or into the lumen of some hollow viscus. Healing of wounds is not
impaired but infections of the skin tend to become chronic and
respond poorly to treatment.

Case Report

Our patient was born of normal parents who had no blood
relationship, on 19 June 1935 at the University Hospitals. There
are several normal siblings and family history is completely negative. The first record we have of anything abnormal was at the age
of four when it was thought he had purpuric spots on the scrotum
when one of the lesions bled spontaneously. He was studied carefully and no blood dyscrasia was found, though he did have a low
hemoglobin. A systolic murmur was heard over the precordium.
X-rays were normal and there were no other positive findings.
Beginning at the age of twelve and continuing now into his twenty-
third year, he has had forty-three admissions to the hospital and
innumerable trips to the Out-Patient Clinic troubled by weakness,
bleeding and anemia. Hardly a week has gone by when he has not
had bleeding. In 1948 the diagnosis of generalized vascular nevus
was made and slightly later, because of the belief that he might
have Banti's syndrome and be bleeding from varices not demonstrated by x-ray, he had a splenectomy. The postoperative course
was smooth. Healing was normal. There was no improvement in
the anemia and he continued to bleed. During many of his admissions he required transfusions and was kept regularly on a program
of iron therapy. He has bled from innumerable places in the skin,
from the urinary tract, from the alimentary canal, regularly from
the nose, had intracerebral hemorrhage, subarachnoid hemorrhage
and hemorrhage into the eye grounds. The generalized vascular
weakness is somewhat reminiscent of Osler's disease though there
is no difficulty whatever in distinguishing the lesions he has from
those of Osler's disease. Since he began to bleed around the age of
twelve, he has had more than fifty transfusions and he has spent

almost as much time in the hospital as out. The skin is described in the text and shown in Figure 66.

8.   Elastic Tissue Disease: Pseudoxanthoma Elasticum

Just as Marfan's syndrome is a disorder of all the miscellaneous tissue and structures of mesenchymal origin which comprise the intricate internal scaffolding of the body, so the syndrome of pseudoxanthoma elasticum is an all pervasive inadequacy of elastic tissue. Since elastic tissue is a vital component of blood vessels, vascular disease is part of the clinical picture. Darier, a dermatologist, was the first to describe a "skin disease" which he named pseudoxanthoma elasticum because of a resemblance of the dermal lesions to xanthoma and xanthelasma. At least the similarity strikes those who look casually at the lesion. Then for a time ophthalmologists, concentrating on angioid streaks, thought that they had a new

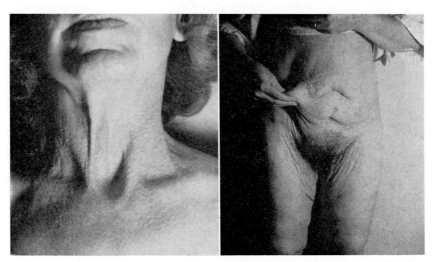

Figure 67.   Pseudoxanthoma elasticum. The skin of the neck reveals somewhat yellowish, wave-like ridges and valleys in skin which is extremely lax and hyperelastic.

Figure 68.   Pseudoxanthoma elasticum. The skin in the pudendal area, abdomen and inner thighs disclosing the exaggerated laxity. The skin falls in sagging ripples resembling those in a patient who has lost much weight though this patient had not lost weight.

disease, but when they came around to look at the skin and when autopsies were done a generalized disease of elastic tissue was revealed. Hemorrhage from the alimentary canal has been reported more often than could occur by chance, though only Kaplan and Hartman established the fact that bleeding was a result of poor elastic tissue in the blood vessels.

Enteric bleeding in this syndrome has been observed most commonly in women during pregnancy. This is another bit of testimony about the widespread vascular alterations in pregnant women, of which obstretricians have selected those of the uterus and fetus as most worthy of study. If physicians had looked at the skin of pregnant women above the lower abdomen as actively as they have observed the belly laced with collateral vessels embroidered with striae and embossed with a pouting navel, it would be easier to decide if this bleeding has a sufficient cause in the frayed elastic tissue and vascular proliferation of pregnant women. Until this is studied carefully, no one can decide with assurance. Hypertension may have a play in this problem too. McCaughey, Alexander and Morrish have reviewed this disorder recently, emphasizing the massive enteric hemorrhage occurring in pregnancy.

Case Report

While this section was being written, we had under observation on the medical wards a woman who first came to the University Hospitals in 1953 because her vision had been poor for three years. A "rash" was described on the neck and the loose skin of the inner thighs was noted. There was no family history of comparable illness. General examination revealed a fairly well developed and nourished woman whose blood pressure was 120/80, pulse 86, and temperature 98.8° F. Her vision in both eyes was approximately ten per cent of normal and there were large central scotomas on both sides. She had the characteristic angioid streaks, hemorrhages, pigmentary clumping and areas of retinal depigmentation. The two years before her most recent admission she had had much pain on the back and outside of the lower part of the right leg and ankle intensified by walking or standing and relieved by lying down. On the present admission her blood pressure was 140/70, pulse 88, and temperature 99.6° F. rectally. She had the same yellowish-pink irregularly papular alteration in the skin on the sides of the neck, the axilla, the thighs, and the lower abdomen. The skin was loose, sagging, and inelastic with pebbly, granular surface (Figures 67 and 68). It could be stretched without pain to a much greater distance than was possible with normal skin. The general appearance of the skin is revealed in Figures 67 and 68. The pulses in both feet were much diminished. The circumference of the right leg was smaller than that of the left. The right calf was flabby and the right ankle jerk hypoactive. There was limitation of straightening the leg raising on both sides because of pain in the right hip but there was no alteration in sensation. Laboratory tests of blood and urine gave normal results.

9. Palmar Varix

Varicose vascularization of the palms is a rare lesion. I have encountered it only four times, and only in relatively old women. They thought that their hands had always been as they were late in life. The lesion is easy to identify. It consists of a network of veins several millimeters in diameter which stand out as soft blue compressible streaks on the palms and palmar surface of the fingers. Though the change is irregularly disposed, both hands have been about equally affected. The hands look like they contain blue worms under a soft pink plastic cover (Figure 69). The veins do not pulsate, and no large sized arteries produce anything like a cirsoid or arteriovenous aneurysm. No symptoms or complaints referable to the hands have been noted in the four persons I have seen with palmar varicosities.

10. Strawberry Nevus, Birthmarks, and the Nape Nevus

Lister's classic observations on the natural history of strawberry nevi are a landmark of observation, in what was a sea of confusion vaguely mapped out by shoals of ignorance and heresay. Lister was impressed by the fact that strawberry nevi, so common in infants, were rare amongst children or adults. He did not believe that they had all been treated successfully in infancy. His impulse to make his study was engendered at a meeting of a dermatological society where a child with a very large number of prominent nervi was discussed. Lister said, "I was struck by the uncertainty of all those present as to the best line of treatment to be adopted, and as to what would happen if nothing were done." He therefore went to the source on which the information in textbooks should be based namely the long-term study of many infants and children who had strawberry nevi, port wine marks, and a few rare vascular tumors. Strawberry nevi, sometimes called cavernous angiomas, are elevated a little above the surface of the skin. They are present at birth or appear shortly thereafter and they grow more or less rapidly during the first six months of life. After this they invariably regress and disappear completely leaving little or no trace by about the fifth year of life. Port wine marks may be called capillary nevi. They are commonest about the face and neck, present at birth, have sharply defined margins, and remain stationary, having neither spontaneous regression or extension except in rare cases. They may become a little more obvious as life goes on, develop some nodularity, and hang as ugly vascular pouches.

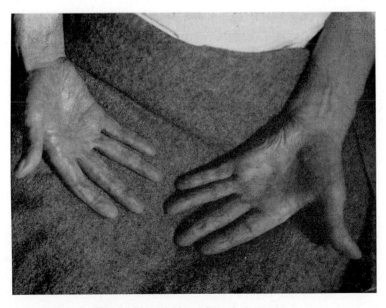

Figure 69.   Varicosities of the palms.

Essentially the strawberry nevus is an area of greatly increased vascularity in the superficial layers of the skin, or more rarely in the deep layers and in the subcutaneous tissue. The surface is finely lobulated. The color ranges from scarlet to deep purple but usually is a very vivid crimson. The nevus increases in size when the child strains or cries in one of the repeated Valsalva manuvers which punctuate early existence. Pressure ordinarily will cause the lesion to fade. In several reported series, there have been two or three times as many girls as boys, which may represent actual incidence or maternal worry. From Lister's observations, he was led to remark that strawberry nevi of infants have a natural history all their own. They enjoy a period of more or less rapid growth during the first few months after their appearance, but this stops within the first year, usually between the sixth and eighth month when regression sets in. Ordinarily all traces of color are gone by the fifth year or before. Only in very prominent and large nevi is a further term of years required for the absorption of re-dundant skin. Lister attributes the aggressive treatment of these lesions to the fact that mothers are likely to be worried by what they think a bad blemish or perhaps a horrible disfigurement of their child and the great relief they experience when it is removed, as it may be by a variety of methods. If it is not very disfiguring, however, time in divided doses will produce the same effect without any risk of radiation burns or scars. Traub submitted a question-naire to pediatricians and dermatologists concerning their experi-ence with vascular nevi. He found that only 10 per cent had observed spontaneous disappearance as a common occurrence and many had never seen it at all. This reflects aggressive therapy. Ronchese has devoted much attention to the spontaneous involu-tion of cutaneous vascular tumors. In the discussion of Rochese's paper, many different points of view were expressed. Despite the realization that many of these nevi disappear spontaneously, there is a widespread belief among dermatologists and pediatricians that they should be treated. There is, however, some danger in x-ray therapy, a danger which apparently is not shared by the technique of radiophosphorus therapy advocated by Roe, Hodges, Innes, and Pope. It would certainly seem wise to leave alone those lesions which do not show, examine the child at intervals and reassure the mother that nature will take care of the strawberry nevus in good time.

A. THE NAPE NEVUS

Even the casual observer is vaguely aware that in healthy adults as well as in persons with various diseases splotchy areas of erythema, paler than the ordinary strawberry nevus or the nevus flammeus but a darker red or reddish-purple than the nearby skin may be found on the back of the neck. Often they extend up into the scalp. As with so many other vascular changes in the skin, since this is without symptoms, little attention is paid to it. Furthermore, since it is ordinarily well within the area covered by the hair, even women with their highly developed cosmetic sense rarely are aware of such blemishes. To find this blotch on oneself requires fair acrobatic skill in manipulating two mirrors unless of course some-one else discovers it. There has been a small flurry of letters in the *Lancet* and *British Medical Journal* about the nape nevus. Obser-vations and detailed study of it goes back to Unna in the 1880's and 90's. He obtained histologic sections of a number of examples. He concluded that it was a birthmark, that the changes were telangiec-tatic and that they were of the same order but of less intensity than those of the nevus flammeus. It has been called Unna's nevus. If either one of uniovular twins has the nape nevus the other practi-cally always does too, but ordinary twins show no such tendency.

There are not many studies of its incidence in children. Bettley, who made an intensive search for such disorders in the newborn, found it in approximately 50 per cent of newborn children, the sex incidence being equal. Sharfar has called attention to the nape nevus as a mark likely to occur in families but since it is so very common in the general population much more evidence will have to be accumulated before we can accept any notion of an unusual hereditary disposition to the disorder. Parkes Weber, whose clinical connoisseurship has illuminated many neglected areas in the bor-derland between general medicine and dermatology, has empha-sized the possibility of the relationship of the nape nevus to such conditions as encephalofacial hemangiomatosis, particularly the type which involves the territory supplied by the trigeminial nerve with an angiomatus disorder affecting the brain beneath the cutaneous angioma.

As for the cause of the nape nevus we have absolutely no notion. Dixey comments that the midwives in his part of England ascribe it to an affectionate peck on the neck by the storks as they are completing their midwifely offices. This seems as good an idea as any. My own observations on what is still a relatively small series of persons makes me believe that the lesion must be much commoner than had been usually thought. I have found it in more than 40 per cent of normal adults. Only by very careful inspection and concentration on particular lesions do we get anything like a true notion of their incidence. They usually turn out to be commoner than was suspected.

The nape nevus may be a single spot, a streak, a cluster, a coast of Maine mapwork, a skewed tracery of red or purple-red marks. It has no extra heat, blanches on pressure and causes no symptoms. The great variability of size, shape and pattern of the nape nevus might stir the imagination of the natural historian of vascular lesions to all manner of fancied resemblances as the eager candidate in the Rorschach test imagines all forms of good or evil from inkblots and is said to display thereby his own deepest secrets.

IV

FUNCTIONAL FLUSHES AND VASCULAR PATTERNS

1. Functional Blushes, Flushes, and Blotches

Full understanding of vascular lesions of the skin depends on a better comprehension than we have now of the intimate details of structure and function of the skin, particularly its vascular system. There are only a limited number of architectural patterns by which a surface area can be furnished with an irrigation and drainage system. The possible patterns in human circulation include a series of parallel vessels, a complex interlocking network or a multitude of end arteries. These three exist singly or in combination. The tiny cone shaped zones of skin supplied by an end artery are too small to produce a macroscopic pattern. If the normal skin is cooled, however, it may exhibit a reticulated pattern of pale islands enmeshed in a darker network. The white central areas have increased flow, slightly warmer skin and increased vascular tone. This pattern may be determined by vasomotor nerves, by anatomical arrangement of the branching arteries or by local metabolic variations. Often but not always spiders form in the white spots. They soon outgrow the small compass of the spot. They push out branches into the anemic halo which expands. The inner and outer dimensions of the halo increase as the spider enlarges. The anemic ring around a large spider leaves the original pale area and encroaches on neighboring ones. Martini believes that the white spots in a cirrhotic patient which stand out clearly when the skin is cooled are not the same as those which determine the markings of the fire strains of *erythema ab igne*. I do not know.

Despite shortcomings in our knowledge of the microphysiology and microanatomy of the skin there are a number of functional changes which may be observed as "spontaneous" events or as reactions to physical and chemical stimuli. We are far from understanding the mechanisms by which they are produced.

A. Blushing

The social blush varies with the mores and manners of each age. By inborn tendency some families have a vasolabile skin. The state of the emotions and the activity of autonomic control of vasomotion alter the circulation of the skin. Increased environmental temperature produces diffuse blushing. If Victorian novelists are to be trusted, our generation is below standard in the frequency and intensity of blushing. Blushing is commoner in the young than the old, rare in the elderly, and is a correlate of embarrassment, true or feigned shyness, modesty or social fear. Though some people, having guilty thoughts, blush in the dark, blushing is par excellence a manifestation of herd existence. It would be expected to flourish in a culture where organized deference to opinion is producing an "other-directed" society, though it seems to be declining.

Blushing may be induced or aggravated by fear of blushing. It may promote anxiety or panic and a strong desire to escape. When extreme it may bring tears to the eyes. Most people outgrow the tendency in its severe form, perhaps as maturity dulls or hides the self-consciousness of adolescence and youth. It has some features in common with the involuntary sneeze, cough, hiccup, seasickness and other forms of paroxysmal autonomic activity.

Anger and emotional outbursts may be associated with blushing, flushing, blinking of the eyes, and patterned motor activity. Parkes Weber has compared the flush of anger to the swelling of the turkey's wattle in anger. He relates the story of a young man posing naked as an artist's model who became intensely angered at some political news. He was observed to flush not only in his face and neck but "to become bright red and lobster-like over his whole body."

Blushing may extend far beyond the exposed areas of the skin though it is most intense over the face, ears, and neck. Observant physicians have described a rectal blush during a proctoscopic examination. Such a procedure is inherently embarrassing. It puts one in an awkward and indefensible position. Though I have seen spontaneous flushing and paling of the rectal mucosa during endoscopic examinations, embarrassment did not seem a likely cause, though perhaps anger or annoyance was.

2. Dysautonomia

The doctrines of vagotonia and sympathotonia went the way of angina vasomotoria, vasomotor ataxia (Solis-Cohen), and related situations with sonorous names. Persons who might have been classified in one of these categories years ago now are found to have pheochromocytomas, diencephalic epilepsy, islet cell tumors, the syndrome of chronic hyperventilation or some other neurosis. Among the functional flushes and specklings of the skin Riley and his associates have described evanescent blotching of the skin, emotional instability, mental retardation, excessive sweating, poor control of temperature and hypertension with postural hypotension in infants and children. This they call dysautonomia. Crying without tears, indifference to pain, hyporeflexia, incoordination of motor activity, and trouble with swallowing round out the picture of physical inadequacy and misery. The preponderance of Jewish children may be an accidental selection of clinical material. Linde has emphasized the vast array of laboratory studies and diagnostic procedures wasted in a search for some more orthodox explanation of the curious cluster of troubles these children have. Treatment is difficult, and needs to be directed towards the parents as well as the child. Chlorpromazine is said to be of some help but the evidence is far from convincing.

I have seen two adults, both young women who may have been suffering from such a condition. They were both puzzling. I did not achieve much success in treatment. Here is the story of one.

Case Report

The patient was twenty-three years old, the oldest child of five in a family of strict Roman Catholics. The past history is uncertain and perhaps untrustworthy, but she was not obviously peculiar, and no one had noticed signs or symptoms until adolescence. At that time she began to have pronounced mottled blushing of the face, chest and upper arms, a sense of apprehension, great sweating, crying without tears, some incoordination, dizziness, and faintness but no actual syncope. There might or might not be headaches. Her menses were normal. We could not be sure that anxiety was part of the trouble since the senses seemed dull rather than alert during an attack. She did not hyperventilate sponta-neously.

The physical examination revealed an apparently healthy young woman, except during an attack when a bright pink mottled flush colored the neck and upper chest. Sweating was general. At times she would weep but we thought she might be feigning it since no tears came. Neurological studies were negative. We did not do an electroencephalogram. Fasting blood sugar and toler-ance tests were normal. Withholding food did not evoke a reac-tion. Tests for pheochromocytoma were negative. There was a pronounced sinus arrhythmia but the normal blood pressure was not erratic either in an attack or at rest. Induced hyperventilation provoked no symptoms of undue magnitude. She would not coop-erate enough to see a psychiatrist. Her whole attitude was negati-vistic. She did not seem retarded mentally though she would not cooperate for special tests. Our conclusion was that she had vaso-motor storms of some sort. We have no evidence for diencephalic epilepsy, pheochromocytoma, islet cell tumor, carcinoid tumor or any other definite clinical entity. She may have an acquired form of dysautonomia, though annexing this title does not really help me understand her trouble. It has continued for several years. The symptoms vary. Months of freedom from attacks are followed by many attacks in a week. She refuses to have further studies.

Without claiming to understand the disorder, I am recording this example of a young woman with a peculiar mottled flushing, a vasomotor squall perhaps related to some special dysfunction of the autonomic nervous system. If others encounter similar persons they may clarify the mechanisms and help provide sensible man-agement. The clinical picture differs from what has been described in infants and children in being late in onset and thus not obviously an inborn error.

3.   The Harlequin Reaction and Unilateral Sweating

Observant physicians who have the care of newborn infants may see a strange vascular phenomenon. This is the "harlequin" reaction, in which there is a sudden paling of half of the body as the child lies naked on one side or the other. The upper side of the body retains its natural pink color, the lower half blanching. The midline neatly separates the pink and white sides. This red and white division is very spectacular. It commences abruptly but usually vanishes more gradually. Close observation of the child does not suggest that it is having any unpleasant sensation. The essential features have been described by Neligan and Strang and verified by Sharpe. I am told by my colleagues, Russell Meyers and Adolph Sahs, that they have never seen a similar phenomenon in adults with various neurological disorders.

The nature of this little one-sided vasomotor squall, putting an infant in the masquerade of a harlequin, is altogether speculative. It must be mediated through the nervous system by some reflex with a central mechanism. The only analogy I know is the unilateral sweating reflex. I have made many observations on the circumstances in which it appears. Whenever the temperature and moisture content of the air are sufficiently high and the body is warm enough, sweating occurs. If one is sitting, standing, lying prone or supine, the body surface becomes moist in more or less uniform fashion all over. If, however, one lies on the right or left side, within a few minutes the lower half of the body stops sweating. This process can be reversed many times by turning over onto the other side. I have made many simple tests on the relation of head position to body position in provoking the response when it is warm enough for the reaction to be evoked at will. For instance, if the position of the body remains fixed while one is lying on either side, and the head is rotated through 150°-180° so that the face looks over the back and shoulder (an increasingly difficult maneuver as the years go by) the lower side remains dry. If, while the head is kept as still as possible, the up and down sides of the body are reversed by turning through 180° (no mean test of agility!) sweating reverses sides. The lower side stops sweating and the upper side begins to sweat. Thus the position of the body rather than the position of the head determines the stimulus. The position of the arms and legs is less important. Twisting the trunk reveals that the bulk of the body must be disposed with one side up and the other down to set this curious gravitational reaction going. As the prone or supine position are approached the reflex fails and sweating becomes evenly distributed. Such diversions may occupy the long nights of a heat wave where insomnia can be so grievous a burden to the incurious.

I have no idea what the mechanism for unilateral vasomotor activity or unilateral sweating may be; nor can I think of any teleological end to be gained. The reactions seem to be inherent in the mechanisms our bodies have for other purposes, or they may exist as nothing more than playthings to stimulate the curiosity of the observant, and delight those still able to wonder. Long after I had noted this unilateral sweating reflex, I found that Kuno in his classic studies of sweating, had described and studied it in wonderful detail. Both sweating and vasoconstriction have a unilateral pattern which probably has the same or a similar reflex mechanism. In the recent edition of Kuno's book in a series of elegant experiments he demonstrated that lateral pressure applied when the sweating subject stands upright will inhibit sweating on that side so the pressure need not be hydrostatic or gravitational. No one has reported lateral pressure on an infant who exhibits the "harlequin" reaction.

4.   Marble Skin, Fire Stains, Chilblains and Livedo Reticularis

With wonderful artistry Nature paints elegant patterns in the skin. Not the leopard and zebra only, but normal human beings and those sick with various troubles may exhibit in their skin constant or changing designs of pigment or vascular marks. Furthermore, man can and does change his spots. Little thought has been given to the reasons for localization of the rashes of the common exanthems, the spots of spotted fever, or the variegated patterns of cutaneous syphilis. Indeed, localization of vascular marks, ephemeral or established, is a fertile field for investigation, since this neat little problem has evaded the zealots in medicine and dermatology.

Fashion may decree tattooing the skin, dying the hair, painting the lips, plastic and polish for nails and different degrees of nudity or complete coverage. Exposure of the skin to the elements may produce its own designs. Suntan, avoided with much forethought fifty years ago, is socially desirable today.

Anyone who looks at the skin of children, or women, with legs and arms exposed to the cold, notices a mottled network—pale islands surrounded by a reticulum of a dark pink or a cyanotic hue

(Figure 70). Marble skin or cutis marmorata is a natural phenome-non and betokens no disease. It may be much exaggerated in chil-dren when they are ill. It is most likely to be noticed at such a time, since then children may actually be examined in detail. The islands vary in size averaging two or more centimeters in diameter. They are elliptical or rhomboidal in outline with the long axis the same as that of the limb. The dividing network is made up of bands varying in width up to several millimeters or a centimeter. At the intersections the strands of dark skin may be much wider. In places the band is as wide as the pale island. Sometimes the dark mottling is much wider than the enmeshed pale spots. The dark strands are irregular with little wisps and bunches branching into the pale

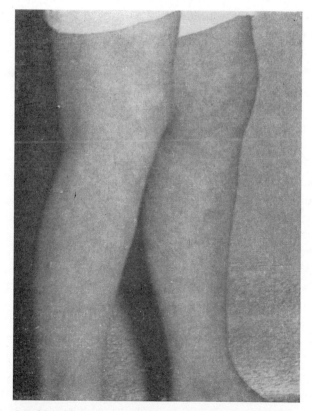

Figure 70. Marble skin. The pattern of reticulated mottling in the lower extremities of a twenty-five-year-old woman who had chilblains every winter.

zones like fraying rope seen in silhouette. Their arrangement over a period of months is fixed, and a general constancy of design may last for several years but it does change somewhat. I have observed this change only in growing children, the only subjects I have followed for any length of time. The color of the reticulum varies with the temperature, being bluish when it is cold. If the temperature is raised the whole pattern is lost and leaves no visible residue in the increasing redness. If skin marbling is known to have appeared or increased recently it may be a clue to minor or beginning illness. The design depends on the anatomical disposition of arteries, arterioles, subpapillary venous plexus and capillaries and the state of the circulation. The depth of color depends on the amount of blood, which may flow fast or stagnate in the little vessels near the skin surface. Thus marble skin is a pattern based on anatomical disposition of vessels, physiological changes in blood vessels and blood flow of the skin.

Thomson described two members of a family with such excessive marbling of the skin that he thought it was severe enough to constitute a disease.

Fire stains may be called *erythema ab igne* but improperly since a suntan is not a sunburn. These marks are brown melanin deposited exactly in the region of the dark network of marbled skin. The pigment develops where the blood flow is sluggish, away from the central pallid spot which is supplied by an artery larger than the end artery of Renaut. Figure 71 shows the characteristic mottled design of fire stain. On the lower legs it may occur as a result of sitting before an open fire, stove, radiator, or furnace. I have seen it in an old woman who sat always with her rocking chair in one position. Only the right side of each lower leg got marked. This result of exposure to heat has been known for years. It was studied carefully many years ago (509-509a). When fire stains occur over the chest or trunk usually a hot water bottle or electric heat pad has been used for a long time because of underlying pain (Figures 72 and 73). As such, it is a helpful clinical clue. In some cases the pigmented areas may develop superficial ulcers and erosions which heal slowly. Carcinoma has arisen in such places (657).

I have studied fire stains in infrared, colored and black-and-white photographs. When the pigment was fading, infrared photographs showed that the pigment occurred where the dark blue venous structures were prominent or the blood flow was sluggish. One additional set of observations was made during a study of the production of unilateral skin lesions in pellagra years ago (75). In several malnourished subjects who did not have or later get pellagra, and in normal controls, the pattern of *erythema ab igne* was induced by the application of stasis and heat. The studies were done as follows. An electric heat pad with the temperature set at 120° F. was held snugly on the forearm by sandbags, the total weighing three and one-half pounds. Pressure and heat were applied for sixty to ninety minutes daily. The earliest fire stain appeared after

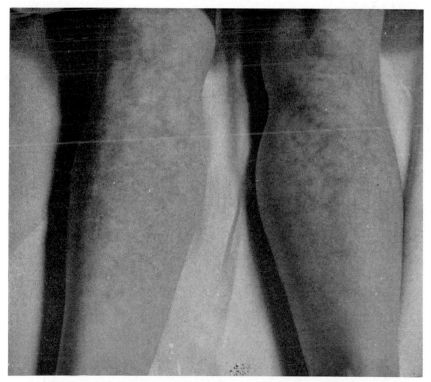

Figure 71.   Firestains. The lower anterior aspect of the legs of a patient who had spent much of the previous winter sitting in front of an open fire. She was healthy and had noticed no ill effects from this exposure.

eight consecutive days of exposures totaling ten hours. One of two women and two of three men got some fire stains though the subject exposed longest did not. These casual observations have not been extended to get more data.

The order of permanence of the fire stains seems higher than that of suntan. They gradually fade out so that a year after induction, if no further stimulus is applied, they have faded substantially, but traces may be seen. Within three years, however, the change has vanished completely and the skin looks normal.

The darker regions of cutis marmorata and marbled skin are refractory to the effects of locally instilled adrenalin or histamine. In the case of fire stain this refractory state is nearly absolute, and so remains for many months after exposure to heat has ended (46).

Livedo reticularis, lupus pernio, and the blains of chilblains all follow the same anatomical pattern of vascular supply to the skin in their distribution and arrangements. Though the classical form follows mild cold injury, another variety may cause trouble only in warm weather (260). Ulcers form and may not heal until cool weather returns. The significance of this rarer variety is unknown.

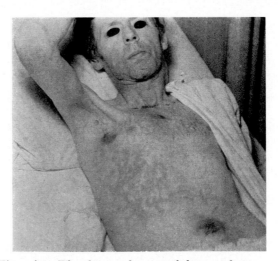

Figure 72.   Firestains. The chest and upper abdomen of a man with actinomycosis. He had used a hot water bottle for many hours every day during the previous six weeks. The wide areas of pigmentation extended far beyond the locus of any vein in the subcutaneous tissue.

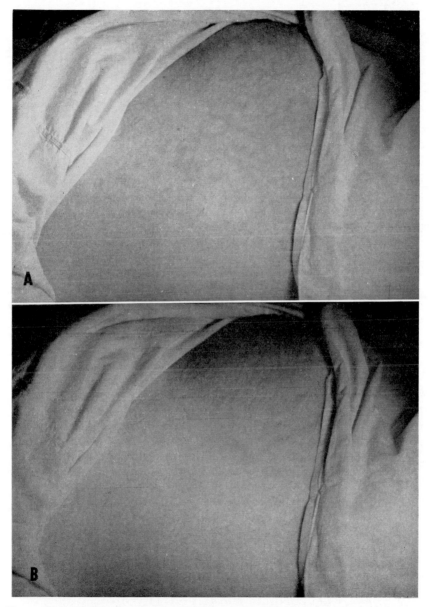

Figure 73.   Firestains. Black and white and infrared photographs of the pattern on the lateral portion of the abdomen.   The patient had used a hot water bottle.   Several of the more prominent marks and lines lie exactly above major veins as may be seen in the infrared photograph.   They do not all do so.

5.   Menstrual Erythema and Menopausal Hot Flashes

Bulkley has described a woman who had erythema simplex with striking red discoloration of the face repeatedly during her menstrual cycle. "Time and again she has noticed the great aggravation of the redness and burning one or two days before the menstrual period and subsidence on the second day of flow." He reported a series of comparable cases some from his own experience and others recorded in medical writings. I have noticed cyclical variation in the redness of spiders; and this phenomenon has been related to me also by observant patients. The pattern has not been consistent enough to make me certain that it has any significance. Presumably the local effect of estrogens or other humoral factors on the skin either sensitizes the blood vessels or in some way enhances neurovascular reactions in such fashion that flushing is sustained for several days.

Menopausal hot flashes, about which there is lurid folklore, tales from the women's clubs, and little careful observation, are paroxysmal vasomotor changes. A sweeping surge of flushing, sweating, and tingling of the skin occurs. Generalized paresthesias or disagreeable sensations are described. The blush of embarrassment may add to the nuisance. Close scrutiny may reveal few signs for many symptoms or the red flush may be spectacular. These phenomena have not been demonstrated to be a result of estrogen deficiency. Indeed many women go through the menopause without having any difficulty of this kind. Others have hot flashes unrelated to the menopause. The nature of the condition is not understood though it is assumed to represent a transitory oversensitivity of the autonomic control of blood vessels of the skin. Emotional factors may trigger it off and at times treatment with sex hormones has been followed by improvement of the symptoms though the results are erratic.

6.   Pheochromocytoma and Thyrotoxicosis

Cutaneous manifestations in pheochromocytoma include all varieties of neurofibromatosis, and there may be paroxysmal episodes of throbbing, palpitation, hyperperistalsis, great increases in blood pressure, tachycardia, anxiety, sweating, nausea, vomiting, headache and blurring of vision. There may be acute alterations in the blood flow in the skin with spells of flushing and warmth. Adrenal catachols cause constriction of cutaneous arterioles with a reduction of the circulation of the skin. Pallor is common during the attack but there may be cold mottling of the hands and feet, blanching of the fingers, and bluish red discoloration of the extremities and less commonly of the trunk together with numbness and tingling. The skin may have the same kind of mottling which occurs particularly in cold weather or during the incipient stage of minor febrile illnesses. It may become established with some constancy in the presence of pheochromocytoma but it is not diagnostic. One occasionally has some difficulty in distinguishing the clinical state of the skin in pheochromocytoma from that of thyrotoxicosis. The hyperkinetic state of the circulation, tachycardia, palpitation, flushing, lacrimation, warm skin, tremor, and anxiety go with both. A useful clinical finding may be the high diastolic pressure which often occurs during a crisis in pheochromocytoma, whereas in thyrotoxicosis the diastolic blood pressure usually does not rise during a vasomotor outburst. Often it falls. Braley has called attention to medullated nerve fibers in the cornea which can be detected by the slit lamp technique as a helpful sign in pheochromocytoma. They are found in neurofibromatosis also and confirm the relationship of pheochromocytoma and neurofibromatosis.

7. Migraine

In migraine the full throbbing felt in the internal and superficial aspects of the head, scalp and brain may be measured and recorded by appropriate studies. Varying degrees of flushing or pallor may attend the headaches, precede or follow it. After severe headaches the scalp may be very sensitive. It feels sore. Sometimes it is actually edematous, and rarely there is effusion of blood which may resemble an ordinary bruise.

8. Diencephalic Blotching

From time to time one encounters a mottled blotchy erythema of the face, upper part of the chest, shoulders, and back, particularly in women who have a florid complexion. Often they have hypertension. Page and Schroeder suggested that a special form of diencephalic hypertension may be recognized. In most cases there is but meager resemblance to diencephalic epilepsy as described by Penfield. Many women who show this mottled flushing have dermatographism. The same kind of blotching may occur in men. It may occur without hypertension. Sometimes it is provoked by eating. Its exact nature is obscure.

Outbursts which have been called diencephalic autonomic attacks include rage, tremor, vasoconstriction of the lower extremities, intense flushing of the face, neck and upper part of chest, lacrimation, tachycardia, transitory hypertension, fever, peripheral vascular collapse, multiple extrasystoles, and increased peristaltic activity. There are changes in libido. Some of the characteristics of such attacks have a close resemblance to symptoms and signs which may occur in patients with pheochromocytoma. A lesion in the diencephalon may be responsible, or the disorder may be analogous to the common forms of idiopathic epilepsy.

9. Flushes Evoked by Pharmacologic Agents

Histamine, a natural humor, produces a characteristic vasodilatation seen as a generalized flush of the skin. It produces this effect so fast that it has been used as a circulation timer (244, 898). Intravenous injection very promptly produces a conspicuous generalized vasodilatation of the skin characterized by a bright beet-red color, a sense of fullness, sometimes lacrimation, a very profound burning and sometimes actual pain or a very disagreeable sensation in the skin. The flush, though most intense over the upper part of the body, especially the face and the so-called "blush area," may spread widely over the whole surface of the skin. To what extent histamine governs the everyday fluctuations in vascular tone in the skin, or how much its local release or suppression determines the intimate variation of blood flow in the skin is not known. Put into an artery slowly it may lose its systemic effect by being destroyed, bound or segregated in peripheral tissues. It is not possible to distinguish a flush induced by histamine from one induced by nicotinic acid, the hectic flush of fever, the transitory blush of embarrassment, or the mild erythema induced by sun or heat.

We do not know to what degree histamine mediates some of the "spontaneous" blushes which decorate the human skin and enliven a social gathering. Such problems, germane to the comfort and repose of the ordinary person, have been beneath the notice of scientists who address themselves to important problems.

Nicotinic acid, one form of a vitamin of the B-complex family, induces flushing of the skin and other vascular reactions (74). One of the curious facts which has not been explained is that an intravenous injection of nicotinic acid produces its vasodilatation after a lag of thirty to sixty seconds. Is this vasodilatation caused by a fundamentally different mechanism from that induced by histamine? Or is histamine released by nicotinic acid? As with so many simple clinical problems, no one has done the work we need to get the answer. In a series of studies in which the specific molecule responsible for evoking the vasodilatation was identified it was possible to show that there were some related pyrazine compounds with lesser effects (74). Furthermore, certain chemicals of the same molecular kindred had toxic effects though it is not certain that this is an example of strife and competition at the molecular level or whether it is effected through some unrelated mechanism.

10. The Auriculotemporal Syndrome

The auriculotemporal syndrome is a curious flushing and sweating of the skin over the area supplied by the auriculotemporal nerve, provoked by eating or by anything which stimulates the flow of saliva. Usually it is a late sequel to injury of the auriculotemporal nerve. It develops after an illness, injury, or operation has damaged the nerve usually in or near the parotid gland. The disorder is caused by misguided reinnervation of sweat glands by regenerating parasympathetic salivary fibers. In this syndrome there is impaired sensation in the distribution of the nerve. Temporary relief of sweating and flushing follows procaine block of the nerve. Cure follows resection. The signs and symptoms fail to respond to procaine block of the cervical sympathetic chain. The elimination of the signs by atrophine, their aggravation by pilo-carpine, and the great sensitivity of affected sweat glands to the intra-dermal injection of acetylcholine characterize the syndrome. Sweating is usually the troublesome feature. This is a remarkable example of vasomotor change induced under peculiar circum-stances by the misdirected regeneration of a nerve.

Parkes Weber has discussed the auriculotemporal syndrome. He presented a case late in the 19th century. Uprus, Gaylor and Carmichael, in their discussion of abnormal localized flushing and sweating on eating, described a patient whose trouble was not the usual surgical or suppurative disorder of the parotid. Their patient was a healthy woman of twenty-two who, at the age of five, had had scrofula and excision of the lymphatic chain on the right side of the neck. A year after operation eating would invoke flushing

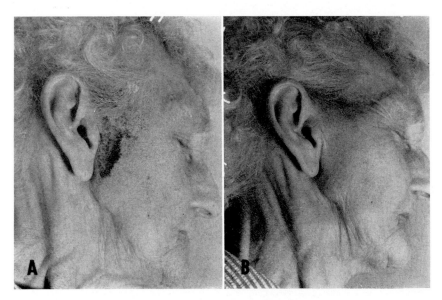

Figure 74. The auriculotemporal syndrome. Photograph with and without iodinated starch illustrating the area of sweating. It extends down in front of the ears and up into the scalp, covering a region roughly the size of the ear and directly anterior to it. Even without such techniques it was easy to see beads of sweat and pronounced erythema during eating. A sharp line of demarcation separated it from the adjacent areas of unaffected skin.

in the right submental region. Two years later, on eating, profuse sweating occurred in the same area.

Occasionally gustatory lacrimation, the syndrome "crocodile tears," occurs after injury to the large or small superficial petrosal nerves. Upon eating, tears well up in one eye, even though the food is good and the occasion merry. The trouble can be corrected by severing the ninth nerve inside the cranium. There is no flushing with the flow of tears in this syndrome. This is the opposite state to a part of the disturbed functions in the dysautonomia syndrome.

V

NEOPLASTIC LESIONS

1. The Glomus Tumor and Related Structures

The glomus tumor is a small bump or nodule, elevated above the surface of the skin, a few millimeters to a centimeter or more in diameter, bluish or red, partly compressible and dreadfully painful. Though it may occur anywhere, the hand and fingers, especially beneath the nail, are favorite sites. The larger lesions may be relatively less painful than the small or tiny ones. For a long time it has been thought that the glomus tumor resulted from a kind of localized gigantism which distorted and ruined a glomus body. Thus the tumor was believed to be absolutely dependent for its origin on a glomus body. The studies of Stout and his co-workers suggest very strongly that such tumors may arise anywhere from the pericyte of Zimmermann in small arteries and veins. The pericyte is related to the cell that surrounds and at times constricts capillaries.

Since glomus tumors are painful, and painful out of all proportion to their size, it is not surprising that their history goes back a long way. One can read into writings we ascribe to Hippocrates a possibility that they were known even in his time. There are medical references to such penomena for several hundred years. The modern era was ushered in by Wood (928, 929) of Edinburgh who in 1812 and later gave a classical and complete description of the clinical features of the glomus tumor. He observed its small size, its firm consistency, the fact that it was benign, its limited growth potential, and the areas likely to be affected as well as the long duration of the symptoms. He mentioned especially the pain which came in excruciating paroxysms. It might wax and wane under circumstances not always clear. In two of Wood's patients he observed an influence of changes in temperature. Either an increase in heat or an increase in cold might provoke symptoms. He made the remarkable observation that one of these painful nodules increased in size during the agonizing attacks of pain. He and his patients alike expressed their satisfaction with the permanent relief which came after simple excision of the tumor.

There are intermittent reports of these tumors in German writings usually under the name angiosarcomas and later peritheliomas. Chandelux, in 1882, published a paper called "Histologic researches on painful subcutaneous tubercle." At least one of his patients almost certainly had a glomus tumor. In 1922, Barré, a French surgeon, had a patient with a very painful tiny tumor beneath a fingernail. He removed it and gave it to Masson for an investigation of the histopathology. Masson's report of this tumor, published in 1924, gave the first full description of a glomic neoplasm. The tumor was blue-red, about four millimeters in diameter, composed of large, clear, round polyhydral cells. It was recognized that these were similar to those in the coccygeal gland or glomus body. In addition to "epitheloid" cells, there was a mass of arteries, veins, smooth muscle cells and nerve fibers scattered around pretty much helter-skelter. Parkes Weber calls the glomus tumor a dysplastic benignant organoid hamartoma. Recent collections of reports culled from medical writings now contain several hundred cases.

The details of the normal glomus body, first described by Suquet in 1862 and later by Hoyer in 1877, were extended by Popoff who, in 1934, gave the classical description of the normal arteriovenous glomus body and its multiple potential avenues for getting blood from the arterial to the venous side of the circulation. He noted, as had been observed before, that glomus bodies were distributed widely in the skin. Their highest frequency occurred in the palmar and plantar surfaces of the hands and feet with emphasis on the hypothenar and thenar eminence and the distal pads of the fingers as well as the skin at the base of the nails. Fewer were found on the trunk.

Extensive work on the physiology of glomus bodies, particularly their role in temperature regulation, is found in the detailed studies of Grant and his collaborators. The peculiar concentration in the palmar and plantar pads, the nail beds, and the ungual phalanx of each digit, is noteworthy in connection with palmar erythema in which these regions become prominently marked with a more or less permanent redness associated with an increase in objective and subjective warmth (46). Studies on the simple arteriovenous shunts and complex glomus bodies have brought to light facts relevant to the vascular spider (357, 358, 674). The simplest kind of shunt is direct, with a single loop between an arteriole and a venule. The structure of the connecting vessel usually changes gradually from that of an artery to that of a vein. The true glomus is a complex series of vascular spaces with several alternate routes for passage of blood from artery to vein. Its essential constituent parts include the afferent artery, the Suquet-Hoyer canal, the primary collecting vein, preglomic arterioles, and an abundance of nerves. The canal, a tortuous, bulbous, modified arteriole, empties directly into a vein. Its lumen is narrow and irregular, lined with endothelial cells in one or two layers, but without an inner elastic membrane. Muscle cells in the wall are interspersed with cuboidal cells whose nuclei are poor in chromatin. These "epithelioid" cells have poorly staining cytoplasm which gives a characteristic appearance. Non-medullated nerves are plentiful in the collagenous peripheral zone.

Remarkable changes in vasomotor reactions associated with glomus tumors have been reported by Stabins, Thornton, and Scott. Their patient noticed an increased warmth in regions where pain was produced by the tumor. They studied chiefly skin temperature and blood flow. Skin temperature after immersion of a limb in cold water returned to the control value in the "glomus tumor" side more rapidly than it did when a similar test was done on the other side. This suggests a reflex, the arc of which is not limited to the peripheral nerve field in which the sensory stimuli arise, but one involving spinal or sympathetic ganglia. The persistence of strong vasodilatation as long as eight weeks after removal of the tumor may have been caused by persistence of discomfort at the site of the operation. Vasodilatation may have resulted from extremely painful sensory stimulation. Thus it differs radically from the usual effect of painful stimuli in the extremities which is spasm or vasoconstriction rather than vasodilatation. Stabins and his associates suggested a possible relationship between the reflex disorders associated with glomus tumors and the painful vasodilatation in erythromelalgia.

Some osteoporosis may disturb the underlying bone; and this may have a bearing on the painful vasoneuroses such as the hand-shoulder syndrome after myocardial infarction, Sudek's atrophy, and the traumatic vasoneuroses.

Gilmer and his associates have laid great emphasis on the relationship of glomus bodies to cutaneous vibration and pressure sensation in the skin, noting particularly the failure to find the expected sensory end organs in the discrete spots at which such sensations are evoked. Gilmer noted that glomus cells were frequently grouped about coils of sweat glands in the subcutaneous stratum of the skin. He emphasized a small canal located on the venous side of the arteriovenous aneurysm with a well developed smooth muscle wall. He believed that this structure might explain the variation in the size of glomus bodies and the fact that some are straight, some tortuous, some coiled, and some tight, ball-like knots. His conclusion was that the skin contains certain structures richly supplied with nerves, surrounded by regions with fewer nerves. Biopsy specimens taken from cutaneous areas highly sensitive to pressure and vibratory stimulation contained a richer cellular, arterial and nerve supply than the specimens taken as controls from adjacent tissue less sensitive or insensitive to pressure and vibration. In several of the biopsy specimens from spots sensitive to pressure and vibration there were straight tubular canals with muscular walls which united the glomus bodies of the stratum subcutaneum with the capillary zone of the stratum papillare and its rich reticular nerve supply. These findings strengthened his postulation that arteriovenous anastomoses in the skin are in some way related to sensory perceptions and interpretations. But as he made clear, a body may serve as *a* receptor rather than *the* receptor of pressure sensations.

Guild has made very extensive studies on the glomus jugularis in the human ear. This structure has not been credited with the production of any symptoms. For some years I have been looking for evidence that glomus tumors might be responsible for many of the paroxysmal pains such as classical trigeminal neuralgia and related clinical states. The possibility that the glomus jugulare may be the site of a glomus tumor in persons with trigeminal neuralgia remains a speculation which has not yet been demonstrated on histological grounds. It would account for the known phenomena of the syndrome as would severely perverted function without a tumor.

The number of persons who have suffered tortures with glomus tumors for periods of many years without diagnosis and the easy relief which removal of the tumor brings, indicate that few physicians know about these tumors. Such patients are heaped on the diagnostic carryall "neurosis." These small lesions may be the source of tremendous trouble and of vast pain. We should not allow ourselves to be misled if we do not find the size of lesions proportionate to symptoms or complaints. Here certainly a very small lesion can produce the most exquisite and disabling pain which has even gone so far as to lead some of its victims to suicide.

2. Angiosarcoma

Among the tumors which may produce vascular metastases in the skin, angiosarcoma ranks high. In addition to such outlandish forerunners as Maffucci's syndrome, angiosarcomas may arise in multicentric foci in the arm edematous after mastectomy for cancer of the breast. Months or years after an operation which has left some residual edema of the arm, one or several purplish vascular lumps appear in the region of persistent lymphedema. These lesions are vascular, compressible and slowly erectile after compression. Satellites may spring up around a primary lesion or several may arise simultaneously, grow rapidly, and become surrounded by expanding clusters of new lesions. In contrast to Kaposi's sarcoma, the course of angiosarcoma arising in the lymphedema which follows mastectomy is acute. Without copious x-rays or a strategically placed and timed operation radical enough to expunge the widely spreading neoplasm, the patient fails rapidly and soon dies in contrast to the much slower clinical course in Kaposi's sarcoma.

The histopathology is similar to that of Kaposi's sarcoma and some students believe they are one and the same.

3. Vascular Metastases from Carcinoma

A number of cancers in various portions of the body may metastasize to the skin, giving rise to rapidly growing very vascular lesions. They may be very painful or completely painless. Often pulsations may be felt in the larger ones. Occasionally in the extremely vascular tumors pulsation may be seen. Lesions tend to occur in multitudes rather than singly. They are illustrated in black and white and infrared photographs displayed in Figure 75. The lesions vary in color from those with the surface coloration of the adjacent skin to reddish, reddish purple, cyanotic, and almost black lesions which may glisten with a shimmering highlight from the thinned out skin overlying them. Occasionally they outgrow their blood supply and become necrotic and develop infarcts. They may ulcerate and sometimes bleed.

Carcinoma telangiectaticum is described by Parkes Weber as being caused by cells from carcinoma of the breast entering blood capillaries which they partially block and dilate. This produces a curious red color of the thorax, which fades, but sometimes only partially, upon applying pressure.

4. Pulsating Metastasis from Hypernephroma

When we encounter a swelling with intrinsic expansile pulsation we assume that the underlying lesion is an aneurysm of a large

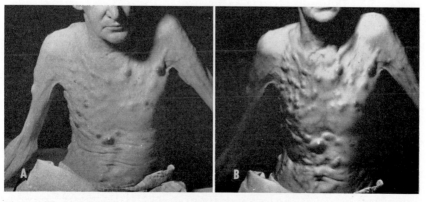

Figure 75.   Metastatic carcinoma. Black and white and infrared photographs of a patient with carcinoma of the lung with widely generalized, very vascular, metastatic lesions in the skin.

artery, or an arteriovenous aneurysm. Rarely a congenital lesion, a cirsoid aneurysm, resembling a bag of seething snakes, presents some of the same general features. Another rarer lesion which reveals itself by expansile pulsation is the metastatic deposit of a hypernephroma lodging in a bone. In recent years I have observed two patients and found the record of another with expansile pulsation in a metastatic deposit from a hypernephroma. During this period more than eighty patients with hypernephroma were seen in the hospital. None of the others had any recorded pulsation. This tumor is the commonest cause of such a sign though rarely other very vascular tumors such as angiosarcomas, either primary or metastatic, may exhibit the same pulsating swelling. Throbbing pain may occur or there may be none. Studies of the circulation may disclose a high cardiac output and rapid peripheral outflow of blood with a low diastolic pressure resembling the circulatory state in arteriovenous aneurysm or Paget's disease (232-242). X-ray therapy directed to the tumor may diminish the pulsation and relieve the pain. Most pulsating metastases from hypernephroma do not grow large enough to produce significant changes in the circulation because the patient dies before this can happen. Metastatic lesions from carcinoma of the thyroid also may pulsate, especially when lodged in bone.

5. Telangiectases in Experimental Neoplasms

Sobel and Furth, Cliffton and Wolstenholme, Furth and Boon, and Selye and Richer have described telangiectases of internal organs associated with granulosa-cell tumors and transplantable fibrosarcomas in experimental animals. Lesions in the skin were not described at autopsy or during life. The skin of experimental animals is mentioned very rarely in such papers. Vascular lesions may fade after death (46). The largest telangiectases were found in the adrenal cortex, ovary and kidney with smaller lesions in the liver and spleen (766). The vascular changes were connected intimately with the tumors, did not occur in parabiotic mates and were not found if the tumor regressed spontaneously. The nature of these changes is altogether mysterious and whether the agent or agents is viral, hormonal, or something else is a guess. It may have no relation to the eruptive telangiectasies of epidemic dropsy or any of the others discussed in this book. They are included here because of their vascular nature and obscure cause.

6. Angioreticulomatosis: Kaposi's Sarcoma

Kaposi's sarcoma is a disease of unkown etiology, and of disputed nature, with a multitude of ineffective therapies. It is a good example of a syndrome where the use of a proper name is justified. At least twenty-five different names have been used to describe it ranging from "angiomatosis Kaposi" to "perithelioma multiplex nodulosum cavernosum lymphangectoides cutaneum" which holds the current indoor record for length. The lesions in Kaposi's angioreticulomatosis are thought by some to be neoplastic; by some infectious granulomas; by some infectious granulomas with neoplastic potential; and finally others believe they represent reticuloendothelial hyperplasia. The multitude of speculations about etiology parallel the very large variety of clinical lesions in the skin. Characteristically the trouble begins with a small brown or bluish red spot. Nodules and plaques later develop. The lesions may be primarily nodules or primarily plaques or the two may be combined in any proportion. They are firm, not tender, and vary from a few millimeters to three centimeters in diameter; and from a few in number to several hundred. They may be widely separated or groups of them close together may coalesce. Telangiectases frequently are present in the skin composing the superficial aspect of the tumor. The lesion may develop in a purpuric area. Deep angiomas may occur as well. The hands and feet are usually first and most severely affected. The characteristic edema of the lower extremities is not associated with congestive heart failure. Presumably it arises because of lymph stasis though this is not certain. The disorder is far commoner in men than in women, occurs with its greatest frequency in the sixth and seventh decades, tends to be symmetrical and painless, though the lesions commonly ulcerate. Involution of the lesions occurs and causes areas of atrophy in the skin. Ordinarily there is slow progress and the patient may go on through months or years without much deterioration until towards the end of the disease. A few patients have been reported who had the disease twenty-five or thirty years or more before they died.

VI

TRAUMATIC VASCULAR LESIONS

1. Radiation Telangiectases

Possible injury of the skin is a limiting factor in standard x-ray therapy directed at the internal portions of the body. Long after the erythema is gone and often enough after the experience of irradiation is forgotten, or nearly forgotten, changes begin to occur in the skin. These are subtle at first. Unless one is looking for them, they will not be recognized by the patient or the physician. Tiny little red streaks, irregularly disposed, appear in the skin. They are confined strictly to the area of the port through which radiation was given. Pressure on such streaks produces complete blanching. With release there is fairly rapid filling. As time goes on this lacework of angiomatous marks may increase until the red portion becomes dominant, occupying most of the region. A capillary microscope or magnification of twenty times reveals such marks to be dilated, coiled and distorted vascular spaces. In gross outline frequently they appear as deformed blunt sausage- or balloon-shaped vessels. Spontaneous bleeding is rare, but a scratch in such regions bleeds much longer than one in adjacent normal skin. There is some atrophy of the skin associated with the telangiectasia. The remarkable pattern of distribution conforming precisely to the pattern of impingement of x-rays on the skin is the most striking feature and serves to identify the mark and tell its tale of previous radiation therapy (Figure 76).

This is a clearcut example of a specific injury of the skin giving rise to vascular lesions. They come always after a latent period measured in months and years rather than days or weeks. The long latency is important in demonstrating that the cause or causes of vascular lesions in the skin may have disappeared long before the lesions appear. This greatly complicates the pursuit of elusive clues. It is not known to what extent the development of cutaneous neoplasms may be related to the telangiectatic disorganization of blood vessels, nor do we know the mechanism whereby this dis-organization is produced. Figure 76 shows a lesion over the lower abdomen in a woman who had received irradiation of the uterus for carcinoma three years previously.

2. Capillary Telangiectases in Tar Workers

Among men who work in the distillation of tar, Fisher has observed many with a large number of capillary telangiectases, far more than found ordinarily in persons not so exposed. The lesions are concentrated in the parts of the skin exposed to tar. The lesions are simply little patches of dilated blood vessels in the skin. The face, neck, hands and forearms have most of the lesions. The only unexposed region where they sometimes occur is the scrotum where the angioma may be an ordinary Fordyce lesion. They do not occur in the palms. In a subject accustomed to stripping to the waist and getting spattered repeatedly with tar, the telangiectases were extensive over the forearms, upper arms, neck and chest. The incidence of capillary telangiectases rose from about 10 per cent to 100 per cent as the length of exposure in years increased. A similar trend was apparent in chronic erythema, hyperkeratoses and freckles. Presumably aging and exposure to tar were the important

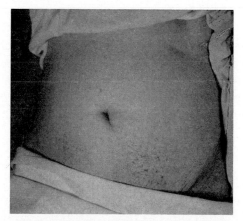

Figure 76.   Radiation telangiectases.   Scattered irregular red spots localized on the right and left sides of the lower abdomen precisely in areas where the x-ray ports had been beamed for irradiation of cancer of the cervex several years before.

elements in leading to the change, but there were no figures of an exactly comparable group not exposed to tar. There was nothing to indicate from the observations that such lesions were precursors of carcinoma though this point can be determined only by subsequent studies. Biopsies are not available. In a photograph kindly sent by Dr. Fisher an anemic halo is seen around several lesions.

3. Telangiectases in Progressive Systemic Sclerosis: Scleroderma

The nature of the disorder called progressive systemic sclerosis, acrosclerosis, or scleroderma and its relation to collagen diseases are not established. Vasomotor, trophic and ulcerative changes predominate in the early stages. Ultimately destructive processes may affect most tissues of the body. It is quite common in scleroderma to encounter multiple telangiectases usually on the face, sometimes the extremities and occasionally on the mucous surfaces. Naegeli has emphasized a prodrome with urticaria, erythema, diffuse pigmentation and eruptive telangiectases, noting the usual localization on the face, neck, and upper part of the chest. Single or multiple telangiectases appear in fast succession often anticipated by febrile episodes. The telangiectases occur in spot-forming patterns, not as diffuse erythematous foci. Sometimes typical spider forms appear but more often there are discrete telangiectatic mats without a large central vessel. Marked dilatation of vessels of the subpapillary venous plexus is noted. There is fragmentation of the elastic membrane and infiltration of round cells and plasma cells. A lumen may be occluded by proliferation of the intima and later undergo fibrinoid degeneration. Some of the telangiectases fade as the disease advances.

4. Telangiectases in Raynaud's Disease

Verel has given a good resume of the problem of telangiectasia in Raynaud's disease and has described his own experience with nine women all of whom had had Raynaud's disease for at least ten years and some for as long as thirty or thirty-five years. He described a variety of telangiectases most of which were capillary dilatations sometimes involving the venules also. He made a number of drawings from observations with the dissecting microscope. He found the lesions constantly present on the lips, less regularly on the forehead, nose, cheeks, hands, and forearms. He did not mention the ears. One patient who had Raynaud's disease for "many years" had lesions on the lips alone. From his photograph of the mouth I suspect that at least some of these may be venous lakes. The nature of others is certainly different though they are obviously dilated small vessels.

I have observed a number of patients with Raynaud's disease who have a variety of angiomas and telangiectases but I have also followed other patients with Raynaud's disease or the Raynaud's phenomenon for periods of more than ten years who have not had such lesions. Their nature, therefore, remains indeterminate. They should be studied further to obtain the necessary information to catalog them appropriately if, indeed, Raynaud's disease is in any way a specific factor in their occurrence. If it is we may suppose that the body injures itself by intermittent ischemia and asphyxia, damaging vessels so that at length telangiectases result.

5. Pigment of the Skin Over Veins

Bass has reported examples of pigment over the veins in a forty-year-old negro millhand who had pellagra. I have seen one example of this phenomena in the same disease. Bass described his patient thus: "While looking at the lesions on the hands and arms, we noticed peculiar dark pigmented streaks running across the backs of the forearms. They are quite distinct and on further investigation we find they are situated over the course of the large veins in this part of the arm. By constricting the arm and distending the veins, we note this quite striking pigmentation over the course of all the large veins in this part of the arm." Bass' explanation was that in the lumber yard the man frequently rubbed his arms against his soiled clothes, especially when he was carrying lumber while the veins were inflated with blood. It is not surprising that there was enough irritation and trauma to produce the pigmentation. The veins on the dorsum were not affected but only those on the volar aspects of the arms as indicated in his photograph. In the pellagrin

I saw there was no recognized background of irritation. Recently I observed another person with heavy streaks of pigment over the veins of the forearm. The following case report describes this condition in someone who did not have pellagra through his nutrition was below normal.

Case Report

A 51-year-old painter had had Hodgkin's disease for two years when admitted to the University Hospitals. He had had five courses of nitrogen mustard resulting in some thrombosis of veins in the antecubital fossa of each arm. At the time of his admission, he had a hemoglobin of 5 grams. The anemia had not improved despite many transfusions. He had much enlargement of the spleen but there was no lymphadenopathy. Venous pressure in the arms and hands was normal by clinical estimation. The striking feature of the physical examination was the deep pigmentation of the veins of both arms from the wrists two-thirds of the way up to the elbows. There had been no recent exposure to sunlight though presumably the venous pressure had been high following the sclerosing of the veins.

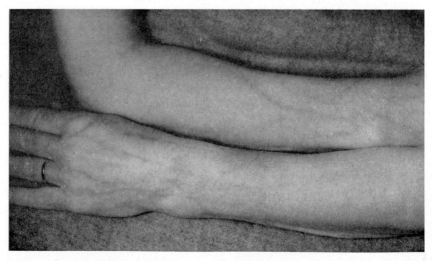

Figure 77.   Pigment over veins. The dorsum of the hands in a patient with advanced Hodgkin's disease showing linear streaks of pigment over veins.

Figure 77 includes several of the larger veins in the forearm with pigmentation of the skin over much of their course. Since the skin on both dorsal and ventral surfaces of the arms was pigmented equally, suntanning seems an unlikely mechanism. Under certain circumstances the temperature of the skin just above superficial veins is one or more degrees Centigrade warmer than the skin of adjoining areas (46). Presumably this small increase in heat might enhance pigmentation if there was a special tendency to pigmentation. If this postulation is correct, this rather rare pigment over veins bears some analogy to the pigmentation of firestains. This seems a somewhat better speculation than the notion that pressure and irritation are causes though both might have some influence.

6. Traumatic Asphyxia or the Ecchymotic Mask

Observant hangmen of olden days and even of today occasionally notice that hanging may produce an enduring lividity of the faces of their victims. Traumatic asphyxia or the ecchymotic mask was a well-recognized and understood phenomenon though it has not figured largely in descriptions of hanging. Today the ecchymotic mask is more apt to be found in people who have been caught between compressing surfaces as when a truck backs someone against a wall, or a large box or barrel wedges one against a resisting surface. What occurs, in effect, is that the Valsalva maneuver and the Rumple-Leede test have been combined. A sudden great pressure on the chest and the abdomen, transmitted to the veins produces hemorrhage which may affect the face and neck generally. Rarely is it significant on the chest, arms, or shoulders, perhaps because the valves are more effective so that the pressure elevation is less intense. The entire face may be livid as it is occupied by a giant purpuric spot or ecchymosis. There is likely to be subconjunctival bleeding; sometimes there is retinal hemorrhage. A much lesser degree of the same phenomenon may occur in whooping cough where subconjunctival hemorrhage is not a rarity. Any sudden straining or coughing may induce small conjunctival hemorrhages. The person with traumatic asphyxia may bleed into the brain or subarachnoid space, though in such instances there may be direct injury to the head. If there is no injury or hemorrhage in the brain the condition is self-correcting. Within two or three weeks the changes in blood pigment have occurred and the lesion vanishes without a trace.

VII

VASCULAR LESIONS WHICH INCREASE
WITH AGING

1. Introductory Comments

A vexatious aspect of the problems of aging has to do with definitions. There is no generally accepted definition of what aging is. Does aging mean more than the passage of time, something like the mere turning of pages of a calendar? Is it an intrinsic deterioration which is inherent in the germ plasm and protoplasm? Or is it the cumulative buffets and injuries of known and unknown kind which increase as time goes on. Most of us tend to look upon aging as a process somewhere in the future. People are old who are a few years older than we are; those are young who are a few years younger. This sliding scale of subjectivity lets the real problem evade us.

The subject of aging has been treated variously by writers and philosophers from Cicero to Ponce de Leon, from Seneca to Browning. Our present preoccupation with gerontology in an aging society casts oblique Darwinian light on those who, growing old, pontificate upon growing old. Gray hair, wrinkles, presbyopia, the menopause, prostatic difficulties, loss of muscle tone, obesity, the burden of disease in later decades and increasing conservatism all have caught our attention. We are troubled in our speculation about disease by the lack of detailed clinical information about aging. Even now it gets only reluctant attention.

It is not possible to say what aging is without a prior definition of *life* and the process of *time*. Should we look at it in the Newtonian sense of an absolute or in the Einsteinian sense as a relative aspect of existence. In short, is aging merely the running down of a wound up clock with doom foreordained? It had only so much time to run and stops like grandfather's clock at a given point. This is the Calvinistic view. Or is aging rather the same process of running down in a clock which is buffeted about and thus does not run as long as its unbuffeted control? We cannot say whether aging can be slowed and prolonged, or perhaps even forestalled. I have spent much time in recent years collecting information about a variety of vascular lesions in the skin which I have been obliged to notice because of my interest in spiders. The vascular lesions which I am considering are mostly well known. Some are undescribed or are little known. Few have been studied systematically. Cherry angiomas are known best though they too have been misunderstood and have been the source of much confusion to the casual observer.

Looked at in a relative way, are the differences between congenital vascular lesions, those of early youth, those of the middle years and those of old age merely the result of the speed with which aging occurs? Is there acceleration of a process which usually goes more slowly? Or are the mechanisms causing the vascular lesions which increase with increasing age of a different nature altogether? The answer will not be found in the following pages, but there are enough observations to provide food for speculation.

2. Cherry Angiomas

Errors in our comprehension of the meaning of vascular lesions of the skin are those of omission, commission, or both. A lesion, unrecognized, does not help us treat a patient though it could provide a diagnostic clue. Even when such a lesion can bring no helpful hint in diagnosis or prognosis, knowledge that it is innocuous may allay fears of some mysterious imagined disease. Actively harmful is the error of attributing to such a lesion or mark significance it does not have, for here lives are warped by adding sorrows without need.

There are few more striking examples of the misuse of observation and generalization than those which mark the medical history of the meager little lesion variously called senile angioma, capillary angioma, capillary angiectasis, papillary telangiectasis, ruby spot, cherry angioma, or de Morgan spot (64). I have described this tale as a collectors item among examples of the melancholy longevity of error. The story goes like this. About eighty-five years ago, Campbell de Morgan wrote a treatise on cancer. In it he called attention to angiomas in the skin in victims of cancer. This was seized upon as an infallible sign of cancer. It is hard to tell how much de Morgan should be blamed for this since his writings are not explicit on the matter. Much more significance seems to have been read into his words than he actually wrote. What he said and taught we do not know.

Anyhow, out of the jumbled chaos of mother's marks, envies and witch's marks, the cherry angioma emerged as a readily identified lesion to which de Morgan's name became attached. We cannot even guess whether the cherry angioma was used by our remote and recent forefathers as an infallible stigma of witchhood. Any mole or wen must have been enough "verification" for a diagnosis already established by passionate belief. I have been able to find no description of witch's marks clear enough to know what they may have been. William Harvey's testimony bespeaks vague definitions. No doubt any blemish would do. It is a somber reflection on the frailty of human intellect to see how readily, on authority rather than on evidence, ruby spots were accepted as a specific sign of cancer. The mental jump from witch to cancer is indeed a short one.

In the dying years of the last century, this error, which was slowly burning out into the ashes of oblivion, was revived by some German clinicians. We do not know whether unacknowledged borrowing or a perverse capacity to repeat errors was responsible. Hollander, Israel, Freund, Lagenbeck and Lesser, in a flurry of papers, stressed the association of cherry angiomas with malignant disease. Some department heads or their too eagerly complying assistants, repeating ancient dogma, even went so far as to suggest that the regional concentration of angiomas, acting as a dermal divining rod, pointed to the site of an internal cancer—X marks the spot!

But this odd blemish on common sense in the heyday of German medical greatness, even with well bolstered authoritarian statements, did not stand unchallenged for long. Carefully selected patients, controls without cancer, were found to have just as many angiomas. There was no relation to cancer though most persons with cancer did indeed have cherry angiomas. So did most persons in the age periods when cancer frequency is high, whether they had cancer or not. In spite of this we can still find such statements as "capillary angiomas are common in persons with cancer" with the explicit or implied addition that the association is somehow specific or has diagnostic significance. An excellent study of cherry angiomas by Murison, Sutherland and Williamson was published in 1947 but I had not read it when I wrote my first paper on the subject. Their findings of a steady increase in size and number of lesions with aging, and failure to find any connection with cancer are in complete agreement with my observations. Howell and Reade made some observations on old women, including the de Morgan spot. Since they observed only women from seventy to one hundred their data do not justify their conclusions about aging, nor do their own figures and tables support their contention that there is no relationship to the aging process. Parkes Weber (891) has emphasized the banal nature of cherry angiomas and lack of any peculiar relation to cancer.

Wagner has made the most comprehensive study of cherry angiomas. He studied one thousand seven hundred and seventy persons, nine hundred and six women and eight hundred and sixty-four men. In general we agree that there is a slight lag in the appearance of these lesions in women compared with men. In my material this is obvious in the twenties and thirties and fades out later. We have some disagreement about the frequency of such lesions as time goes on to advanced old age. I have observed only four of more than a hundred persons older than seventy who did not have cherry angiomas. If, however, we attempt to measure what we might call the volume of angiomas by a calculation of the number of lesions multiplied by size there is a distinct decline, certainly after seventy, perhaps beginning near the age of sixty. The implication of such a decrescent process is that there is senile involution of lesions. This I have established by observing a secular change, a decline in size of lesions in individual persons advancing into old age, and by the detection of atrophic lesions, small, with few vessels for the size of the angioma and with some light brown pigment. A final point which I have emphasized in several publications is that the occurrence in one person of several kinds of vascular lesions, mostly telangiectatic, relates to the basic process of aging rather than indicating that one kind of lesion somehow influences the development of another or that they have some other subtle connection. They all seem to be comparable results of the processes of aging which vary because of the nature of the tissues and vessels which are affected. One biological force may produce different effects as it works on different anatomical substrates.

DISTRIBUTION OF CHERRY ANGIOMA
Adults 50-80

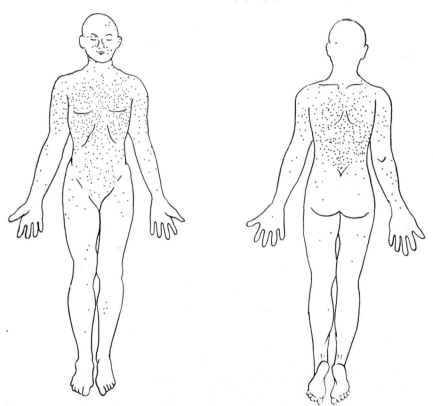

Figure 78. Cherry angioma. Distribution indicating the occurrence on the lower portion of the body and the relative rarity on the neck and face.

In a more detailed statistical analysis of the mutual association of senile angiomas, essential telangiectases, varices and gray hair, and their relationship to aging, Wagner discovered good correlations with increasing age and all four conditions. He believed that aging rather than such a diathesis as Curtius' "status varicosus" was the primary etiologic factor. The very extensive material and detailed statistical treatment leave little room to argue with his conclusions.

A. OBSERVATION

Now for the lesion. I began to notice ruby spots during early studies of arterial spiders. I wondered about them. I read much. I found few facts. Dermatologists have described them, named them with Latin names and noted some of their histological features. To get more information I was reluctantly forced to collect it myself. I have looked for these lesions systematically for the last eight years in more than two thousand patients.

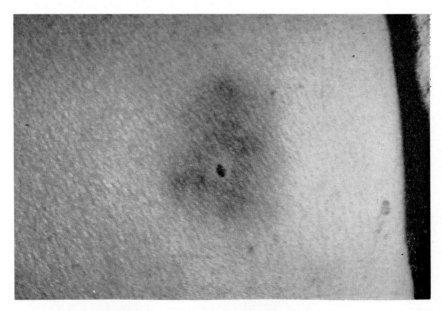

Figure 79.   Cherry angioma. Five ml. of the patient's blood had been injected under the skin.   The artficial bruise so created avoids the area of the anemic halo immediately adjacent to the lesion.

What is this much maligned lesion? You are all familiar with it, or should be. The cherry angioma is a well circumscribed, discrete ruby-red lesion in the skin (Figures 80-84). It is composed of an overgrowth of dilated vessels. Bright cherry red color is a salient characteristic. Usually cherry angiomas are roughly circular in outline but may be irregular. The larger lesions may be elevated one or a few millimeters above the surface of the skin. As they grow they rise from the level of the skin. Very large ones may expand and overhang resembling a miniature mushroom or puffball, attached by a relatively small stem. Small lesions, consisting of only one or a few capillary loops, invisible to the naked eye, can be found in most persons who have many ordinary ones. A magnifying glass reveals that the angioma is composed of numerous vascular loops,

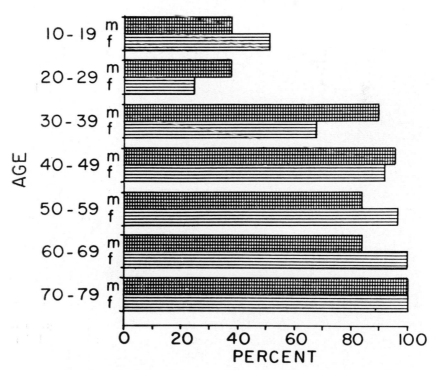

Figure 80. Cherry angioma. Age and sex distribution.

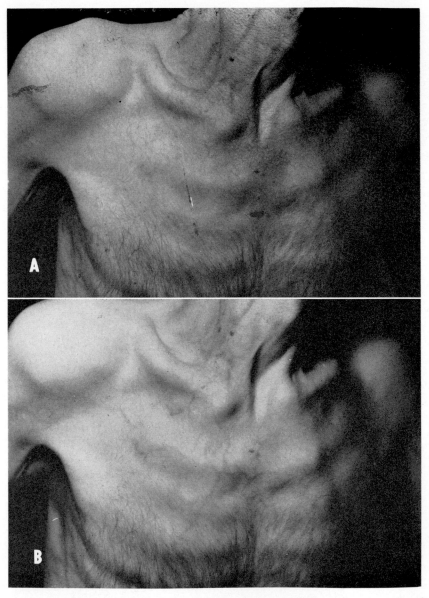

Figure 81. Cherry angioma. Black and white and infrared photograph of typical cherry angiomas arising in a birthmark (nevus flammeus). These lesions did not have an anemic halo.

discrete and easily identified at the periphery, jumbled together at the center (Figure 83). It is suggestive of looking at a huge renal glomerulous end on, or folded hands with fingers interlocked in miscellaneous confusion. Pressure on an angioma usually induces only a little blanching. After sustained squeezing it may take a minute or more for blood to return slowly and refill it. Pulsation I have not observed. The skin temperature is slightly lower over the lesion than over the adjacent skin, but the difference is negligible. The bright cherry or ruby red of the angioma differs distinctly from the fiery erythema of the arterial spider. In persons with cyanosis who have cherry angiomas the lesion may be cyanotic over much of the body though some may retain the cherry red color. In very old people and in very old lesions, there is much fading and some atrophy. The color then may be tinged with brown. Distribu-

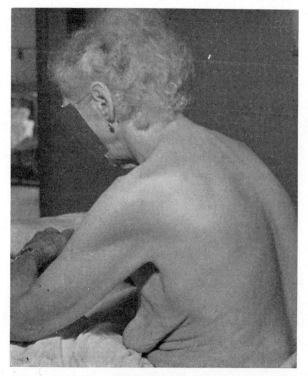

Figure 82.   Cherry angioma. The back, arm and side of an elderly woman. Lesions on the lateral portion of the upper arm have anemic halos.

tion of cherry angiomas is consistent from person to person. The highest concentration is on the trunk, then on the limbs with relatively few on the face (Figure 78). I have found none on the hands or feet. They are common over the abdomen and lower part of the back. Though they are rare in the hairy portions of the body, they have occurred in the scalp. I have observed extreme variations in number ranging from none to more than three hundred. One patient was literally covered with them; she was disfigured and had much concern about their significance. They may bleed persistently if injured. There is not much blanching after hemorrhage unless it is extreme. No connection has been found with any disease, unless aging is a disease.

One remarkable example of a woman developing two crops of eruptive cherry angiomas was related to me by Dr. Harold W. Morgan. He had in his care "a maiden lady school teacher approximately fifty-five years of age, who on two occasions in her life has developed crops of cherry angioma type lesions on the chest and face. Each time it followed surgery, the first for an appendectomy and the second for a gallbladder. Shortly after each episode the angiomas appeared and these are typical cherry type. However, on each occasion she also developed small angiomatous type lesions, not typical cherry angiomas, of the vulva. I biopsied the larger lesion which was 4 to 5 mm. in diameter, and it shows only a typical angiomatous structure with no pigment cells and no evidence of malignancy. Following the surgery some twenty years ago for appendectomy, similar lesions occurred and were cauterized. The patient gives no history of any other illnesses. There is no history of liver disease at any time during her life, and I am certain there has been no pregnancy." This is unique, and unless there be some curious relation to the eruptive angiomas of epidemic dropsy, I am aware of nothing like it.

One of the salient features of the cherry angioma is the anemic halo of pale skin immediately surrounding the lesion. It calls to mind the anemic halo which close scrutiny reveals around arterial spiders especially the small rapidly enlarging ones. Such halos are seen most readily when the skin is cooled by fanning. The reality of this halo was denied by some of my skeptical associates. In a patient with spontaneous bleeding, I found a large purpuric area surrounding an angioma; but the blood did not infiltrate into a pale island more than a centimeter in diameter around the angioma, thus elegantly demonstrating the halo which framed the lesion. We then brought art to the aid of nature by injecting 1-5 ml. of blood just below the skin surface near a number of angiomas, invariably demonstrating a halo around the angioma into which no blood would go (Figure 79). Study of serial sections of such artificial bruises has not given me a clear understanding of the anemic halo. I cannot say whether a certain spot of skin, pale and relatively avascular, is a fertile site for the angioma to grow, or whether the angioma alters its immediate environment by reducing the vascularity or changing the structure of the neighboring parts of the skin. Finding cherry spots at times in the pale central islands of skin marked with fire stains or with livedo reticularis suggests that there are special loci in skin with an affinity for the development of angiomas. A study of the smallest lesions might help clarify this point.

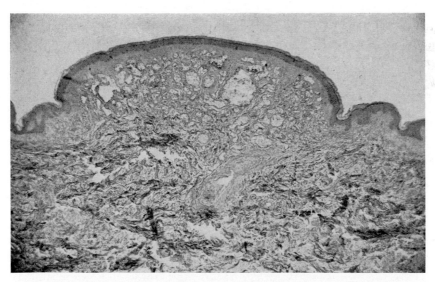

Figure 83.   Cherry angioma. Histologic section of typical lesions showing a network of intercommunicating, dilated varicose channels, vascular spaces with small thin walls and scant supporting tissue. Note how the rete pegs have been lost in the thin skin overlying the lesion.

In view of the appearance of these lesions in many persons at an early age and their relative frequency during and after adolescence, it is hardly polite to call them *senile* angiomas. The descriptive term cherry angioma or ruby spot is preferable. Since persons in later years are almost universally affected, investigation of family tendencies is futile. I have observed several kindreds where members of three generations were affected, the youngest being in the teens. In other instances they have been found in a young person but not in a parent. They are very rare before the age of puberty. Figure 80 and Table V show that the incidence rises sharply in the thirties so that approximately three-fourths of the people observed in the thirties have such lesions. Thereafter they occur with greater frequency until in the sixties and seventies they occur almost universally. As they increase in number they grow in size. The size and shape vary considerably.

Among the observations made on the cherry angioma, these may be noted:

1. The incidence rises with the intensity of the search.
2. They may occur in old scars, birthmarks, the areola of the nipple or in silver striations over the abdomen.
3. There is no relation to health, disease, or any type of disease.
4. There is no relationship to cancer or other neoplasm.
5. They increase in frequency, size and number with advancing age as do other vascular dilatations such as caviar lesions and venous stars.
6. Some atrophy occurs in advanced old age.

The need once again to exorcise the ghost of cancer illustrates the ratio between the small work of making a positive but wrong assertion and the effort needed to demonstrate its invalidity, since science can never prove a negative. Someone with authority and enthusiasm makes an uncontrolled observation, or an eager assistant makes it for him. It becomes enmeshed in what with innocent euphemism we call "the literature." It carries the mystical potency of the written word in an age when mere literacy exposes the uncritical to the hazard of believing whatever they read. No one has calculated the counter effect, the sad series of negative reports needed to bury the error. No doubt it will crop up again.

TABLE V

FIGURES IN THE FIRST FIVE COLUMNS INDICATE THE PERCENTAGE OF PERSONS BY DECADE HAVING ONE OR MORE CHERRY ANGIOMAS. THE LAST TWO COLUMNS ARE FROM PERSONAL OBSERVATION ON MORE THAN 1,000 SUBJECTS

Age	Raff	Symmers	Rosenbaum	Wagner	Beam	Average Number Per Person	Average Size mm.
0-10	0	0	—	2	0	—	—
11-20	13	5	22	11	33	2	1
21-30	19	25	52	22	31	3	1.5
31-40	45	40	86	35	75	6	1.7
41-50	54	61	94	63	93	13	2.3
51-60	60	75	91	74	90	14	3.5
61-70	65	78	100	77	91	38	3.5
71-80	75	82	100	76	100	39	3.2
80+	75	75	—	72	96	—	—

B. Conclusion

I have tried to demonstrate once more that the cherry angioma is not a latter day imprint of witches and not the hallmark of cancer which naive and too hopeful physicians have desired. As such it exemplifies the tragic longevity of error, what Trotter has called "the mysterious viability of the false." Instead, along with venous stars, venous lakes, Fordyce lesions and the caviar lesions, it is a trivial and clinically inconsequential correlate of the inexorable aging process. Its standard pattern of distribution, the strange anemic halo which indicates a close meshed state of dermal tissues, the association with aging—all must have interest for the curious and significance for the perceptive. What is Nature up to in the modest vascular anarchy of the cherry angioma? What is she trying to tell us? Are there lessons here before us every day for those to read who will? Could we but comprehend in full the meaning of this least of clinical signs who knows but that those older and too casual observers may have stumbled on a tiny sign, compact of significance, of why vessels depart from the rule of patterned conformity, and, now with restraint, now with malign wildness, leave the order of health to attain benign or fatal neoplasm. Its present significance is that it is insignificant. I hope, but hardly dare trust, that no one who reads this chapter will think he has learned of a new sign for cancer.

3. Venous Stars

Venous stare are memorable to me as the theme of my first paper before the Association of American Physicians and a passport for an excursion into mildly satirical verse. This section is taken largely from a paper published in the *Transactions of the Association of American Physicians* in 1951.

The doctrine of signatures, a philosophic concept arose in antiquity to justify some of the paradoxes of God's ways to man. This doctrine held that, having created man and then creating disease to plague him, God relented and gave signatures or signs in the fabric of man's body as clues to the nature of disease, and provided in the world about signatures of palliative or curative essences and processes. Man was supposed to see these and thus apply them to the curing or easing of disease. The fact that many of the clinical observations recorded in this book are original suggests that devotion to the signatures of the laboratory in modern days has gone on at the expense of thoughtful contemplation of signatures written for us to find in man himself, and displayed so lavishly in the skin.

Venous stars came into my field of vision when I began to find that occasionally they were mistaken for arterial spiders. A motley array of small but easily seen venous structures has been encountered. Sometimes they are strikingly similar to the arterial spider in superficial appearance. To distinguish them from spiders, I called them venous stars, thus easily shifting from entomology to astronomy. A fairly extensive survey of medical writings indicates only vague familiarity with these structures. The observations here reported are fairly systematic and now include studies done over a period of about twenty years with more intensive study during the past eight years. Even such simple recording of bedside phenomena

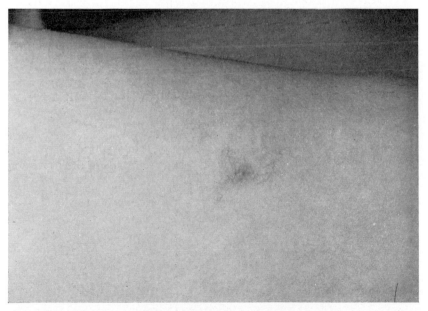

Figure 84. Venous star. Black and white photograph of a lesion situated over the confluence of two collecting veins in a woman with varicose veins. Note the small adjoining cascades.

demonstrates that a modest clinical observer can find fields left fallow by his brothers whose devotion to science is measured by increasing attention to the paraphernalia and rubrics of the laboratory rather than to the pleasant fields of natural history in clinical medicine. Occasionally the laboratory Alexander does a service by standing aside and letting a little sunlight shine, not on Diogenes, but on the patient.

The basic structure of the venous star is the ordinary small vein in the skin. It enlarges and becomes readily visible when subjected to prolonged increase in intravascular pressure. It is a correlate of stasis. Small veins of like nature have been recognized by various specialists when they occupy their special fraction of the human body. They have been called brushes, chaplets, and knots. Osler's description of a spider nevus as a collection of *veins* converging upon a "central bright red nodule projecting a little beyond the skin" suggests a venous star rather than an arterial spider (Figures 84-88). About fifty years ago, dermatologists thought that these structures and senile capillary angiomas might imply hidden

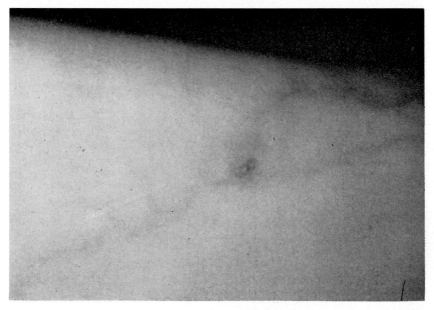

Figure 85. Venous star. Infrared photograph of the same lesion emphasizing location of the vessel at the confluence of several veins to which it is tributary.

neoplasm. Vascular surgeons and varicose vein ligators have mentioned venous stars but apparently not studied them much beyond the warning to leave them alone, an ominous warning from surgeons. Apparently no one has studied a normal control group or observed the seeming unity of such changes and their simple mechanical cause. A most elegant example of these vessels appears when obstruction to the superior vena cava detours blood back to the heart near the surface of upper parts of the trunk where small vessels of the skin are readily available for examination. The coming and going of venous stars under the influence of sudden rise and fall of venous pressure are seen best in such circumstances.

Venous stars may occur in the skin in association with elevation of venous pressure wherever it happens. They are common on the dorsum of the foot, the lower leg, both front and back, and above the knee, especially on the medial aspect of the thigh in association with varicose veins. In cirrhosis of the liver they occur, though rarely, on the belly in patients with ascites and collateral

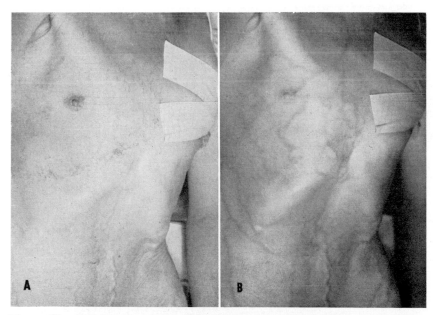

Figure 86. Venous star. Black and white infrared photographs of the chest and abdomen revealing stars directly over large collecting anastomotic veins in a patient with obstruction of the superior vena cava.

vessels. They are especially numerous in persons whose superior vena cava has become obstructed. The back of the neck may be occupied by a star. It is common, particularly in middle aged and elderly women who are somewhat obese, to find them in the small of the back overlying the region of the lower lumbar vertebrae and the upper part of the sacrum. In size the venous star may be just visible or go to make up a telangiectatic lattice work several inches in diameter. The star shape is over idealized since linear, angular, and polymorphous ones, or those arranged like a cascade, flare, rocket or a tangle may embellish an otherwise undecorated leg.

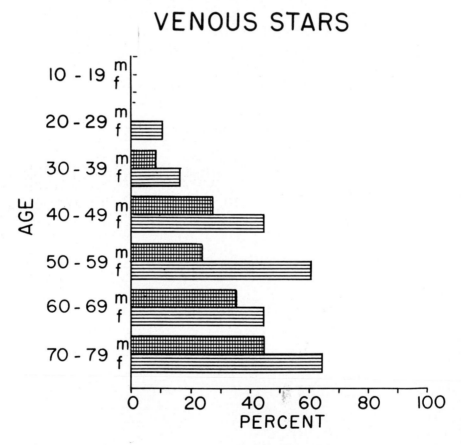

Figure 87. Venous star. Age and sex distribution. Note the preponderance of women, particularly in the fifth and sixth decades.

I have seen these lesions only in persons well past adolescence, usually in the thirties and with increasing prevalence as age increases. Pregnant women often have them in the legs even before the uterus has enlarged to oppress venous return in the pelvis. The increasing frequency with which these structures are encountered in increasing years is illustrated in Figure 87. One sees also their preponderance in women.

Many stars have intimate and direct connection with an underlying large vein to which they are tributaries. The vein may be demonstrated by infrared photography if it is not clear on inspection (Figure 85) There is a dramatic difference in the relationship of the arterial spider and the venous star to the major underlying veins, the spider being widely separated from veins, the star being directly or nearly directly on top of them, particularly at their confluence.

Digital pressure easily squeezes blood from the star. When suddenly released, the star fills from the center just as the arterial spider, the color spreading rapidly towards the periphery. This is the opposite direction from the natural course of blood in stars. The rate of refilling varies with the pressure in the column of blood in the large vein. Usually it takes longer than the spurt of blushing which recolors an arterial spider when pressure is suddenly released. If the subadjacent large vein can be obliterated by pressure above and below, the blanched star recovers its color by filling from capillary blood suffusing towards the center from the periphery at a slower rate. This centrifugal flow is the ordinary direction in which the blood moves. If the point of a pencil is pressed upon the center of a venous star the collecting radicals do not blanch much in contrast to the arterial spider which fades out with such pressure (Figure 88). Infrared photography has been used in various ways to make an attempt to discriminate between red arterial, and blue venous structures in or near the skin. With such a technique, the arterial spider suffers photographic obliteration and its tendency to occur away from large cutaneous veins is readily demonstrated. Contrary to my early expectation the sometimes dusky blue lesion of Osler's disease usually disappears in infrared photographs. In comparing colored, black-and-white, and infrared photographs, venous stars are absent from infrared photographs while appearing blue in the colored picture. Thus the infrared technique does not provide for invariable photographic differentiation between arterial and venous lesions in the skin. But it has demonstrated clearly

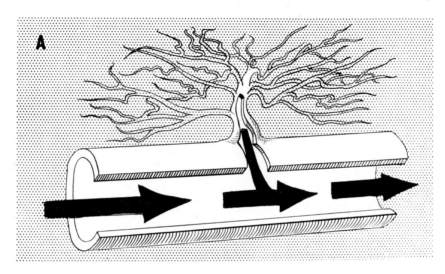

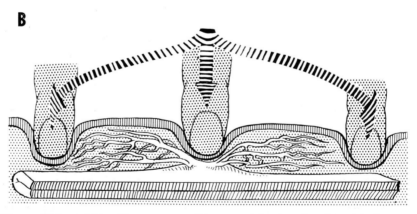

Figure 88 (a and b).   Venous stars.   Diagrammatic view showing: (a) close connection with cutaneous collecting veins and the centrifugal direction of blood flow. In the arterial spider flow is centripital; (b) complete obliteration of the vascular structure by pressure on the central vein of the star with one finger and on both sides of the underlying collecting vein with other fingers.

that the venous star has intimate connection with the large underlying veins.

Several victims of superior vena caval obstruction have provided an opportunity to observe the comings and goings of venous
stars. Two lesions were observed to double in size from 1.5 to 3.0
cm. within ten days. In another patient a star increased from bare
visibility to a diameter of 5 cm. over a nineteen day period, and

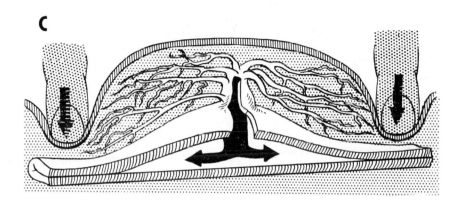

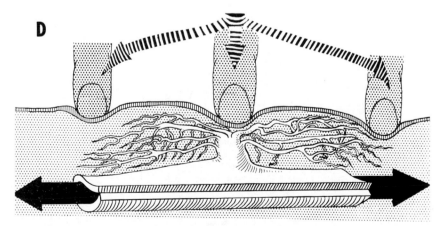

Figure 88 (c and d).   (c) Slow filling in the usual direction of capillary blood
flowing from the periphery; (d) obliteration by squeezing blood from an underlying vein with the two fingers followed by pressure with the central finger.

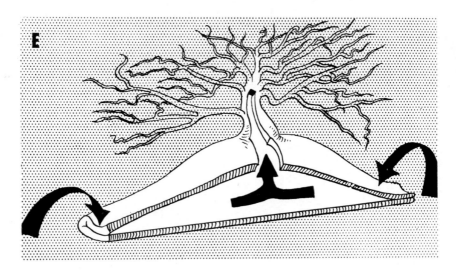

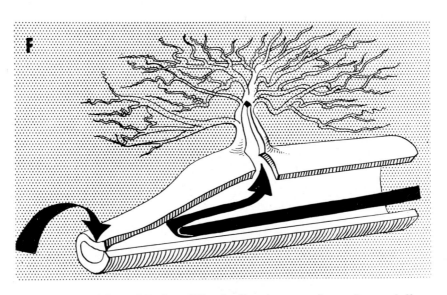

Figure 88 (e and f).   (e) Reflux filling in direction opposite to the usual direction of flow; (f) reflux filling when only one end of the collecting vein is obliterated.

another reached the size of 7 cm. during an unobserved interval of three months. In two patients whose vena caval obstruction was relieved, venous stars on the thorax disappeared within four weeks and seven weeks respectively. They may remain for at least six months if the obstruction persists and the patient survives. They do not enlarge after adequate collateral circulation has become established. I have not seen them on the upper part of the body in patients with congestive heart failure and chronic elevation of the venous pressure.

The skin temperature is no higher over a venous star than over adjacent skin. This is in contrast with arterial spider which is warmer than the adjacent skin. Stars do not pulsate or twinkle. When arterial inflow to a limb is poor, a star obliterated by manual pressure may stay blanched for many seconds, refilling slowly from capillary blood.

A. SUMMARY

Venous stars are little varicules or varicose veins in the skin. They occur when venous pressure has been elevated over a long period of time. An array of venous stars may first call attention to obstruction of the superior vena cava. Differentiation from the arterial spider sometimes presents slight difficulty but the absence of pulsation, the absence of elevated temperature, and the generally bluer color as well as the distribution on the lower extremities and in direct communication with large underlying veins suffice to differentiate them. Thus the meaning of their signature is high pressure in superficial veins, often of sudden appearance, sustained or intermittent. There is a basic unity among the miscellaneous chapulets, brushes, mats, telangiectatic networks of neck, thorax, back, and legs. They are little dilated veins.

4.   Venous Lakes

In recent years I have encountered a structure which I must have looked at many times in the past but did not see perceptively. It is a collection of venous blood off the main line of flow of the circulating blood. I have called it a venous lake. Walsh and I have described the main features of this vascular structure (76). We have not found any medical writings dealing with it though some record of such lesions may exist.

The venous lake looks like a blood blister produced when the skin is pinched or mashed. Its favorite site is the ear which only rarely is pinched or mashed, at least in older persons. The surface of the lesion may have a gray highlight. Unlike a blood blister, it is not tense with its contained blood. The surface is more or less elevated and irregular because it is composed of a network of interlocking contiguous, vascular bubbles of different sizes. This design of irregular surface and margin results from the varying degrees of

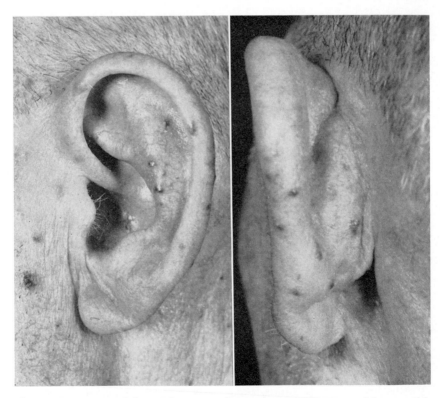

Figure 89. Venous lakes. The external ear of a sixty five year old man with many venous lakes and some dilated blood vessels. The lesions of the rim of the ear may be seen in silhouette showing very slight elevation above the skin.
Figure 90. Venous lakes. Posterior aspect of the ear of the same subject with many venous lakes.

multilocularity of the interconnecting venous spaces. The characteristics of the macroscopic structure are detailed in Figures 89 and 90.

The color is dark bluish, almost black at the center, and sometimes fading into a claret red at the edge. A faint residue of the same reddish color may be all that remains after most of the blood is expressed from the lake by steady pressure with the finger or a glass slide. The purplish blue color is given to the lesion by the large accumulation of venous blood. Purpuric spots have much the same color from their extravasated blood. Some variation in quality and depth of color occurs in different lesions, or even in parts of the same one. Unevenness in thickness of endothelium and the thin layer of overlying skin and the depth of the accumulated blood account for this variability.

There is but frail supporting tissue for this little bag of blood. Steady pressure empties the lake of blood; completely in small ones, incompletely in the larger, more complex structures. Pressure between finger and thumb readily squeezes blood from those on the ear or lip. Sustained pressure usually indents the surface, depressing it in an irregular saucer shape below the surface of the surrounding skin. Transillumination with a small flashlight reveals the gradual refilling. This is slow as would be expected in a structure containing stagnant blood. Blood may enter from vessels hidden deep in the bottom, or seep in from a network of vessels reaching the margin at the surface of the skin. Within ten to twenty seconds the crumpled surface slowly swells out again much like the gradual inflation of an empty balloon. Temperature of the surface of the lesion is the same as that of adjoining skin or at times a trifle below.

Histologic study shows the lake to have very thin walls with relatively little muscle or elastic tissue, and sometimes little more than a layer of endothelium one or two cells thick. There is scanty supporting fibrous tissue. Lakes lack elements which would enable them to contract (Figure 91). They can scarcely serve as tiny reservoirs on call for service in the regional economy of blood supply and demand. There are many connections with small veins. In some specimens small arteries apparently feed the lake. They

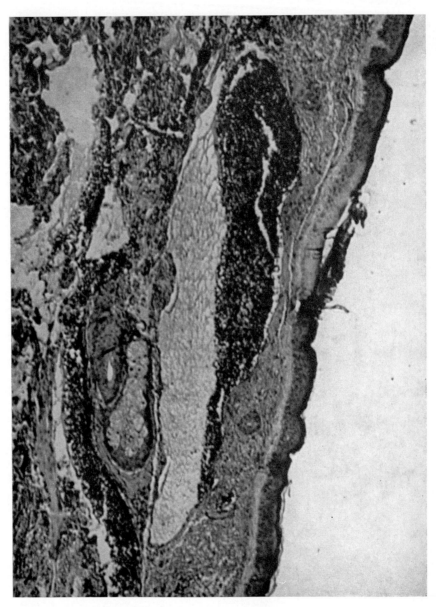

Figure 91. Venous lakes. Microscopic section revealing dilated vascular structures with thin wall, atrophy of overlying skin, and loss of the rete pegs. There is no obvious elevation of the skin as is seen during life because the wall collapsed in obtaining the biopsy specimen.

give the impression of being varicules, venous aneurysms of some magnitude, rather than overgrown or hypertrophied venous structures. Such lesions appear to begin as dilatation of veins at or near the skin surface. They expand freely above the skin surface as their size increases.

A. CLINICAL OBSERVATIONS

Some of our observations on venous lakes are detailed in Table VI. I have observed now more than two hundred persons with such lesions. The great majority were found in men, elderly or old men, although some were found in women and occasionally in younger men. I have seen none in any women under the age of fifty-five. The question we keep asking about these lesions is, do they have a purpose. Are they related to any particular kind of disease? I have observed them in healthy old men, seen for annual physical examinations, and in patients with most of the diseases common to the elderly and the old. Perhaps their neglect hitherto reflects the lack of interest of the young in our society for

TABLE VI

VENOUS LAKES

Sex:	
Men	95%
Women	5%
Average age	65
Age range	34-88
Average number of lesions	4
Number of lesions, range	1-27
Diameter of lesions	1-5 mm.
Associated diseases	No apparent relationship to any disease
Frequency in men 60 years and older	±5%
Location of venous lakes:	
Ears	50%
Face	20%
Lips	15%
Neck	10%
Miscellaneous	5%

their elders. From information available at present, I conclude
that they have significance only from their association with aging.

The fact that these little lakes may be numerous and the ears
and face liberally peppered with them (Figures 89 and 90) makes
their neglect seem even more surprising. They cause no symptoms
unless traumatized. Those on the face may be nicked in shaving.
When injured, they bleed with nasty persistence, since they are
little and have none of the self-sealing mechanism of sticky vasoconstriction available in such high perfection in the small vessels
of normal skin and of the interior of the body.

The localization is peculiar. About half are found on the
ears, in fact so many that they are entitled to be called earmarks.
The face, lips, and neck provide most of the remaining sites.
Rarely have they been noticed except above the level of the shoulders. Whether the anatomical substrate of the skin of the ears has
some peculiar structure with an affinity for such lesions or whether, as I suspect, exposure to sun, wind, and cold damages the
vessels, is only a guess. Perhaps cosmic rays or radiant energy in
other forms may be causal factors. We have no knowledge whether
such vascular structures on the surface have any counterpart inside
the body. Might such thin-walled venous lakes in the brain be an
anatomical basis for some forms of cerebral hemorrhage? Such
speculation merely indicates the scope of our ignorance.

B. SUMMARY

The venous lake is a banal vascular structure of the skin
found most often on the ears of elderly men. It differs from the
senile angioma or ruby spot, the venous star, the spider, the caviar
lesion, the telangiectasis of hereditary hemorrhagic telangiectasia
and other superficially similar marks, moles and nevi. Its gross
physical characteristics and microscopic morphology have been detailed. I have found no connection with any special disease to
which old people are liable. Knowledge of it at present adds little
to our therapeutic power except reassurance that the venous lake
seems to be an innocuous mark in elderly people and that it should
not be traumatized. Such is my present concept. As to what extent it results from the unopposable forces of the aging process,
tissue integrity dissolving with the inevitable running down of

the metabolic clock, to what extent it results from the cumulative minor trauma of exposure to physical elements, known or unrecognized, observations made so far give no final clue. My impression is that both factors are important, with the external environment playing a more important role than internal environmental factors.

5.   The Caviar Lesion Under the Tongue

In clinical medicine the tongue has been the cynosure in deficiency disease, the weathervane of fluid balance, the milestone in estimating anemia, the landmark of cyanosis, and the traditional beacon for the diagnostic efforts of our medical forefathers. Thus one would suppose the tongue to be barren of new clinical interest. Strangely enough, the lower surface of the tongue has scarcely had any attention, certainly not as much as the more readily inspected tip, dorsum, and sides. Hidden along the under surface of the tongue may be found small clusters of dilated and varicose veins which occasionally reach large size and may occupy almost the whole soft underbelly of the tongue. For many years I have paid attention to them and have collected figures on their incidence as well as taken photographs of a considerable number of them. They look grossly like BB's, buckshot, or to the more expansively imaginative, like black caviar. The lesion itself is a roughly spherical, varicose enlargement of a small vein in the collecting system of veins coursing along beneath the tongue (Figures 92-93). The caviar lesion usually occurs in one of four sites. The commonest is along the large superficial veins on the under surface of the tongue lateral to the sublingual vein. The next is in the small connecting channels which link the ranine veins to the lateral lingual veins. The next location is on the floor of the mouth near the ostia of the sublingual glands. A fourth site is the under surface of the lateral portions of the tongue. Singly, by twos, or in any combination these regions may be involved. It is rare for caviar lesions to occur on the lateral aspects or near the ostia of the ducts unless more plentiful and bigger ones exist along the main collecting system of veins. The earliest sign which one can find is a small outpouching at a branch of one of the communicating

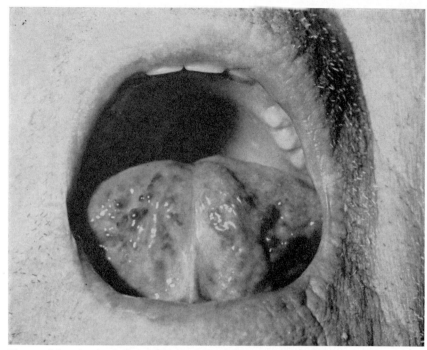

Figure 92.   Caviar lesion. There are several small buckshot sized dilated veins in the collecting veining system most prominent on the left side.

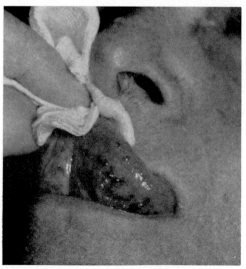

Figure 93.   Caviar lesion. This reveals strands of beads disposed laterally.

veins, but with no displacement of the overlying mucosa. Later such small varicosities become numerous. When they reach the size of an ordinary pinhead they may begin to distend the glistening mucosa.

Observations of this lesion are difficult because most patients find it almost impossible to follow instructions about elevating the tongue; and it will surprise no one that many persons cannot hold the tongue still. Grasped gently in a tenaculum, it may be manipulated with ease; but the tension introduces artifacts. If the tongue be lifted up and a glass slide pressed against the under surface, the caviar lesion disappears as the blood is squeezed into

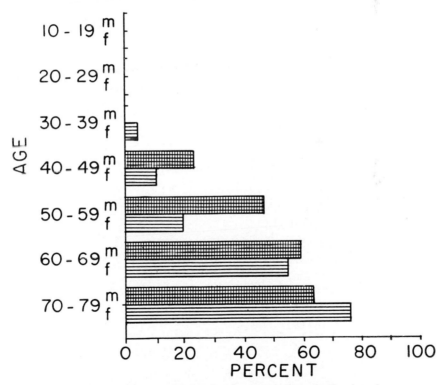

Figure 94.   Caviar lesion. Distribution by age and sex indicating the percentage of people having any lesion at all.

one of the connecting veins. As soon as the pressure is released, the varicule refills. Within a few seconds the external silhouette has resumed its natural contour. Figure 94 indicates the increasing incidence of such lesions particularly in men as age increases. Nearly half of the patients observed in their sixties and seventies were found to have one or several characteristic lesions. Such changes may be extensive with knots and clusters of caviar lesions found along both sides of the under surface of the tongue. Although very large numbers of people are affected, only about five per cent of those with lesions have large, spectacular ones.

Infrared photography has given somewhat uncertain results. Sometimes the lesions show up well and sometimes they do not.

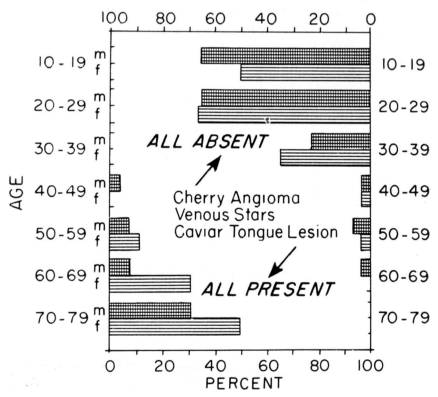

Figure 95. Vascular lesions and aging. Diagram showing the generally reciprocal relation between the incidence in younger persons who may have no lesion at all and older persons who may have all three.

The quantity and oxygen content of the blood within the vessels account for such variation. Histologic study shows simple dilatation of veins with no inflammatory changes. The endothelium especially may be hypoplastic or the wall may be fairly thick and cellular. I attribute these sublingual varicules to aging and the concomitant relaxation of tissues generally. My notes do not exclude the possibility that cough, with intermittant rises of pressure in a venous system undefended by valves, might be a contributing cause. This was suggested by da Costa and Cremer whose interesting report was called to my attention some time after my own observations were made.

A person rarely looks into a mirror and sticks out his tongue at himself and sees the caviar lesion to his great astonishment, embarrassment, or fright. At least two of my patients confessed this to be the origin of their great worry about the black lumps under the tongue. Both feared cancer. But the lesion is bland; it does not become malignant. Knowing this the physician may bring comfort and relief. No treatment is needed since the caviar lesion does not show and does not produce symptoms.

6. The Costal Fringe

In a great many persons in or past the middle years of life the lower chest wall anteriorly is marked with a pattern of branching veins irregularly disposed but usually running in the same general direction. They terminate along a line which may be straight or curved but it has no necessary relation to the skeletal or supporting structures of the rib cage, nor with the diaphragm. Careful observation and photographs with the infrared technique reveal that the border towards which a fringe drains is directly over a collecting vein. Such a vein may appear anywhere over the chest. It may even follow rib margins. There may be almost any variety of twisting, turning, and meandering of the vein (Figure 96).

Casual references contain nothing but bits of material copied from ancient text books on the basis of authority rather than evidence. Apparently Solis-Cohen first called it the costal fringe in 1894. Osler, Rollston and Parkes Weber have commented on it. Dr. Ulrich tells me that Osler used to call it the "zona corona."

There is a recurring indication of the illusion that the costal fringe
has some peculiar connection with emphysema, tuberculosis, or
congestive heart failure. Having now made observations on more
than 2,000 persons with this point in mind, I can find no connection with any underlying disease. Undeterred by observation or
deceived by bizarre recollections of anatomy, writers have even
stated that the diaphragm was somehow responsible for the distribution of the costal fringe. It has been called Franckes' stria and
by some mysterious microcosmic horoscopy has been said to indicate which lung was diseased in pulmonary tuberculosis. The
fringe is more likely to be seen in men, in the elderly, and in thin
persons. There is some association with emphysema and congestive heart failure because they too increase in incidence with ad-

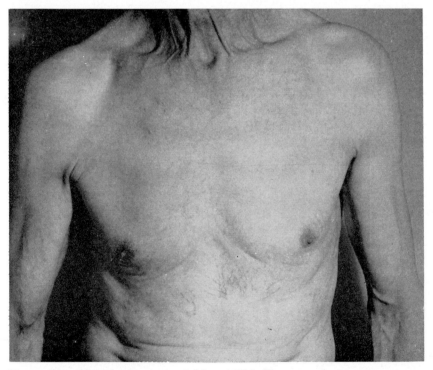

Figure 96. Zona corona or costal fringe. This illustrates the irregular scatter-
ing of vessels. Many drain into a common large collecting vein which runs at
right angles to their long axis and occupies the clear skin at the end of their
course.

vancing age but since the costal fringe may be seen without any evidence of either condition there is no reason to connect them. I have no evidence suggesting that vigorous muscular people who depend on their muscles for a livelihood have either a greater or smaller risk of developing such vascular changes. Parkes Weber thinks that a dysplastic tendency underlies the lesion.

The costal fringe is another indication that dilatation of veins is commoner with increasing age. The skin becomes thinner and thus little veins are more readily seen, but they are larger too.

7. The Cervical Fringe

Readily visible veins in hair-like whisps or linear strands which differ from the ordinary nape nevus are common at the base of the neck posteriorly. They may extend down between the shoulder blades or occur only in these regions. Rarely do they form dilatations sufficiently large or organized to be called venous stars.

A series of letters was published in the *Lancet* in 1916 concerning the significance of cervical capillary markings. Holt, Chisholm, and Hughes believed that they were diagnostic of pulmonary tuberculosis, and somehow related to disease in the lung. Indeed some also said that lesions were more plentiful on the side with tuberculosis. Parkes Weber and Riviere thought they were not pathognomonic of tuberculosis. At least half of the affected persons they had seen were healthy and normal. It was finally agreed that these markings were neither characteristic nor diagnostic of pulmonary diseases.

The relation to age is more obvious in men for I have observed a number of young women in the late teens and twenties with them though they are commoner in elderly women. In men they are rare before the fifties.

8. Capillary Telangiectases of the Face and Nose

Nasal and facial telangiectasis range in one direction toward severe acne rosacea and rhinophyma, and in the other to the fine networks of vessels seen beneath the thin almost transparent skin of the elderly. The vessels of the skin of the nose, cheeks, and face may have lesions comparable to those elsewhere in the body. It is not always easy to tell whether these vessels are venous or arterial. A series of observations has demonstrated that the great majority of them are merely dilated veins, sometimes caught and immobilized in the meshworks of connective tissue in the skin. These vascular changes of the face ordinarily signify nothing. They may occur in persons who are rarely exposed to sun, wind, rain or the elements so aging without much exposure is an adequate explanation. They are often very pronounced in persons with cirrhosis of the liver. The forces which give rise to arterial spiders and palmar erythema seem to affect facial vessels too, in many persons.

9.   Angiomas of the Scrotum: The Fordyce Lesion

Angiokeratomas or angiomas of the scrotum seem to have been unveiled for comment in the medical world for the first time by Fordyce in 1896. Many subsequent papers indicate that such lesions have confused not only their owners but sometimes physicians and dermatologists who have taken notice of them. I came across them for the first time in my intensive survey of the body for vascular spiders. I fancied that a spider of the scrotum would present a number of interesting opportunities for observations on pressure, transillumination, and the like. I found no spiders but sometimes I did find little venous angiomas, perhaps strung like pendants or beads on a strand along the little collecting veins which run approximately at right angles to the raphe on both sides of the scrotum. With all the confusion about nomenclature and the significance of angiokeratomas of the scrotum, it is well enough to call it the Fordyce lesion until there is agreement on the subject. Scrotal angiomas differ not only in location but in their natural history from the angiokeratomas of Mibelli which occur on the extensor surfaces of the extremeties in association with frostbite. Angiomas of the scrotum have no relation whatever to cold injury. Indeed the histological picture is also different as was pointed out by Wile and Belote in 1928. Excellent photographs are found in the thoughtful review of Robinson and Tashen. Head depicted a fabulous example where angiomas had reached the proportions of a caricature, festooning the scrotum in ornate draperies as if a vari-cocele had set up business on the outside.

At times there may be similar lesions on the penis and fore-skin but I have seen them only twice, both times in association with more numerous lesions on the scrotum. In only three of my seventy examples has there been any hyperkeratatic element so the term used by Parkes Weber and others confuses the lesions with Mibelli's lesions which are entirely different.

An unflattering commentary on our atrophied talent for ac-tually seeing the skin is the fact that so many reported cases of scrotal angiomas were found in patients with anal pruritus. The scrotum intruded itself upon the physician's half averted glance and the lesions were discovered. For several years I have looked at the scrotum of all the old or aging men seen in private consulta-tion, much to their amusement. Two patients, however, had been alarmed at the thought of cancer. A poignant note about one of them indicates that successful dieting induced loss of much ab-dominal corpulence, bringing the scrotum once more into pur-view. This led to the anguished discovery of the scrotum peppered with dark red marks. Still another patient, a judge, after sitting in tight pants in a movie theater on a hot day discovered when he made his dramatic exit that it was blood, not sweat, which had drenched his legs. His family doctor found that a scrotal angioma had burst. Gentle pressure stopped the hemorrhage, and put an end to an alarming and spectacular episode. Recently I saw a man whose lesions bled after a careful examination of the lesions, and another who induced bleeding by scratching.

In a total of five hundred men fifty years or older, I have observed scrotal angiomas in seventy. One man of forty-seven had them, but no other younger than fifty. Except for the three which bled, they produced no symptoms.

The lesion is rarely larger than 3-4 mm. in diameter. Usually it can be seen to arise in connection with a vein, frequently one of some prominence, and usually running at right angles to the scrotal raphe. It may be elevated in a lentil-like shape. The color is dark red, sometimes blackish. Gentle pressure evacuates the blood into the vein to which the angioma forms a sluggish varicose tributary. Rumpling of the scrotal skin by contraction of the dartos may hide an angioma in a valley or leave it exposed on an elevated fold. Transillumination may disclose the vascular connections in handsome detail (Figure 97).

I can find no evidence that the scrotal angioma constitutes anything more than another fruit of aging, associated with weakening of the walls of the little veins. These varicules should be known so that we can allay the fears of old men many of whom have worries enough already. To understand the true causes of such lesions would give us a better clue than we yet have of the significance of the aging process.

10.   Temporal Arteritis

Temporal arteritis is rare until the years of middle and later life so I have included it in the chapter on aging. In the almost inexhaustible motherlode of clinical ore which Jonathan Hutchinson stored in his *Archives of Surgery* he recorded what is probably the first published case of temporal arteritis under the heading of "Diseases of the Arteries" in a paper entitled "On a Peculiar Form of Thrombotic Arteritis of the Aged Which is Sometimes Productive of Gangrene." He described a patient as follows: "The subject of this case was an old man named Rumbold, the father of a well-remembered beadle at the London Hospital College thirty years ago. He was a tall, fine looking man, rather thin, and quite bald. He had been a gentleman's servant, having lived in the family of the Earl of Dundonald, and he had, I believe, suffered from gout. At the time that I saw him he was living with his son near to the London Hospital College. He was upwards of eighty, and almost in his dotage. I was asked to see him because, as I was told, he had red 'streaks on his head' which were painful and prevented his wearing his hat. As I have said, he was bald, and his scalp was thin. The 'red streaks' proved, on examination, to be his temporal arteries, which on both sides were found to be inflamed and swollen. The streaks extended from the temporal region almost to the middle of the scalp, and several branches of

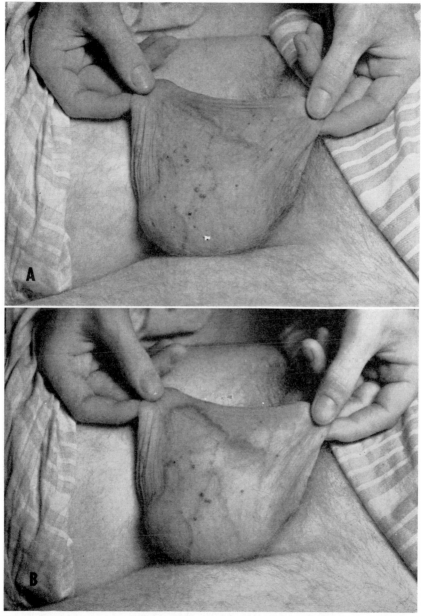

Figure 97.   The Fordyce lesion.   Black and white (A) and infrared (B) photographs of angiomas of the scrotum showing their tendency to follow the course
of the major collecting veins.

each artery could be distinctly traced. The conditions were nearly symmetrical. During the first week that he was under my observation pulsation could be feebly detected in the affected vessels, but it finally ceased; the redness then subsided, and the vessels were left impervious cords. At no time was any gangrene of the skin of the scalp threatened. The old gentleman lived, I believe, several years after this without any other manifestations of arterial disease. It was thought that the pressure of his hat on his temples had been the exciting cause of the arteritis. At any rate it was on account of the tenderness produced by the hat that he first sought advice. We appear to have in this case an unquestionable example of an arteritis which spread along the affected vessels, causing swelling of their external coats and adjacent cellular tissue with congestion of the overlying skin, and which resulted very quickly in occlusion of the vessels. It is not proved that there was any thrombosis; it is, indeed, certain that in the first stage there was not. That there was no gangrene of the skin supplied is not perhaps very surprising when we remember the other smaller sources of supply which the scalp possesses, and reflect that it probably needs a very small quantity of blood to keep it alive. Had similar changes occurred in the main arteries of one of the limbs the result might have been very different."

In 1907, Rivolta described another possible case, one overlooked by later writers. The patient was a young man of twenty-nine who had never had syphilis and was not addicted to alcohol or tobacco. He was seen in consultation because he had hurt his head in a fall from a horse. He vomited and was unconscious for ten days, and remained confined to bed for twenty-five days in all. A month after he was up and about, it was noticed that his temporal arteries were increased to the dimensions of a goose quill, and the walls were thickened and very tortuous. Even his friends noticed the changes in the temporal arteries which are very prominent in the illustrations. What is even stranger is that six months later all signs of the arterial lesions had vanished. There was no report of a subsequent follow-up.

The syndrome was established by Horton, Magath, and George Brown in 1932. Since then it has been recognized in increasing numbers of patients. It is an uncommon but by no means rare disease which usually affects older people. The term temporal arteritis is a bad one since the disease is a generalized vascular trouble. It is one of the few, however, in which cutaneous manifestations of a granulomatous inflammatory process in accessible superficial vessels permit it to be included with vascular lesions of the skin.

A. Clinical Observations

While the first manifestation may be pain in the head, usually described as merely a headache, actually the pain is in the scalp (175). The time of origin of the disease may have been forgotten in a somewhat ill-defined pattern of general malaise, loss of appetite, and loss of weight, together with aches in the muscles and joints. Headache and mental confusion may occur. Loss of vision is common and it may become established as permanent blindness (121). In fact, the occurrence of visual difficulty not otherwise explained, which progresses or does not respond to treatment, should call attention to the possibility of granulomatous arteritis. The disease usually occurs in the elderly, and women have outnumbered men in reported series. Various signs and symptoms arising from vascular lesions in the brain and central nervous system have been reported. Phlebitis of retinal veins has occurred. Occlusion of the retinal artery or its branches has been reported in several instances, but diminution of vision may be out of proportion to the retinal vascular changes. The temporal artery is thick and there is reddening of the overlying skin. Pulsation commonly is absent but may return after the inflammation subsides. Ultimately thrombosis is likely to occur. Fever of unexplained origin is sometimes the early masquerade. There is no perfect treatment although good results have been obtained with steroid hormones. Relief of pain may occur if a portion of the inflammed artery is removed.

Although blindness is not rare and the disease may actually prove fatal, in many it is self-limited, and after a period of one or two years of considerable disability patients may improve spontaneously and the clinical signs may disappear. The characteristic histopathology is that of a granulomatous arteritis in which there are numerous giant cells. Some patients with "temporal arteritis" develop arterial aneurysms because of weakening of the artery wall from the chronic inflammatory process.

VIII

ABDOMINAL AND THORACIC VENOUS STRUCTURES

1. Caput Medusae and the Cruveilhier-Baumgarten Syndrome

Almost everyone who writes about cirrhosis of the liver pays a compliment to the caput medusae. Even those who omit spiders, palmar erythema and gynecomastia dote on the caput. Perhaps some secret guilt that they no longer know any Latin gives a Freudian urge to display defunct knowledge and use Latin words, or perhaps the serpentine mysteries of some ancient mythology only vaguely remembered have distracted them. The caput is a very rare lesion and one of extreme rarity in Laennec's cirrhosis of the liver. In nearly a thousand persons with disease of the liver, I have seen three typical and two atypical examples of the caput medusae. These occurred in the Cruveilhier-Baumgarten syndrome. Most textbooks repeat with childlike amiability the erroneous notion that caput medusae is a common sign of cirrhosis of the liver. Trousseau described an obvious case of the Cruveilhier-Baumgarten syndrome. The autopsy by Sappey revealed that the hum and thrill were caused by dilated abdominal veins and not by a patent umbilical vein. No one should be confused by the caput medusae after reading the observations of Armstrong, Adams, Tragerman, and Townsend who reviewed the medical reports, distinguished between the very rare Cruveilhier-Baumgarten disease and the not so rare Cruveilhier-Baumgarten syndrome, and reported observations of their own. The essential feature of the *disease* is that at necropsy patency of the umbilical vein must be demonstrated together with atrophy but little or no fibrosis of the liver. On the other hand, the Cruveilhier-Baumgarten *syndrome* includes a miscellaneous collection of cases with signs and symptoms of portal hypertension and evidence of excessive umbilical circulation such as a venous hum and thrill. The enhanced umbilical collateral circulation which comes as a sequel to portal hypertension can result from a variety of factors. The resultant medusa head has a great many different subvarieties depending on the anatomical disposition of the umbilical circulation. A single snake or many may issue from the omphalic scalp of this ancient goddess. It is obvious that it is not possible to distinguish between the disease and the syndrome without autopsy. The clinical features of the Cruveilhier-Baumgarten syndrome include abdominal distention, digestive disturbances, hematemesis, varices of the esophagus and bleeding from them. Commonly enough, just as in certain examples of Wilson's disease, the underlying liver trouble may not be evident from history and examination; or laboratory studies may be trivial compared to the clinical findings. The principal physical signs are the venous hum, the thrill, the enlarged spleen, and the dilated anterior abdominal and thoracic veins (Figures 98 and 99). Though the liver is enlarged during life it may shrink down at autopsy since part of its enlargement comes from vascular con-

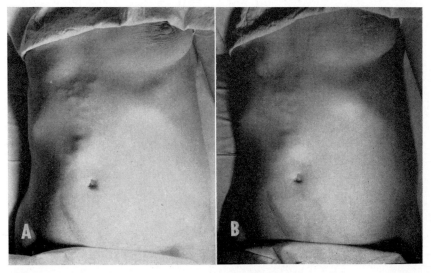

Figure 98.   Portal anastomotic vein. It courses upward toward the costal margin in a woman with advanced atrophic cirrhosis. A loud hum could be heard and a thrill felt over the large vessel. Where such a structure emerges from the umbilicus it is called a capu medusae. B. Infrared photograph.

gestion. The venous hum may be obliterated by pressure on the central vessel or one of the small legs.

Portal anastomotic veins may exist without the Cruveilheir-Baumgarten syndrome. Single vessels of large size may present

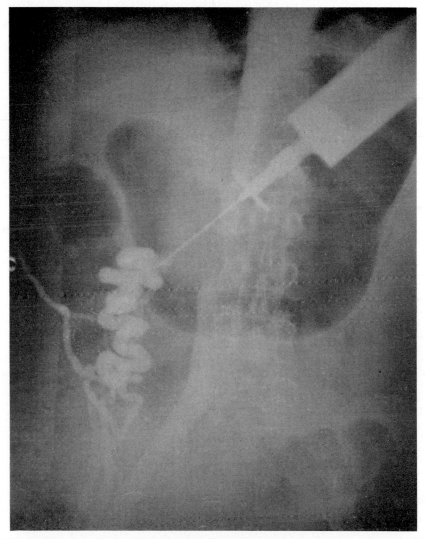

Figure 99.   Portal anastomotic vein. X-ray after injection of opaque material into the vein demonstrating its surprising course downward to make connection with the femoral vein and inferior vena cava.

themselves at various points on the abdomen, but not necessarily at the navel (Figure 100). They give an opportunity to sample portal blood and study absorption (70).

2. Vena Caval Obstruction

When the upper or lower vena cava becomes obstructed, blood must find its way back to the right atrium through collaterals which develop over the surface of the body as well as by old and new channels inside. The external vessels are visible for inspection, palpation and various tests of circulation and pressure. Several clinical patterns may be identified. The progression of signs and symptoms presents a model of the natural history of vascular lesions of the skin. Two hundred years ago William Hunter described obstruction of the superior vena cava caused by an aortic aneurysm. Obstruction of the inferior vena cava was recognized later. Despite the many collections of cases not much has been

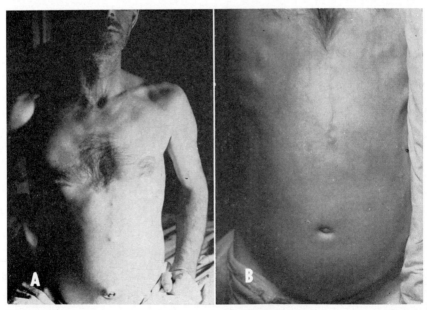

Figure 100.   Portal anastomotic vein.   The black and white photograph (A) shows how the vein stands out when the patient strains with his glottis closed; the infrared photograph (B) shows it in its natural state.

written of the sequences of change which begin as soon as the vena cava is obstructed and follow a predictable course. Studies of the altered venous circulation with accurate techniques only now are beginning to appear.

A. Superior Vena Caval Obstruction

Stokes, describing a man aged thirty-three, discussed the change which has been called Stokes' collar. "The first appearance of the disease took place about four years ago, when he found that

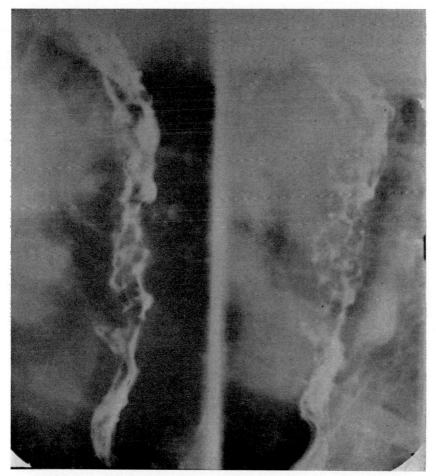

Figure 101.   Esophageal varices.   Outline following a barium swallow.

his neck was gradually enlarging. This patient was of a nervous temperament, and had been exposed to much mental annoyance. His health, too, had suffered from intense application to study. Under the influance of change of air and occupation the swelling of the neck gradually disappeared, and in about a year subsided. Thus he continued until six months since, when, after severe mental exertion both by day and night, the symptoms returned, and he began to suffer from difficulty of breathing, and a feeling of constriction in the neck. The circumference of the neck progressively increased, so that he was obliged to enlarge his shirt-collars again and again. His eyes were suffused and red, but he did not suffer from palpitation of the heart nor from dysphagia. At this time, in consequence of being informed by his medical attendants that his disease was aneurism, a great increase of nervous excitement, and consequently of the local disease, took place. When I saw him, the circumference of the neck was greatly augmented, giving something of the tippet-like appearance which is occasionally observed in aneurism of the aorta; but this was not produced by oedema. The thyroid gland was greatly enlarged, forming a flat tumour, on each side of which vast dilatations of the veins, forming elastic swellings having a sacculated appearance, could be seen. I could not find any fremitus, but the central portion of the tumour had a

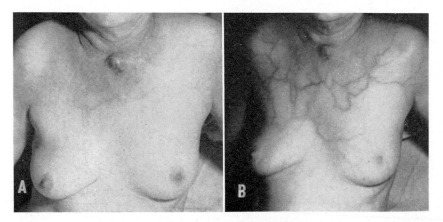

Figure 102.   Obstruction of the superior vena cava. Black and white and infra-red photographs of a woman with carcinoma of the thyroid. The veins disappear beneath the breasts and do not go down over the superficial epigastric region to join the inferior vena cava. Presumably they get blood back to the right auricle by way of the azygos vein.

diastolic pulsation, which anticipated the pulse of the radial artery by a short but distinct interval. A deep systolic murmur, loudest at the top of the sternum, and feebly heard under the clavicles, was perceptible. The heart's action was excited but regular, and no valvular murmur could be found."

When the superior vena cava is blocked, symptoms may occur before any objective sign. The first complaint is a sense of fullness in the head and suffusion of the eyes. At times a feeling of giddiness is troublesome. Rapid development of complete obstruction leads to edema of the eyelids, a sign which occurs early because of the lax support of the skin around the eyes. If the obstruction is not complete, swelling subsides promptly after assumption of the erect posture in the morning. Another complaint may be the unpleasant sensation of "red-out," a feature of the circulatory plight familiar to flyers who do an outside loop. The centrifugal force of deflection from linear motion raises the blood and spinal fluid pressures to high levels within the fixed confines of the cranium. Congestion and stasis produce a dimming of consciousness, a visual sensation of redness and the physical feeling of fullness, tension and pain. A feeling of suffocation and heaviness is another unpleasant aspect. These may all increase. Syncope follows. With partial or early occlusion of the superior vena cava, leaning, bending, or lifting may produce these same manifestations of the red-out. The victim may first suspect that something is wrong when changing tires on his car, or lifting a child.

Sometimes symptoms are meager. The first indication of trouble may be edema of the face and neck. The patient notices the swollen facies, the full neck, the collar suddenly too tight, the flushed, florid or cyanotic look described so well by Stokes. As a rule, the cyanosis, blood-shot eyes and engorgement of face and neck progress slowly. They may produce a sadly grotesque caricature of the former appearance. The edema and cyanosis may remain stationary; but if the collateral circulation develops effectively many of the signs and symptoms change. The edema recedes, the cyanosis declines or vanishes and the recurrent symptoms of red-out abate. The same improvement, without the rapid changes in skin

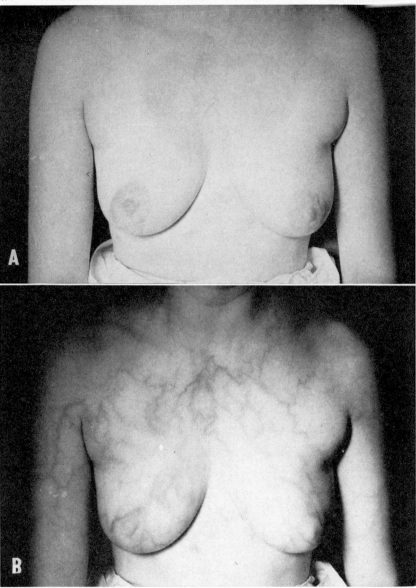

Figure 103.   Obstruction of the superior vena cava.   In the black and white
photograph the conspicuous lesion, striking on physical examination, was the
cluster of blue venous stars along the lower portion of the sternum and rib
margin near the costochondral junction.   There were superficial abdominal
veins indicating that the obstruction by large lymph nodes of Hodgkin's disease
included the azygos vein.   This required blood to make its return to the heart
by way of the inferior vena cava.

vessels, occurs when the obstruction of the superior vena cava is released surgically, or x-ray therapy reopens natural channels.

If the obstruction persists, within one to three weeks from the assumed time obstruction is complete, small blue punctate or linear vessels appear in the skin of the upper chest, rarely of the back, neck, or shoulders. These are the venous stars described in Chapter VII, Section 3. Within days to weeks, usually within two weeks, the first stars enlarge, expand in clusters and tend to extend down the chest. Thus a necklace at the level of the upper sternum may be replicated in additional festoons, clusters of blue or purple vessels, varicose, tortuous, elevated a little above the surface of the skin and attached to larger underlying veins which are establishing their new vascular detour around the roadblock. After the cluster of stars is fully established larger veins may become prominent, growing slowly, and sometimes reaching the thickness of a finger. These may come down over the chest, back and abdomen in varying profusion (Figures 102-105). If there are large internal anastomotic channels the veins over the surface may be developed only a little beyond the normal. Since most persons with vena caval obstruction have cancer or lymphoma, weight loss and lack of superficial fat enhance the accessability of the superficial veins and make it easy to observe their distribution.

Over the back one may see a few blue stars but the veins are not as prominent as they are over the front of the chest and the abdomen. They may be revealed by infrared photography where not apparent to inspection (see Chapter XII). If one is aware that they may be present, palpation often discloses veins which cannot be seen.

The course of the veins is irregular with many twists, turns and buckles. If they become a permanent fixture, as they may with a bland thrombosis of a vena cava, a few large channels finally carry the returning blood in vessels which stand out as much as two or three centimeters. They have taken over the function of the occluded vena cava. For reasons which are obscure, the collateral veins may pulsate in rare instances.

If the intrathoracic obstruction happens to occur above the entry of the azygous vein the new collateral veins do not extend over the surface with such extensive tracery as when all the blood from the upper part of the body must course down over the surface and gain entry to the inferior caval system via the femoral veins. Here the collaterals may develop only over the chest as a vascular vest or breast plate. The connection is made by way of the intercostal and internal mammary veins to the azygous vein which may become as large as the superior vena cava, carrying its load from a shunt of only moderate extent. When the superior vena cava is blocked near the right atrium, or when the azygous vein is caught up in the process all venous blood must reach the right antrim by way of the inferior vena cava. This is reached by a rope-work of veins over the abdomen which go down below Poupart's ligament or connect with the superficial branches of the inferior epigastric veins (Figure 104). A casual observer might suppose that the anastomotic channel resulted from obstruction of the inferior vena cava. It is a traditional statement that one can establish the direction of flow in superficial veins over the abdomen by stripping blood from a vein and releasing upper or lower end and estimating the speed of filling in the two directions. Since there are no effective valves in large collateral veins reflux may be about as rapid as the flow of blood going in its natural direction so this test must be made with care. It is better to establish the site of the obstruction by an analysis of the geography of the new anastomotic vessels.

In a few patients rather severe pain may occur with the development of collaterals. It is described as a dull, heavy, hard pain such as may occur when the arm vein clamps down on the cardiac catheter. Unpublished studies by Eckstein indicate that venomotor tone is increased in the upper extremity of persons with obstruction of the superior vena cava. My impression is that the venous pressure falls after the collaterals are well established. Edema usually disappears.

B. INFERIOR VENA CAVAL OBSTRUCTION

Obstruction of the inferior vena cava is much rarer than obstruction of the superior vena cava. If obstruction between the heart and the renal veins occurs rapidly survival is short. Obstruction below the renal veins may not produce signs since most lesions which can occlude the inferior vena cava near the pelvis are malig-

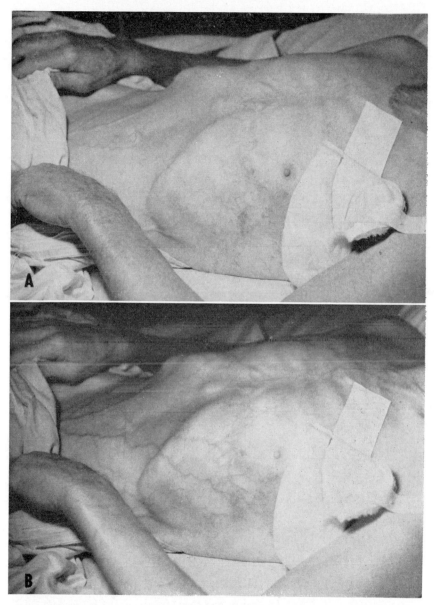

Figure 104 (a and b).   Obstruction of the superior vena cava.   (a) Black and white photograph with a sprinkling of venous stars and dilated veins; (b) the connection of the veins and the venous stars as indicated in an infrared photograph.

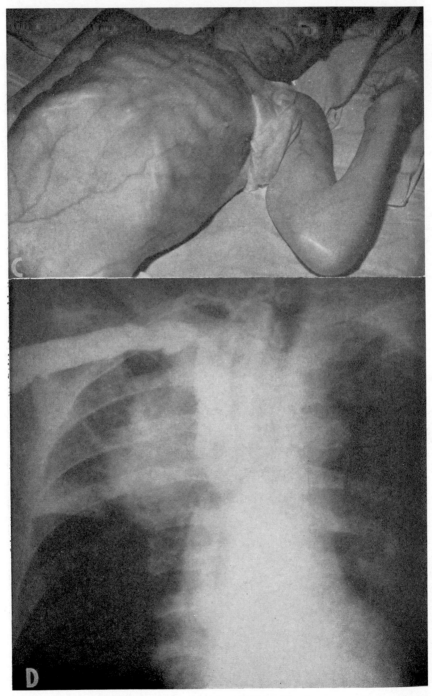

Figure 104 (c and d).   (c) The asymmetry of the collecting system in the lower abdomen and (d) an angiogram revealing obstruction of the superior vena cava near the right auricle.

nant tumors which may prove fatal before collaterals have much chance to develop. The same factors govern the emergence of superficial collaterals here as in obstruction of the superior vena cava.

One point which is emphasized in my own experience with inferior vena caval obstructions is the number of patients with a high degree of asymmetry in the pattern of lower abdominal veins (Figure 107), though this may be true in superior vena caval block too (Figure 104). Presumably when collateral channels are developing, a single one may reach a large size before the others, thus lowering the pressure and reducing or ending the stimulus to further collateral vein enlargement and formation.

The design of new veins over the abdomen varies from patient to patient. In some the large abdominal veins vanish beneath the ribs, finding connection with intercostal and internal mammary vein systems. In other patients the veins may course up over the front and back of the chest, carrying blood to the heart by way of the superior vena cava. As in obstruction of the superior vena cava it may not be possible to be sure of the direction of blood

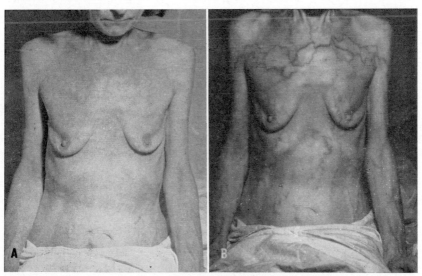

Figure 105.   Obstruction to the inferior vena cava. Black and white and infrared photographs. There are no large vessels over the shoulder. The abdominal veins do not disappear at the level of the ribs.

flow. There is no increase in veins over the shoulders or arms, though the chest may be well marked with new veins.

Edema is conspicuous in obstruction of the inferior vena cava but since congestive heart failure may have such a debut, the cause of edema may remain unidentified for some time. Eventually edema may clear up completely when collateral circulation is

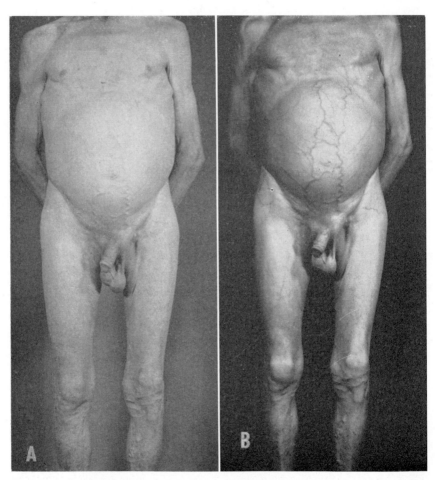

Figure 106. Functional obstruction of the inferior vena cava. Infrared and ascites. The course of the veins over the middle of the abdomen and their black and white photographs of veins in a patient with cirrhosis of the liver and connection with the femoral vein is seen in the infrared photograph.

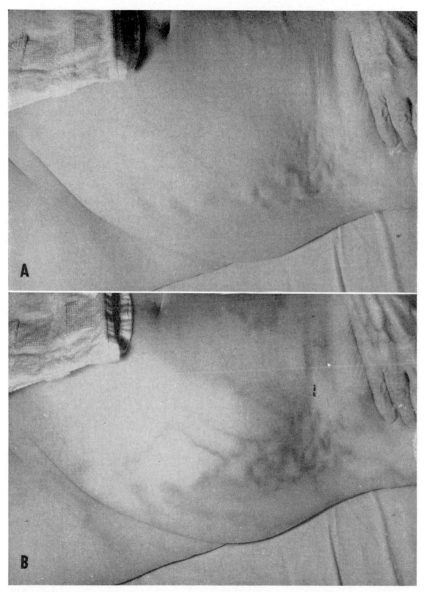

Figure 107. Obstruction of the inferior vena cava. This patient had the entire collateral circulation from both extremities carried up in superficial abdominal veins confined to the left side as seen in black and white and infrared photographs. No venous hum or thrill was found in this very vascular and readily compressible area.

established. Venous stars may be seen, but rarely in the same profusion as when the superior vena cava is obstructed.

3. Abdominal Collaterals

A. CIRRHOSIS

Most books dealing with disease of the liver and monographs on cirrhosis describe the venous networks over the belly as a manifestation of collateral circulation from the portal system. To some extent, and in some cases this is accurate, but it is only a partial explanation. I have examined many patients with cirrhosis before and after ascites appeared, or was removed and cleared, to study the abdominal veins. Therefore I have wondered whether the same force which leads to vascular proliferation of spiders might not occasionally affect the large veins too. I have no evidence one way or the other. Abdominal collaterals were not seen in persons with extrahepatic portal thrombosis.

The prominence of abdominal veins is influenced by the thickness and translucency of the skin, the amount of subcutan-

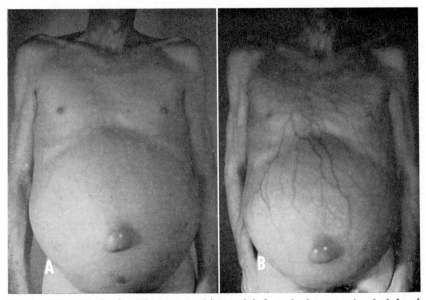

Figure 108.   Cirrhosis. Black and white and infrared photograph of abdominal veins.

eous tissue, and tension from the distended abdomen (Figures 108-109). When these are taken into account, it can be demonstrated that much of the collateral circulation over the belly results from compression and partial obstruction by ascites of the inferior vena cava and its pelvic and intraabdominal tributaries. In some cases mechanical encroachment of the liver on the vena cava is another factor. Then in many cirrhotic patients abdominal veins are prominent because of a partial inferior vena caval syndrome. I have observed three instances of well developed abdominal collaterals in patients with severe cirrhosis, plentifully decorated with spiders and liver palms, who had no evidence of or history to suggest ascites, esophageal varices or portal hypertension. They are rare.

B. PREGNANCY

Texts of obstetrics often repeat the logical belief that the prominent veins of pregnancy result from pressure by the gravid uterus upon the pelvic veins and the inferior vena cava. The same reason is given as an explanation for the varicose veins which often develop or grow worse during pregnancy. The only trouble with

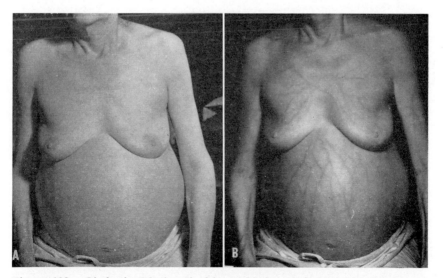

Figure 109.   Cirrhosis. Black and white and infrared photographs of collateral vessels over the abdomen.

these traditional ideas is that the varicose veins, abdominal veins and engorged veins draining the breasts may appear before any functional vena caval obstruction could occur. McCausland in 1939 suggested that progesterone might be a humoral agent responsible for the development of varicosities in pregnancy. Fried, Pulstein and Wagner have emphasized the 'angiectid' of pregnancy as a vascular structure different from the ordinary varix of the saphenous system. They suggested that it might be caused by estrogens and used the testimony I had adduced for the spider and palmar erythema as support for their thesis. The problem needs to be studied in the earliest stage of pregnancy with excretion of steroid hormones to be compared with the time of appearance or increase in new vascular formations, to see whether there are any differences between women with and without varicosities.

Piulachs and his associates have studied the peripheral circulation in pregnancy using angiograms to demonstrate the increased size and number of open arteriovenous shunts in the legs. It is their contention that the great increase in the *vis a tergo* rather than stasis accounts for the varicosities of pregnancy. Among correlary points they observed that the dilated veins were taut, warm and often associated with distal ischemia. Venous pressure was increased before mechanical obstruction could be an important factor. Many of the veins had valves. The oxygen content was much higher in the angiectid varicose veins than in veins at the elbow. These observations of open systemic arteriovenous shunts are of interest in the light of Burwell's views of the opening of arteriovenous shunts in the lungs in pregnancy.

The photographs of the changing patterns of the veins of the thorax and breast so elegantly depicted by Massopust with infrared technique display a progression of enlargement of veins already well established by the tenth week of pregnancy. They enlarge throughout pregnancy, and regress after lactation is over. There is no mechanical obstruction to the superior vena cava to account for the increase in these veins. This is the most convincing clinical fact to support a humoral rather than a mechanical cause for the increase in size and capacity of the large superficial veins in pregnant women. This still is an unproved hypothesis.

IX

A DIGRESSION ON NAILS IN LIVER DISEASE

The fingernails in cirrhosis of the liver may be perfectly normal. In many patients they are. Several abnormalities may be observed. A serious study of the fingernails in cirrhosis has been published recently by Martini and Hagemann in which they have emphasized clubbing, nails with watch glass deformity and white nails. All modern considerations of the nail and particularly of clubbing must lean heavily on the classic observations of Mendlowitz who has demonstrated that, whatever the disease process behind acquired clubbing of the nails, there is an increased flow of blood through the terminal phalanx. The gradient of pressure normally diminishing towards the periphery of the finger is lost. Lovell demonstrated hypertrophy of connective tissue between the nail and the bone in clubbing. He described two types of clubbing. One was associated with a great increase in connective tissue, occurring primarily in patients with pulmonary disease. The other was a more vascular variety associated with striking vasodilatation and increased blood supply. It was found primarily in infants with congenital cyanotic heart disease. In keeping with the increased blood flow Lovell found the caliber of digital arteries to be increased. This idea was expressed many years ago by Bier who observed more rapid growth of nails and hair with hyperemia. Likewise hair and nails grew faster in summer than in winter.

I have been keeping detailed observations of my fingernail growth for more than fifteen years. I attribute my failure to find any consistent increase with the summer and decrease in the winter to the fact that the actual climate to which I am exposed most of the hours of the day and night is not remarkably different in the two climatic extremes of the year (60).

Unilateral clubbing or clubbing confined to one finger in association with arteriovenous aneurysm and a deranged circulatory state with increased pressure on the venous side of the circulation give further evidence that increased blood flow is important in the production of clubbing. I have seen unilateral clubbing occur in association with thrombosis of the axillary vein, arterio-venous aneurysm of the upper arm, and aneurysm of the arch of the aorta without conspicuous difference in the blood pressure in the two arms. It has been described as a sequel to the accidental introduction of metalic mercury into an arm artery during blood sampling.

Fifteen years ago I described the association of clubbing of the fingers and palmar erythema and pointed out that the clubbing in cirrhosis was not necessarily confined to Hanot's cirrhosis, or to the cholangiolitic or cholangitic form of biliary cirrhosis. Mild degrees were not rare in alcoholic or Laennec's cirrhosis. Since there is an increase of blood flow in the digital vessels as well as in the red areas in palmar erythema, the basic arrangements postulated by Mendlowitz prevail. Presumably if this forced irrigation of the tissues lasts long enough, typical clubbing will occur (Figures 110 and 111). If this state is terminated, as in pregnancy, the palmar erythema recedes and the nail does not become clubbed.

The whole problem of clubbing has had new attention in the demonstration of Hansen, Flavell, and others of very prompt improvement in clubbing and osteoarthropathy, particularly the severely painful variety, almost immediately after section of the vagus nerve entering the hilum of the lung. This was dramatic in instances of inoperable carcinoma of the lung where section of a branch of the vagus produced very rapid improvement in the joint and bone pain. Flavell was of the opinion that pulmonary hypertrophic osteoarthropathy must be caused by neural reflex arising in the affected lung which could be terminated by severing the vagus even though nothing was done with the primary bronchogenic carcinoma. I have observed many times what is well known to thoracic surgeons,—that the pain of pulmonary osteoarthropathy may be relieved promptly by surgical removal of a primary tumor or metastatic tumor in the lung. During the operation the vagus is cut. A similar mechanism may explain the prompt relief of symptoms which has followed ligation of the pulmonary artery without removal of an inoperable tumor.

How these data relate to other forms of pulmonary osteoar-thropathy, notably clubbing and osteoarthropathy in cirrhosis and ulcerative colitis, and the meaning of Lovell's two varieties of clubbing are yet to be determined. I have observed one patient who developed remarkable clubbing of the fingers on the side that

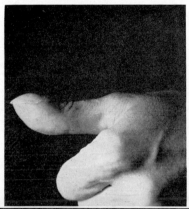

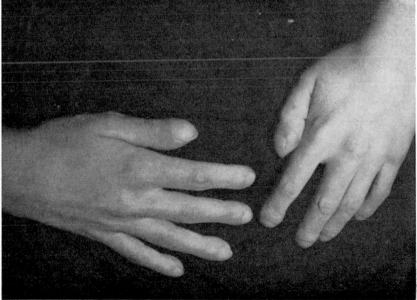

Figure 110.   Clubbing. The thumbnail in a patient with cirrhosis of the liver.
Figure 111.   Clubbing. Watch glass deformity of the nails in a patient with cirrhosis.

had undergone sympathectomy. One assumes that the normal vasomotor control of the circulation was removed and that clubbing
occurred. While we no longer believe in a precise antagonism
between sympathetic and parasympathetic nerves it is very important to consider alterations of reflex control of the distal circulation
in all circumstances in which clubbing may occur.

The relation of increased flow of blood and the growth of tissues is revealed in the clubbing and bone growth which may occur
with arteriovenous aneurysm, Maffucci's syndrome and some of
the congenital dysplastic angiectases. We know so little of the
governors which call a halt to growth when a "normal" state is
reached, which determine the exquisite symmetry of structure and
the complex mutual balances which keep the heart, lungs and vascular system in harmonious function for their small basal needs or
for extremely heavy work. In clubbing and these other examples
of tissue overgrowth with forced feeding by an increased flow of
blood we learn of one mechanism which acts as a governor of
growth. Whether this is a simple result of food and oxygen or
whether the richer abundance of growth hormone which is available, determine the result, are questions for the future.

A. White Nails

Terry observed white nails in eighty-two out of one hundred
consecutive patients with cirrhosis of the liver and described this
condition in detail. He also pointed out that it might be seen under
other circumstances and apparently in normal persons. Since I
have been on the lookout, I have found it in 8 per cent of a miscellaneous group of patients seen in the office but in only 25 per cent
of all patients with cirrhosis. In cirrhotic patients, however, it may
reach a very high degree. The whiteness of the nail is caused by a
ground glass opacity which covers the entire nail bed. If there is
doubt about the finding it may be disclosed by squeezing blood
into the distal portion of the finger. This ordinarily makes the
nail bed appear red and cyanotic. In Terry's observations the only
correlation he was able to find was that 37 per cent of patients with
spiders had grossly white nails whereas only 22 per cent of those
without spiders had white nails. He did not record any observations
on the relationship with palmar erythema. These white nails are

different from the so-called leuconychia striata and punctata in which the white streak or spot is within the nail itself. The opacity results from some change immediately subadjacent to the nail bed since the nail itself is transparent and the tip of the nail bed near the free edge of the nail is normally pink. Terry thought that perhaps this change in the nails might be a manifestation of disturbed steroid hormone function.

The white appearance of the nail is attributed by Martini to an early overgrowth of the connective tissue between the nail and the bone which reduces the amount of blood in the subpapillary plexus of this region.

X

ENTERIC BLEEDING IN PATIENTS WITH DIAGNOSTIC SKIN LESIONS

1. X-ray Telangiectases of the Bowel

Persons who have had x-ray therapy, particularly women who have had radiation for carcinoma of the cervix, may develop telangiectatic lesions in their rectal mucous membrane similar to those in the skin. Radiation telangiectases have been discussed in Chapter VI. Atrophy, stricture, polyposis and sometimes carcinoma may develop in a bowel exposed to the very large amount of x-ray or radium necessary to control the carcinoma. In a sense it is a sign that therapy has succeeded, since it usually takes long survival for telangiectases to develop. The finding of a pattern of dilated vessels of the skin at the site of former x-ray treatment is a good clue about the nature of a rare form of bleeding which then may be diagnosed by endoscopic examination of the rectum and lower colon.

2. Scurvy

Occult blood in the feces may occur in persons with scurvy who have swallowed blood which has oozed from the gums. Actual bleeding from the gut is rare in scurvy but an occasional patient with the oral, cutaneous and subcutaneous manifestations of scurvy bleeds from the bowel. Scurvy is another disease with enteric bleeding whose nature is revealed by characteristic skin lesions. Subcutaneous bleeding in scurvy follows three distinct patterns. In the most characteristic form, perifollicular hemorrhage occurs. This is seen first around the hair follicles on the lower extremities, but the same sort of lesion may appear over the belly and elsewhere. Figure 112 reveals typical small punctate perifollicular hemorrhages of scurvy. One must be careful to examine the individual lesions to detect their connection with hair follicles.

The second form of cutaneous bleeding is seen in widely spreading subcutaneous hematomas which may run the entire length of the leg or cover a large section of the abdomen or back. Their appearance is that of an extravagant bruise though no injury may have been recognized.

The third form is associated with bleeding into a joint space giving rise to a large hematoma, a painful, warm joint stretching the skin, with later discoloration as the blood pigments diffuse out into the subcutaneous tissue. It is important to recall that the gum lesion of scurvy will not occur in persons with no teeth. It is found commonly only in those with teeth who have neglected their oral hygiene, derelict owners of the charnel house mouth.

3. Mucocutaneous Melanin Pigmentation and Intestinal Polyposis

There is little to add to the analysis of gastrointestinal polyposis with mucocutaneous pigmentation given in classic form by

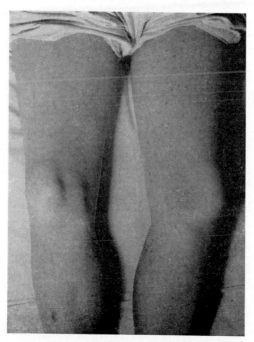

Figure 112.   Scurvy.   Appearance of perifollicular hemorrhage of the legs.

Jeghers, McKusick, and Katz, and the recent extensive review of the same topic by Dormandy. It is included for a brief word in this section because, though the cutaneous lesions are not vascular, their distribution suggests a probable vascular determination. The photographs of the young girl in Figure 113A and B show the major clinical features of this syndrome—the concurrence of melanin pigmentation in excessive freckles disposed in unusual positions, melanin pigmentation of the mucocutaneous junctions of the lips and mouth; and intestinal polyposis. The disorder is transmitted as a mendelian dominant of high penetrance. The main importance of this disorder to the physician is that the mucocutaneous lesions may give the necessary diagnostic clue in persons with unexplained anemia or bleeding from the bowel. Usually the polyps are confined to the small intestine. They are always most numerous there even if they occur in the colon also.

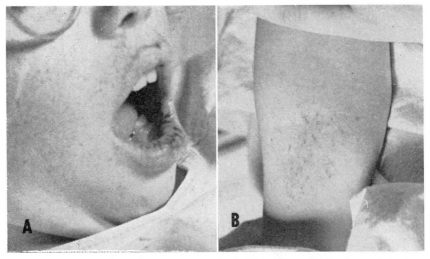

Figure 113 A.   Melanosis of skin and intestinal polyposis. Lesions of the lips and extensive freckling in a patient with bleeding from the small intestine. 113 B.   The extensive and unusual pigment in the antecubital fossa in the patient with polyposis of the small intestine and melanin.

XI

MISCELLANEOUS

1. Vascular Lipomas, Ophthalmoplegia, Steatorrhea, and Phlebectasia

W━hen one encounters an unfamiliar combination of signs and symptoms in a person he must decide whether it is a mere coincidence, an assemblage of unrelated lesions collected by chance in one person, or whether it deserves to be called a syndrome. Uniform groups of signs and symptoms which we encounter with regularity may arise in two ways. A genetic or metabolic error may produce a number of lesions affecting several different organs

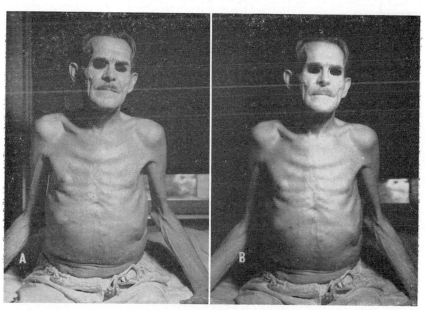

Figure 114. Vascular lipomas, opthalmoplegia, steatorrhea, and phlebectasia. Black and white and infrared photograph illustrating the distended veins, the small elevated vascular lipomas connected with veins, muscle wasting and gynecomastia.

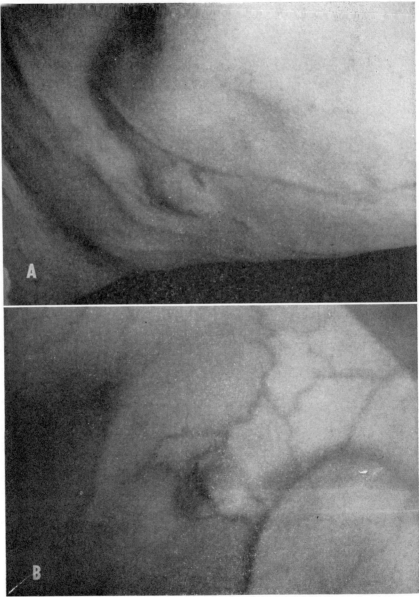

Figure 115.   Vascular lipomas, ophthalmoplegia, steatorrhea, and phlebectasia.
Black and white photograph of the anterolateral aspect of the lower abdomen
on the left showing the large veins and the subcutaneous lumps.
Figure 116.   Vascular lipomas, ophthalmoplegia, steatorrhea, and phlebectasia.
Infrared photograph of the same lesion as in Figure 115.

or systems. On the other hand, a disorder of one system or organ may affect others in turn and thus disturb function or distort tissues removed in locus or differing in primary function from those at the origin of the underlying disorder. This is not just a matter of musty academic interest or imaginative speculation. Insight into the processes of disease may come from intense scrutiny of the rare as well as the multiplication of large collections of the common-place. In this book curious and unusual disorders have been emphasized because of the light they may throw on more common-place or clinically more important conditions. I have reported a patient who had the remarkable combination of ophthalmoplegia, steatorrhea, phlebectasia, and vascular lipomas (68). The general characteristics of this condition are to be observed in Figures 114 to 117.

Case Report

A fifty-one-year-old man, a clerk, was admitted to the Medical Service of the University Hospitals, 9 July 1951 with the story that for the last twenty years he had had fluctuations in a chronic illness characterized by abdominal distension, loose and foul stools, and weakness. Many programs of therapy had been used without con-sistent benefit. The year before admission his left eyelid began to droop and he had increasing difficulty in focusing his eyes. There was diplopia on lateral gaze. His hands and feet felt numb and cold. His main difficulty was overwhelming and progressive weak-ness, so bad that he was unable to walk. Examination disclosed a man who was emaciated and pale. The right pupil was slightly smaller than the left. Both reacted to light. Convergence was im-possible. There was extreme drooping of both lids. He could elevate his gaze no higher than the horizontal (Figure 114). His tongue was slightly smooth. Very prominent veins coursed over his abdomen, chest, back, and extremities; and scattered at various points between the veins were disc- and button-like lesions which felt like lipomas or fibromas (Figures 115 and 116). Sustained pressure would flatten the elevated vascular areas partially. He had bilateral gynecomastia, a few small scattered palpable lymph nodes, wasting of the muscles, but no tenderness or fibrillation. He could not lift his legs when he was lying flat on his back. No tendon reflexes could be elicited. Although he was extremely weak, no

movement was completely absent. He retained some vibratory
sense in the hands but there was complete loss in the legs. Libido
and potency were much reduced. The hemoglobin was 8 gm. per
100 ml. Red cell count was 3.25 million per cubic mm. Leukocyte
count was 13,000 with 52 per cent segmented polymorphonuclear
leukocytes, 2 per cent eosinophils, 42 per cent lymphocytes and 4
per cent monocytes. The stools were clay colored and fatty. Gastric
juice contained free hydrochloric acid. Lumbar puncture was normal as was the spinal fluid. X-ray of the alimentary canal revealed
a "deficiency pattern" of the small bowel. There was a suggestion
of increased fibrosis in the lungs. The stool contained excessive
amounts of fat. Tests of liver function were fairly normal. There
was no response to large doses of thiamine, vitamin B-12 or other
vitamins. There was no response to several different experimental
diets. Biopsy of the partly compressible tumors revealed them to
be vascular lipomas which consisted of numerous interconnecting
vascular spaces containing red cells in areas with increased fat
(Figure 117).

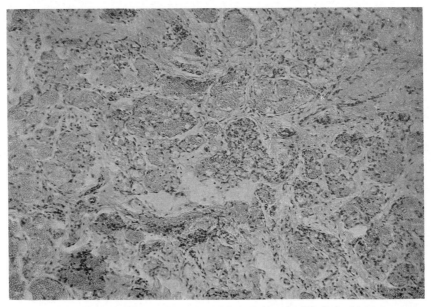

Figure 117.   Vascular lipomas, ophthalmoplegia, steatorrhea, and phlebectasia.
Microscopic section of one of the subcutaneous lesions with numerous intercommunicating vascular spaces containing red cells and areas with increased
fat.

I have been informed by Dr. Edward Shambrom that he has a case under observation with chronic lymphocytic leukemia, steatorrhea, phlebectasia, and vascular lipomas. The relationship of such lesions one to another is still obscure.

2. Pulseless Disease

While pulseless disease perhaps is paradoxical in a book on blood vessels of the skin, this curious condition, sometimes called

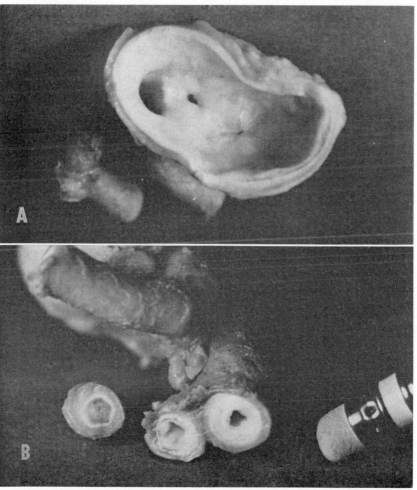

Figure 118.   Pulseless disease.   (a) the obliterative occlusion of vessels in the arch of the aorta; and, (b) the endarterial obliteration of the carotid artery.

reversed coarctation, may be associated with much collateral arterial circulation of the upper part of the body. Often this compensatory supply is inadequate to take care of the circulation to brain or muscle. The disease consists of a throttling of the large branches of the aorta going to the shoulders, arms, neck, and head. A hyperplastic occluding arteritis blocks off the vessels. The disease occurs almost exclusively in relatively young women. Ophthalmologists may be the first to discover it by finding typical retinal arteriovenous aneurysms in persons with visual difficulties. The blood for the retina has to come in by collateral arteries rather than through the central retinal artery. Atrophy of the muscles, various symptoms of cerebral disorders including syncope, mental deterioration, epileptic convulsions and paralysis, and atrophy of the brain, may result from ischemia. Syncope may occur because of the very sensitive carotid sinus reflex. Pulses in the hands, axilla, neck, temporal region, and elsewhere in the upper part of the body are not to be felt at all in fully developed examples of this disease. A picture of the lesions of the large vessels leaving the aorta is seen in Figure 118 kindly provided me by Dr. Sahs of the Department of Neurology. The microscopic picture of the typical lesion is in Figure 119.

3. Janeway's Lesion

Eponymic immortality may reflect the boasting or promotional activity of one's friends and associates or pure chance rather than important discovery or valuable contribution. Fame's fickle finger points erratically. Janeway's lesion is an excellent example of Osler's dictum that "it is strange how the memory of a man may float to posterity on what he would have himself regarded as the most trifling of his works" (45). Janeway no doubt emphasized in his teaching the lesion which bears his name. I have found only two brief references to it in his published work, almost casual asides. They are:

"Several times I have noted numerous small hemorrhages with slight nodular character in the palms of the hands and in the soles of the feet, when possibly the arms and the legs had but a scanty crop in malignant endocarditis whereas this has not been my experience in the processes likely to be mistaken for it."

"There existed a very profuse reddish eruption on the palms of the hands and the soles of the feet which was slightly nodular."

I have looked for Janeway's lesions repeatedly; and have seen but one instance in the last ten years in more than one hundred patients with bacterial endocarditis. For reasons not clear to me many of the nodes, nodules, and cutaneous lesions now are rarer

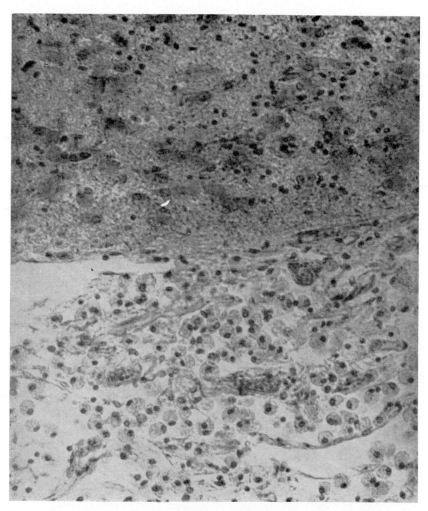

Figure 119.   Pulseless disease. Microscopic section of the proliferative inflammatory endarterial lesion in pulseless disease.

than they were in the past, or we miss them. I think that they are rarer.

The essential features of the lesion are depicted in Figure 120. The vascular alteration beneath the skin is irregularly nodular, with a reddish purple color. It may be tender, or spontaneously painful. A few days after it appears the purple color fades into brown and slowly the irregular lumpy texture is lost and the skin resumes its normal softness.

4. Tuberous Sclerosis

Tuberous sclerosis is hereditary. It is an obscure disorder of the growth of tissues affecting many portions of the body. Because of the associated mental deterioration, the disorder accounts for perhaps one in two hundred and fifty patients in mental institutions. It has been called "adenoma sebaceum," and "epiloia." As long ago as 1838, Rayer portrayed the characteristic facial eruption in color and gave it the title "végétations vasculaires." Addison and Gull described a peculiar eruption "extending across the nose and slightly affecting both cheeks. It consisted of shining tubercles, varying in size . . . to that of ordinary acne. They were of lightish color with . . . superficial capillary veins meandering over them giving them a faint rose tinge." Renal lesions, pulmonary lesions, cardiac tumors, lesions in the brain and in many other tissues occur.

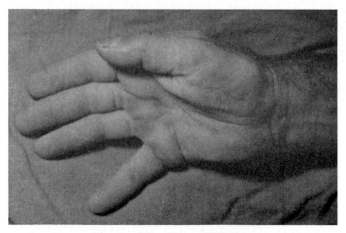

Figure 120.   Janeway's lesion.

The photograph (Figure 121) illustrates the deformities of the nails as well as the lesions of the face. Though the disease is inherited, it does not seem to be a simple mendelian dominant or if it is, penetrance is not regular since generations may be skipped. While tuberous sclerosis is not primarily a vascular lesion of the skin,

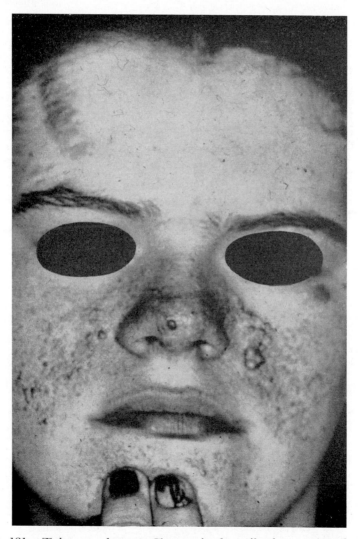

Figure 121.   Tuberous sclerosus. Changes in the nails, the vascular adenomas of the nose and face and the placque-like lesion of the forehead.

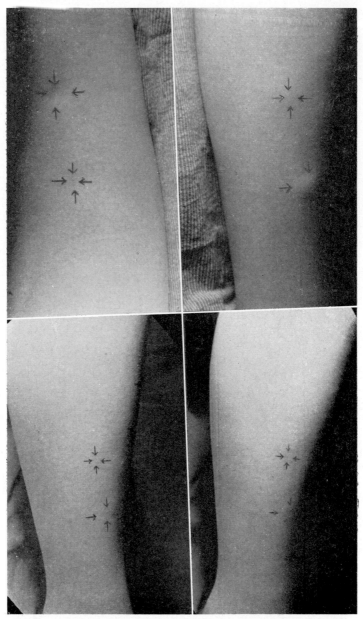

Figure 122.   Fascial hernias of the legs. The upper portion indicates the areas where the hernias appear in the skin while the patient is straining.   The lower picture shows their absence during relaxation.

there may be various angiomatous plaques as well as much vascularity of the cutaneous adenomas. It is important to recognize this symptom complex and to realize that it may explain cerebral disorganizations with epilepsy, mental deterioration, and focal neurologic signs; renal disease with ultimate renal failure; or obscure pulmonary disturbances (195).

5. Fascial Hernias

Among the small bumps which, though not vascular, may be mistaken for vascular lesions because they are easily collapsed, are small fascial hernias. They are seen to best advantage in the legs (Figure 122) though they may appear in other parts of the body. A similar phenomenon is revealed in Figure 123. They result from the transmission of pressure through a small opening in a fascial plane with superficial tissue bulging through the opening. They may occur at the site of a connection of a vein in one fascial plane with a vein in another plane. They should not be confused with valves in veins which they somewhat resemble. They may be demonstrated in the legs by doing the Valsalva maneuver but they are not produced by constricting the leg with a cuff inflated to a level between systolic and diastolic pressure. Figure 122 shows a patient with fascial hernias as they are disclosed by straining and their disappearance when straining is relieved. Figure 123 demonstrates a similar pleural fascial hernia. These lesions have taught me to listen to patients when they tell me that they can produce little bumps in the skin by holding their breath.

6. Purpura

Few contemporary textbooks describe purpuric lesions accurately, and some not at all. It is assumed that everyone knows what purpura is. In the first edition of his textbook of medicine, Osler described purpura as follows: "Purpuric spots vary from 1 to 3 to 4 mm. in diameter. When small and pinpoint like they are called petechiae; when large they are known as ecchymoses. At first bright red in color, they become darker and gradually fade to brownish stains. They do not disappear on pressure."

The difficulty of finding a good definition and description of purpura and the necessity of going back to Osler to get a satisfactory discussion illustrates the decline of interest in purely clinical phenomena. Concentration on so many other problems has displaced the attention of hematologists and clinicians from essential descriptions of minor lesions.

Humble studied the process of formation of petechial hemorrhages because he was dissatisfied with the shortcomings of histologic preparations which usually show merely an exudation of red cells, sometimes with polymorphonuclear neutrophile leukocytes around the tiny vessels in the dermis. The walls themselves appear intact. Humble used a tourniquet to increase intravascular pressure and observed the skin with a capillary microscope in patients with a variety of bleeding diseases. He found that regardless of the underlying disease the site of capillary hemorrhage was localized in the arteriolar end of the capillary loop. He postulated some selective damage to the arteriolar-capillary junction which would be exposed to the highest concentration of any known or hypothetical poison which might be giving rise to purpura.

The diagnosis of purpura is not simply a question for casual discussion. Within the last ten years I have seen twenty-nine patients who were thought to have purpura but the lesion was entirely different. Several had Osler's disease. Others had an extensive crop of tiny cherry angiomas, occasionally scattered widely throughout the skin. They might have been present for a long time but were not noticed until something caused the skin to be examined minutely. Other patients had peculiar telangiectatic lesions, dilated blood vessels, venous stars, the Fordyce lesion, venous lakes, and of course all manner of bruises. The same mistake has been encountered in Fabry's syndrome. The purpuric lesion is a hemorrhage, an extravasation of blood out of the blood vessel. It can reach macroscopic proportions very speedily. The lesion is not elevated except in rare instances. It begins with a bright red spot which quickly becomes dark. In the larger lesions especially, the dark color prevails until the slow destruction and removal of blood occur. The color changes from purple-black to green, becoming copper-yellow and fading out with a faint lemon yellow. A hand

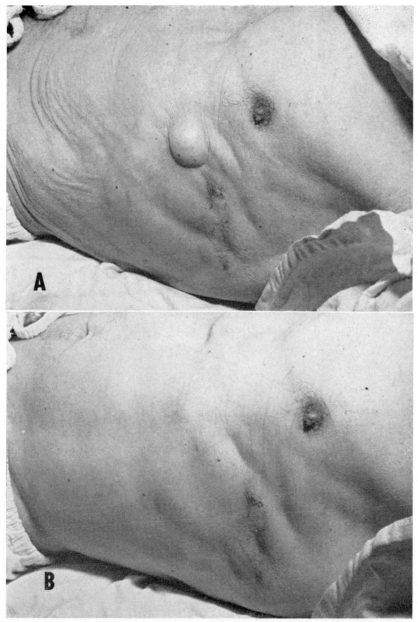

Figure 123.   Fascial hernias.   Herniation of a small portion of the lung through a defect in the intercostal muscles.   Photographed during exhalation (above), and inhalation (below).

lens should enable one to decide the nature of red specks in the skin. Pressure does not cause them to blanch. Angiomas do not undergo the sequence of color change seen in purpura. There is a tendency for purpuric specks to occur where gravitational forces make hydrostatic pressure high so that crops on the legs may occur in persons who are up and about. The splinter hemorrhage is a purpuric lesion beneath the nail. It has no obligatory connection with bacterial endocarditis, though this is a common underlying cause.

The distribution of purpuric lesions with concentration in the lower portion of the body in ambulatory patients and the well-known relationship to increased local vascular pressure in the Rumpel-Leede test stress the importance of gravitational and hydrostatic forces. Among many patients with purpura I have made detailed observations on four in whom black and white and infrared photography during and after the active phase of purpura, and subsequently the use of mild venous stasis, demonstrated that the purpuric spots usually occurred in the central pale area of the mottled skin. This was not invariable. A few perfectly classical purpuric spots occurred in the dark or reticulated regions.

1. TELANGIECTASES ASSOCIATED WITH PURPURIC LESIONS

Wissman and Tagnon have described hemangiomas and thrombocytopenic purpura in two infants and reviewed five other cases in infants. It was their belief that this was a special syndrome. There was a regular recurrence of a period of low platelet counts before the development of the telangiectases, and the simultaneous regression of the hemangiomas and thrombocytopenia. Since healing of a hemangioma usually is preceded by thrombosis within it, it may be that a normal platelet supply is needed for healing (631-633).

Parkes Weber called attention to the fact that with hypostatic forces, toxic or inflammatory conditions which cause hemorrhagic lesions by local diapedesis may also cause local dilatations by weakening the vessel walls. Majocchi described purpura annularis telangiectoides as such a lesion; and Gougerot and Blum have described a somewhat similar lesion which they call purpuric pigmented lichenoid dermatitis. These all are different from the syndrome Wissman and Tagnon described.

7. "Venous Spider"

Juniper has described "venous spiders" in a patient with chronic lymphatic leukemia. The photographs and description suggest to me that the lesions may have been cherry angiomas, some of which either because of leukemic infiltration or for other reasons, became thrombosed. The histologic picture which he gives in his Figure 3 much resembles that of a cherry angioma. There may be many somewhat nondescript lesions of this kind which defy classification in any of the now fairly numerous categories of vascular lesions of the skin. It may be that a whole array of lymphatic vessel disorders exists in addition to the few recognized tumors and dilatations of lymphatic vessels.

8. Striate Atrophy of the Skin

I do not recall seeing described in textbooks of dermatology or elsewhere a condition which I have called striate atrophy of the skin. Characteristically it occurs in older persons. I have observed

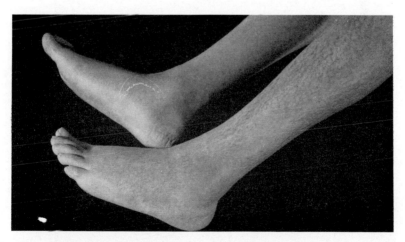

Fig. 124. Striate atrophy of the skin. Demonstration of the linear arrangement of such atrophic changes following the long axis of the extremity.

it only in those confined to a hospital. I have often wondered if it had anything to do with the simple irritations of the skin or sensitivities to linens, laundry soap, or detergents, but this point I have never established. Characteristically the skin shows innumerable linear striations which tend to be pink and are not bluish or cyanotic looking. They are common on the back of the upper arms or the lower legs but may occur in any portion of the body. They may occur in the distribution which striations have in Cushing's syndrome. Ordinarily the condition is not painful though the skin is likely to be atrophic and shiny, with a tendency to become chapped and irritated very easily. The salient features are seen in Figures 124 and 125. Histologic sections reveal something of the same kind of splitting or dissolution of the skin seen in the striae

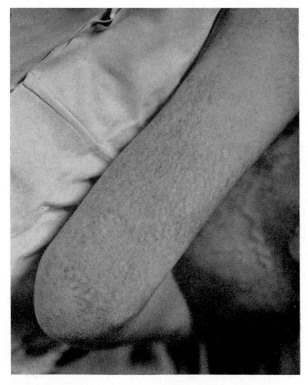

Figure 125.   Striate atrophy.   Skin of the arm and elbow.

of pregnancy. Healing of wounds may be very slow in such skin but this may result from the associated chronic disease.

9. Aneurysm

Vascular lesions of the skin ordinarily would hardly include aneurysm but the illustration in Figure 126 reveals that occasionally the cutaneous manifestations of aneurysm are not only spectacular but may give a clue as to the rate of progress of the patient toward death. Those whose clinical memories go back twenty or thirty years will recall many examples of syphilitic aortic aneurysm presenting as a pulsating tumor stretching the skin and finally rupturing in a dramatic tragedy. Fortunately such examples are rarities nowadays though one occasionally sees such a lesion in persons with untreated syphilis.

10. Telangiectasia Mascularis Eruptiva Perstans

This syndrome is described by Parkes Weber as eruption of generalized telangiectasia with permanent red macules over the trunk and extremities. Obese middle-aged women are the usual

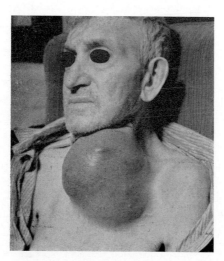

Figure 126.   Luetic aneurysm of the aorta.   It has eroded through the ribs and sternum, and presents a large pulsating mass in the anterior chest.

victims. Individual dilated blood vessels ordinarily cannot be distinguished by naked eye inspection. There is some tendency as time goes on for this disorder to undergo spontaneous remission in contradistinction to congenital generalized telangiectasia which remains static or progresses rather than involutes. Parkes Weber gives a number of other titles which have been used by different dermatologists presumably dealing with this one disorder. The grouping of mast cells around the blood vessels may relate the lesions specifically to a telangiectatic variety of urticaria pigmentosa.

11. Periocular Hyperpigmentation:

The "Masque Biliáre"

The association of dyschromia or pigment anomalies with general systemic conditions is neglected by clinicians. Aldercreutz has discussed dark skin around the eyes in relationship to biliary and genito-urinary disease. Though there was some variability in his data he found hyperpigmentation around the eyes mainly amongst women who had pyelonephritis. Many of them had gynecological diseases also. An almost equal number had biliary dyskinesia or stones and inflammation of the gall bladder. Men were much less commonly affected than women. It was Aldercreutz's impression that chronic infection was the important antecedent in this situation.

While the clinical designation masque biliáre is too specific, there is no doubt that the sign is real. By some curious quirk of fashion such a phenomenon is thought by some women to be alluring, indeed seductive, and art aids nature, producing this surprising replica of a sign which has uncertain connection with disease. Even its relation to bilious and pyelonephritic old women is unsettled.

XII

SPECIAL STUDIES AND OBSERVATIONS

1. The Anemic Halo

The anemic halo is a roughly circular pale region which may surround an agioma, telangiectasis, or purpuric spot in the skin. Excellent examples of the anemic halo may be seen around arterial spiders. In several pregnant patients and in others with progressing cirrhosis of the liver, I have observed pale spots appearing in the skin. This pattern could be provoked or accentuated by exposing the skin to a breeze from an ordinary electric fan or having the patient partially unclad in a cold room. Obstructing the outflow of venous blood may reveal red and white spots on a background of cyanosis but I am not sure that the two patterns are the same or depend on the same mechanism. When spiders make their first appearance, the earliest indication is a small red spot which usually but not invariably appears at the center of one of the pale islands (Figures 23, 24, 25). Pulsation may be demonstrated from the very first. In a few observations I have found that the pressure is 10-30 mm. Hg. lower than in the full-sized spider. In one or more days, small legs appear to grow out from the central punctum; the enveloping erythema appears and the pale margin moves peripherally so that when a spider is two cm. in diameter it is occupying and has extended beyond the locus of the original anemic halo. This leads me to believe that the "lifesaver" frame or anemic halo initially represents an anatomical or physiological arrangement of normal skin vessels. The pale perimeter around larger spiders must be different since it no longer occupies the same area. Martini has suggested that the peripheral arteriovenous shunt he has found beyond the margin situated somewhat more deeply than the spider may drain the edges. Unless they are scattered strategically all around the circumference it is difficult for me to understand how they could produce pallor in a ring if there is only one eccentrically placed and beyond the margin.

The occurrence of cherry angiomas in pale spots and the small well-developed anemic halo around them brings up the question of whether it is the same phenomenon with spiders. Does the cherry angioma grow in a particular area in which the blood flow is so disposed that there is increased vasoconstriction of the subpapillary venous plexus around it or does the blood flow to the adjacent skin become altered after the cherry angioma appears? In patients with cherry angiomas, I have injected a few ml. of blood from an antecubital vein into the skin beneath the angioma. Invariably this revealed the anemic halo. The blood so injected did not permeate the tissues just under the skin in the region around the cherry angioma. Thus what many of my colleagues had called a figment of my imagination, was revealed by this method. From histologic sections taken after such a procedure it was not possible to determine any obvious difference in blood vessels, connective tissue, or other structures in the region which the blood did not enter in comparison with the neighboring skin where it did. The cherry angioma therefore does not give us the answer about the anemic halo. Does the cherry angioma produce a circulatory change or does the region provide a peculiar opportunity for such an angioma to develop?

In the elegant colored photograph of Snyder and Doan's patient with hereditary hemorrhagic telangiectasia there are pale zones around the lesions. I have noticed this same phenomenon in a few patients with Osler's disease. But these observations merely extend the evidence that the anemic halo is a real phenomenon of altered blood flow around a variety of vascular lesions of the skin. But how it is related and whether it is primary or secondary remain unsolved questions.

2. Infrared Photography

The employment of infrared photography has long been recognized as a helpful method of recording vascular lesions and other structures in the skin or mucous membranes where there is a blue or bluish color (449). Massopust has contributed many distinguished papers on this subject. Some years ago I took advantage of the fact that the infrared technique obliterates red structures from photographic representation, in order to demonstrate that arterial spiders could be obliterated photographically by this technique (Figures 3, 51, 52). Since the spider has a bright crimson color it does not show up by the infrared technique. I had hoped that perhaps the lesions of Osler's disease might remain visible in infrared photographs because many of them are purple and cyanotic looking, but the vast majority of all such lesions also undergo photographic obliteration with the infrared method. Occasionally venous stars may be bright red (Figure 130) though usually they are blue or dark blue. By the use of the infrared technique it was possible to demonstrate clearly the close association of the venous star with the underlying system of collecting veins to which it is tributary (58). On the other hand infrared photographs of spiders ordinarily reveal that spiders occupy areas away from the main venous collecting systems which appear in infrared photographs of the skin. While there should rarely be any difficulty in differentiating venous stars and arterial spiders on clinical grounds,

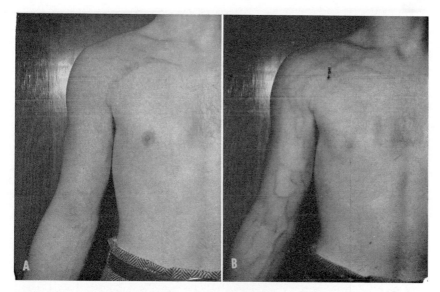

Figure 127. Venous star. Black and white and infrared photograph of a large star on the ankle. This lesion was bright red which may account for the fact that in the infrared photograph it faded completely though others with a blue cast may fade also.

occasionally the infrared technique might help to make this differentiation.

Use of infrared technique has been employed in taking photographs of the abdominal veins in pregnancy, cirrhosis of the liver, and cancer of the breast. These have been discussed elsewhere. Details of the cutaneous circulation, and of many kinds of vascular lesions may be revealed by infrared technique when they are not disclosed by ordinary black and white or color photography. Some of the phenomena are illustrated in the many comparisons of infrared and black and white photographs seen in Figures 3, 34, 35, 52, 73, 75, 77, 81, 84, 85, 97, 98, 100, 102, 103, 104, 105, 106, 107, 108, 109, 127, 128, 129, and 130.

3.   An Aside on Teleology

I have recurring thoughts and speculations about vascular spiders and many other lesions in the skin. Might they serve some function beyond that of stimulating curiosity and providing clues

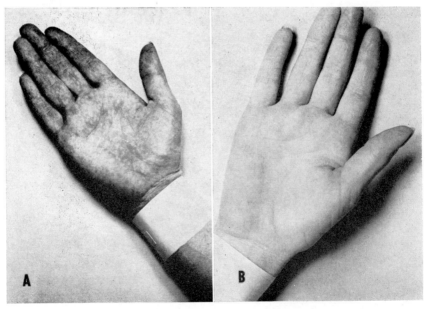

Figure 128.   Diffuse speckled palmar erythema.   A pregnant woman illustrating the complete loss of the pattern in the infrared photograph.

about health and disease? Could spiders, for instance, serve for losing heat as glomus bodies do? The structure of the spider is ideally suited to getting a lot of blood to the surface in a hurry. Thus they might expedite cooling the body. The same is true of the physiological state in palmar erythema. Whether purposeful or not, heat is lost readily in such circumstances. Since heat production is increased in pregnant women and fever is common in cirrhosis, the notion might be put forward that this is an adaptive response to the stimulus for heat loss. No one has ever described spiders appearing in persons going to hot environments after being in a cooler environment. I did not see any such phenomenon in many hundreds of persons I have observed in various desert and tropical regions to which they were not accustomed or in experiments lasting weeks or months in a laboratory hot room. The idea of an adaptive mechanism should not be pushed too far even though Clark and Clark have demonstrated that repeated exposure to unseasonable heat causes the formation of a great many new arteriovenous anastomoses in the rabbit ear. They tend to disappear gradually when the stimulus is removed. I have no evidence to suggest that vascular spiders or any other related lesions have any-

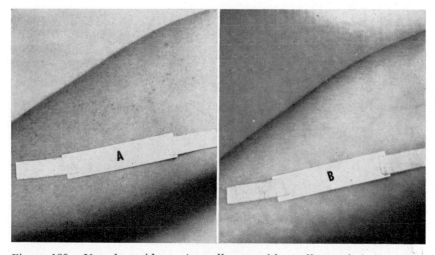

Figure 129. Vascular spiders. A small crop with small anemic halos on the forearm of a pregnant woman and the failure of such lesions to show in an infrared photograph.

thing to do with cutaneous sensation particularly of temperature and vibration, as has been suggested by Gilmer for the glomus body.

If any of the vascular lesions of the skin have pragmatic value, useful function of some kind, it will not be discovered until the lesions are known widely and studied in all aspects from many vantage points. At present they are signs or signatures. The doctrine of signatures, justifying some of the paradoxes of God's ways to man, held that having created man and diseases to plague him, God relented and gave signatures or signs in the fabric of man's body to provide clues to the nature of disease; and in the world about were signatures indicating curative or palliative essences and processes which man could find for the cure or easing of disease. All the vascular lesions gathered in this book recall for us the value of looking for signs and trying to learn their significance. Even such simple recording and contemplation of bedside phenomena demonstrate that the most modest clinical observer can find not just gleanings but whole fields left unharvested by his brothers whose devotion to science has become more abstract.

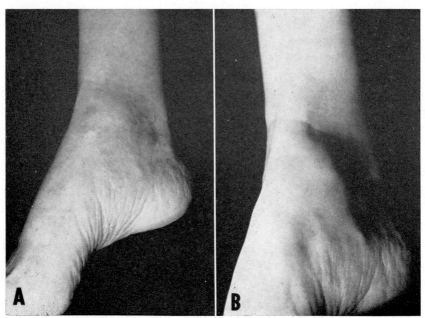

Figure 130.   Traumatic occlusion of the axillary vein.   Black and white and infrared photograph of the venous collecting system.

XIII

CONCLUSIONS

*"No mother's mark is more permanent than the mental nevi
and moles, and excrescences, and mutilations, that students
carry with them out of the lecture-room, if once the teeming
intellect which nourishes theirs has been scared from its
propriety by any misshapen fantasy."*

—OLIVER WENDELL HOLMES

I add these words in conclusion. The quotation from Holmes
has made me wonder about the use of hypothesis, remembering the
tentative value of signs and the provisional nature of ideas. I have
used hypotheses since they help hold ideas together despite the
prevalent tendency of too many writers on medical topics to solidify
somebody's hypothesis into dogma. I have not emphasized the vast
variability of some of the lesions and the possibility of intergrades
between some of the distinct ones. The patterns of distribution
are striking but have not challenged anyone with curiosity, imagination and ideas. Perhaps my effort to put down in readily available form so many of my observations comes from my feeling that
though it is not now fashionable, natural history in medicine must
not go out of style or physicians will be caught and crushed betwixt
bureaucracy and automation. We risk becoming the little middle
men, bewildered by all the chits from the laboratory and all the
newspaper clippings in the eager hands of patients.

One of the unlooked for byproducts of the rise of the laboratory age in medicine has been some decline of the personal side.
This grows. When will such growth reach the logarithmic phase
and get out of control? A curious result of over-emphasis on techniques and laboratory studies which have yielded a marvelous and
wonder fruit — health giving, pain relieving, and life promoting
skills and knowledge — has been the rediscovery by persons trained
in the laboratory that the patient is a person. One of the reasons
why psychosomatic medicine has made older physicians uneasy is
the naive and starry-eyed rediscovery by physicians, either young

319

in years or immature in experience, of many things well known to good physicians and to wise laymen also. When these were announced as new discoveries, perceptive physicians became suspicious of the enthusiasm. The intrinsic nature of clinical medicine is forever introducing difficulties. A dilemma recurs whenever one tries to plot on coordinates, figures of numerical precision like arterial blood pressure, against the subjective symptoms like bellyache, anxiety or anger. To put points where wavy and erratic lines or zones best illustrate the data is an error often buried in the illusion enhanced by an elegantly drawn figure. This is not to say that such elements in medicine defy our understanding, merely that the laboratory methods, so handsome for determining electrolyte concentration, may give us false security when we read more into a number or a chart than the method allows.

The use of scientific techniques in sundry fields of medicine has been going on at an accelerated pace for the past fifty years or more. Its spread suggests the irresistable movement of lava covering old land, changing it into new patterns and contours. Time must pass before vegetation can use the latent fertility of the lava to make a productive crop. There is danger that the vegetation will be burnt out and the seeds will not survive unless cultivated carefully. Physicians must remember that the practice of medicine combines not only scientific method, the discipline of the laboratory, but observation, study and contemplation. These constitute the less well-defined arts of medicine. Such arts comprise its proper practice. Fascination of the present day undergraduate medical student and his teachers with the routines, rubrics and rituals rather than the ideas of science, with techniques and laboratory procedures rather than their critical understanding and evaluation, has left unharvested the less spectacular gleanings of observation. In short, this book embodies an approach to medicine now in low esteem.

Clinical research is the systematic study and contemplation of men, women and children who are sick. It must be done with knowledge of their proper functions when they are well. Despite a numerous company claiming devotion to clinical science, very few have the practical dexterity, the will to work, the feeling for craft, or the capacity to collect and systematize knowledge which enable

them to pass out of the novitiate of clinical research and make original contributions. Though each of the requirements is meager,
the assemblage of the essential needs in any one person is rare.
Progress is slow. This in sharp contradistinction to the rate of
advance by which an inveterate laboratory investigator in a sharp
and narrow salient may move far enough beyond the front lines
of knowledge to attract notice and gain fame. A mature *observer*
is likely to ripen slowly. The *worker in the laboratory* at least has
the opportunity of hitting a ten-strike early in his career. Unhap-
pily the academic field is not without its accretions of one day wonders, early bloomers who have wilted on the vine after an early
blossom dazzled everyone with great promise.

Clinical research in this country, running a course generally
parallel to that in Britain, has followed two lines. One is the
method of piece work, using the expression in its good sense. It is
concerned with processes, the clinical significance of levels of blood
pressure, mechanisms of arrhythmia or sodium retention, rather
than with the disease or the special person who has the particular
phenomenon. To followers of this school we owe the most dramatic
advances which clinical research has brought to modern medicine.
It is an oversimplification to say that investigators of this school
are concerned only with the phenomena of disease. Nonetheless,
the major interest is in mechanisms and their clinical significance.
This group is exemplified by Soma Weiss and a whole school of
clinical investigators striving to follow him in obvious if not always
conscious emulation.

The other method is more ancient and traditional. It thinks
of disease in terms of the broad picture. What is the constellation
of phenomena which appears when noxious stimuli are applied to
a person, sick or well, responding in accordance with his present
fabric as determined by genetic makeup and old and new environmental stimuli? Too facile generalizations have been great impedi-
ments to progress of this school. One virtue of men using this
method is that they are aware of powerful though scarcely measure-
able forces which older physicians called temperament, diathesis,
or disposition. Where such workers have flourished and obtained
useful results they have been explorers and prospectors, uncovering

new terrain, mapping, and staking out claims which the laboratory investigator, as mining engineer, comes in to exploit later. Peabody may be taken as an American exemplar of clinical investigation intent on sick people. Without comparing Weiss and Peabody in intellect or accomplishment, for both were truly great, it is a measure of the temper of our times that Weiss' influence prevails while Peabody's it at a low ebb.

Clinical science of either kind has to be based on clinical observation. The hardest lesson to learn, and too few ever learn it, is that we see not what we look *at* but what we look *for*. It takes intense cultivation of complete concentration to be able to grasp the significance of apparently unimportant signs and symptoms. It is almost too hard to find new and juster significance for phenomena already given fixed meaning in the dogma and doctrine of our texts and teachings.

Clinical research must embody the following sequence: (1) A question is raised by a new or established observation. (2) The question must be worth asking. (3) It has not been answered, and (4) is potentially answerable. (5) An attack is planned using (6) techniques; (7) apparatus to obtain data which might give an answer; (8) work continues, or (9) ends, given up because of distraction, fatigue, loss of enthusiasm, or because the first premises were in error. Or, (10) the question is answered or (11) a new idea arises from an unexpected result which suggests more questions and the cycle begins again.

Another kind of observation forms the basis of all clinical practice. We learn the signs and symptoms of disease from our texts, our teachers, and our growing experience. This corpus of hard won knowledge and skills constitutes the arts of medicine. Like any craft, it becomes an efficient process in the hands of some and remains a crude process in the hands of others. Many are fitted for it not at all. It has a reciprocal relationship with exuberant verbosity. It recognizes signs and symptoms for what they are, understands them, takes appropriate measures, or if such happens to be wiser, leaves well enough alone. We call this clinical intuition or bedside manner, according to whether we admire or mistrust it. This talent resembles that of a well-trained bird dog at a point as well as the mysterious orienting skill of the homing pigeon. It consists mainly of arriving at conclusions by a series of steps, many of which have become so automatic that they are made without conscious awareness. It is the tool and method of practice but rarely that of discovery or clarification.

The third element is truly intuitive. It is compact of imagination and inspiration. It comes we know not whence and we know not why. Hard work cannot achieve it, money cannot buy it, thought cannot command it. It is incomprehensible. We may recognize it, cherish it when it appears in others, and hope that in due course some may come to us. It consists of the rearrangement of established or observed facts so that they reveal a new truth. It is likely to be recognized, perhaps better in the painter or poet, than in the investigator. As an example of it, we may take Castle's brilliant conception of intrinsic and extrinsic factors in pernicious anemia and deficiency disease. Ultimately it led to the isolation and identification of vitamin B_{12}. Such events are so rare that we can count on our fingers the important ones that occur in medicine during any lifetime. They are the flaming torches that light the way for us around corners, bringing into sight new vistas, where again for a time progress may be simple because it is a natural development. The basis for all such spectacular advances lies in natural history, the phenomenology of disease, which poses questions for the more exact science of the laboratory to try to answer. And even the simplest of us can cultivate this field, and have great pleasure in doing so. At length we may be able to say modestly with the Sorcerer in Anthony and Cleopatra, "In nature's infinite book of secrecy a little I can read."

REFERENCES

1. ARBAMI, P., in discussion on Aubertin, C., and Lévy, R.: Angiomatose hémorragique familiale. *Bull. Soc. Méd. Hôp. Paris, 53*:1332, 1931.
2. ADAMSON, H. G.: Livedo reticularis. *Brit. J. Dermat., 28*:281, 1916.
3. ADAMSON, H. G.: A note on multiple small angiomata: angiokeratoma and multiple telangiectases. *Brit. J. Dermat., 30*:85, 1918.
3a. AGUILERA MARURI, C.: Erythema palmare symmetrique, Syphilique? *Ann. de Dermat. et Syph., 10*:415, 1939.
4. AKERS, R. P. AND LEE, R. E.: Nutritional factors in hemodynamics: III. Importance of Vitamin C in maintaining renal VEM mechanisms. *Proc. Soc. Exper. Biol & Med., 82*:195, 1953.
5. ALBAN, H.: Hereditary hemorrhagic telangiectasia. *Northwest Med., 40*:86, 1941.
6. ALDERCREUTZ, E.: Periocular hyperpigmentation (masque biliáre) and its relation to biliary and genitourinary tract diseases. *Acta, Medica Scandinavica, 135*:63, 1949.
7. ALESSANDRINI, G., AND SCALA, A.: *Pellagra.* Translated by Perdue, E. M. Kansas City, Mo., Burton, 1916.
8. ALLEN, R. A. AND DAHLIN, D. C.: Glomus tumor of the stomach: report of 2 cases. *Proc. Staff Meetings of the Mayo Clinic, 29*:429, 1954.
9. ALLISON, S. D.: Psychosomatic dermatology circa 1850. *A.M.A. Arch. Dermat. & Syph., 68*:499, 1953.
10. ALTHAUSEN, T. L., AND KERR, W. J.: Hemochromatosis. A report of three cases with results of insulin therapy in one case. *Endocrinology, 11*:377, 1927.
11. ALTHAUSEN, T. L., AND KERR, W. J.: Hemochromatosis. II. A report of three cases with endocrine disturbances and notes on a previously reported case. Discussion of etiology. *Endocrinology, 17*:621, 1933.
12. ALTSCHULE, M. D., IGLAUER, A., AND ZAMCHECK, N.: Respiration and circulation in patients with obstruction of the superior vena cava. *Arch. Int. Med., 75*:24, 1945.
13. ANDERSON, M., AND PRATT-THOMAS, H. R.: Marfan's syndrome. *Am. Heart J., 46*:911, 1953.
14. ARMENTROUT, H. L., AND UNDERWOOD, F. J.: Familial hemorrhagic telangiectasia with associated pulmonary arteriovenous aneurysm. *Am. J. Med., 8*:246, 1950.
15. ARMSTRONG, E. L., ADAMS, W. L. JR., TRAGERMAN, L. J., AND TOWNSEND, E. W.: The Cruveilhier-Baumgarten syndrome; review of the literature and report of two additional cases. *Ann. Int. Med., 16*:113, 1942.
16. ARON.: Teleangiektasien. *Zentralbl. F. Haut—u. Geschlechtskr., 18*:755, 1926.
17. ARRAK, A.: Zur kenntnis der teleangiectasia hereditaria haemorrhagica. *Deutsches Arch. klin. Med., 147*:287, 1925.
18. ASHBY, D. W. AND BULMER, E.: Hereditary haemorrhagic telangiectasia with hepatosplenomegalgy and ascites. *Brit. M. J., 1*:1059, 1951.
19. ASHE, W. F., PRATT-THOMAS, H. R., AND KUMPE, C. W.: Weil's disease. *Medicine., 20*:145, 1941.
20. AUBERTIN, C.: Deux cas d' angiomatose hémorragique familiale à prédominance linguale. *Presse Méd., 2*:1273, 1933.

21. AUBERTIN, C., AND LÉVY, R: Angiomatose hémorragique familiale (1). *Bull. Soc. méd. Hôp. Paris, 47*:1327, 1931.

22. AUBERTIN, C., LÉVY, R., AND BACLESSE: L' angiomatose hémorragique familiale. *Presse Méd., 41*:185, 1933.

23. AUDRY, J.: Familial diseases. *Lyon méd., 129*:469, 1920.

24. AUDRY, J.: Forme familiale d' épístaxis récídivantes. Associées à des télangiec tasies multiples de la peau et des muqucuses (Osler). *Rev. de Médecine. 31*:22, 1911.

25. BABINGTON, B. G.: Hereditary epistaxis. *Lancet., 2*:362, 1865.

26. BAEHR, G., KLEMPERER, P. AND SCHIFRIN, A.: Diffuse disease of the peripheral circulation (usually associated with lupus erythematosus and endocarditis). *Trans. Assoc. Am. Phys., 50*:139, 1935.

27. BAER, R. W., TAUSSIG, H. B., AND OPPENHEIMER, E. H.: Congenital aneurysmal dilatation of the aorta associated with arachnodactyly. *Bull. Johns Hopkins Hosp., 72*:309, 1943.

28. BAER, S., BEHREND, A., AND GOLDBURGH, H. L.: Arteriovenous fistulas of the lungs. *Circulation, 1*:602, 1950.

29. BAILEY, O. T.: The cutaneous glomus and its tumors—glomangiomas. *Am. J. Path., 11*:915, 1935.

30. BAKER, C. AND TROUNCE, J. R.: Arteriovenous aneurysm of the lung. *Brit. Heart J., 11*:109, 1949.

31. BAKER, G. P.: Hereditary haemorrhagic telangiectasia with gastrointestinal haemorrhage and hepato-splenomegaly. *Guy's Hosp. Rep., 102*:246, 1953.

32. BALLANTYNE, A. J.: Multiple telangiectases: three cases in one family. *Glasgow M. J., 70*:256, 1908.

33. BALLANTYNE, A. J.: Retinal changes associated with diabetes and with hypertension. A comparison and contrast. *Arch. Ophth., 33*:97, 1945.

34. BALPH, J.: Multiple hereditary telangiectasis: report of five cases in one family. *Boston M. & S. J., 197*:1177, 1927.

35. BANYAI, A. L., AND CADDEN, A. V.: Changes in the fingernails in pulmonary tuberculosis. *Arch. Derm. & Syph., 48*:306, 1943.

36. BANYAI, A. L. AND CADDEN, A. V.: The lunula of fingernails in tuberculosis. *Urol. & Cutan. Rev., 48*:330, 1944.

37. BANYAI, A. L. AND HIRSH, L. H.: Acroerythrosis with associated analogous palmar changes in pulmonary tuberculosis. *Urol. & Cutan. Rev., 50*:282, 1946.

38. BARROCK, J. J.: Hereditary hemorrhagic telangiectasia. Report of case with review of literature. *Wisconsin M. J., 43*:805, 1944.

39. BARTELMEZ, G. W.: Histological studies on the menstruating mucous membrane of the human uterus. Contribution to Embryology, No. 142, Pub. 443. Carnegie Inst., Wash., D. C., 1933.

40. BARTELMEZ, G. W.: Menstruation. *J.A.M.A., 116*:702, 1941.

41. BARTELMEZ, G. W.: The human uterine mucous membrane during menstruation. *Am. J. Obst. and Gynec., 21*:623, 1931.

42. BASS, C. C.: Pellagra. *Med. Clin. No. America, 9*:869, 1926.

43. BATEMAN, T.: *Cutaneous Diseases,* 2nd Am. ed. Philadelphia, Crissy, 1824.

44. BAUER, E.: Ein beitrag zur kenntnis der "oslerschen krankheit." *Wien. klin. Wchnschr., 58*:778, 1946.

45. BEAN, R. B. AND BEAN, W. B.: *Sir William Osler, Aphorisms from His Bedside Teachings and Writings.* New York City, Schuman, 1950.

46. BEAN, W. B.: Unpublished observations.
47. BEAN, W. B.: A note on the development of cutaneous arterial "spiders" and palmar erythema in persons with liver disease and their development following the administration of estrogens. *Am. J. M. Sc., 204*:251, 1942.
48. BEAN, W. B.: The relationship of estrogens to certain signs in hepatic diseases, pregnancy and vitamin B complex deficiency syndromes. *Proc. Central Soc. Clin. Research, 15*:24, 1942.
49. BEAN, W. B.: Relationship of estrogens to certain signs in hepatic diseases, pregnancy and vitamin B complex deficiency syndromes — (abstract and discussion). *J.A.M.A., 121*:1412, 1943.
50. BEAN, W. B.: Acquired palmar erythema and cutaneous vascular "spiders". *Am. Heart J., 25*:463, 1943.
51. BEAN, W. B., SPIES, T. D., AND BLANKENHORN, M. A.: Secondary pellagra. *Medicine, 23*:1, 1944.
52. BEAN, W. B.: A note on infrared photography of cutaneous arterial "spiders" and hereditary hemorrhagic telangiectases. *J. Lab. & Clin. Med., 30*:190, 1945.
53. BEAN, W. B.: The cutaneous arterial spider: a survey. *Medicine, 24*:243, 1945.
54. BEAN, W. B., JOHNSON, R. E., HENDERSON, C. R., RICHARDSON, L. N.: Nutrition survey in Pacific Theatre of operations. *Bull. U. S. Army Med. Dept., 5*:697, 1946.
55. BEAN, W. B.: An analysis of subjectivity in the clinical examination in nutrition. *J. Applied Physiol., 1*:358, 1948.
56. BEAN, W. B. AND FRANKLIN, M.: Hepatitis and jaundice: a review of 119 cases. *Am Pract., 4*:148, 1949.
57. BEAN, W. B.: Control in research in human nutrition. *Nutrition Rev., 8*:97, 1950.
58. BEAN, W. B.: A note on venous stars. *Trans. Assoc. Am. Phys., 64*:100, 1951.
59. BEAN, W. B.: The caviar lesion under the tongue. *Trans. Am. Clin. & Clim. Assn., 64*:40, 1952.
60. BEAN, W. B.: A note on fingernail growth. *J. Invest. Dermat., 20*:27, 1953.
61. BEAN, W. B.: The natural history and significance of certain vascular changes in the skin and mucous surfaces. *Q. Bull. N. W. Univ. Med. School, 27*:89, 1953.
62. BEAN, W. B.: The arterial spider and similar lesions of the skin and mucous membranes. *Circulation, 8*:117, 1953.
63. BEAN, W. B.: Clinical pathologic conference. *J. Iowa St. Med. Soc., 43*:107, 1953.
64. BEAN, W. B.: Cherry angioma: a digression on the longevity of error. *Trans. Assn. Am. Phys., 66*:240, 1953.
65. BEAN, W. B.: The changing incidence of certain vascular lesions of the skin with aging. *Ciba Foundation Colloquium on ageing, 1*:80, 1955.
66. BEAN, W. B.: Dyschondroplasia and hemangiomata (Maffucci's syndrome). *A.M.A. Arch. Int. Med., 95*:767, 1955.
67. BEAN, W. B.: The changing incidence of certain vascular lesions of the skin with aging. *Geriatrics, 11*:97, 1956.
68. BEAN, W. B.: Ophthalmoplegia, steatorrhea, phlebectasia and vascular lipomas. *A. M. A. Arch. Int. Med., 98*:284, 1956.
69. BEAN, W. B., COGSWELL, R., DEXTER, M., AND EMBICK, J. F.: Vascular changes of the skin in pregnancy: Vascular spiders and palmar erythema. *Surg. Gynec. & Obst., 88*:739, 1949.

70. BEAN, W. B., FRANKLIN, M., EMBICK, J. F., DAUM, K.: Absorption studies using portal anastomotic veins. *J. Clin. Invest., 30:263*, 1951.

71. BEAN, W. B. AND PONSETI, I. V.: Dissecting aneurysm produced by diet. *Circulation, 12*:185, 1955.

72. BEAN, W. B., OLCH, D., AND WEINBERG, H. B.: The syndrome of carcinoid and acquired valve lesions of the right side of the heart. *Circulation, 12*:1, 1955.

73. BEAN, W. B. AND SPIES, T. D.: Vitamin deficiencies in diarrheal states. *J.A.M.A., 115*:107, 1940.

74. BEAN, W. B., AND SPIES, T. D.: A study of the effects of nicotinic acid and related pyridine and pyrazine compounds on the temperature of the skin of human beings. *Am. Heart J., 20*:62, 1940.

75. BEAN, W. B., SPIES, T. D. AND VILTER, R. W.: Asymmetric cutaneous lesions in pellagra. *Arch. Dermat. & Syph., 49*:335, 1944.

76. BEAN, W. B. AND WALSH, J. R.: Venous lakes. *A.M.A. Arch. of Dermat., 74*:459, 1956.

77. BECKER, S. W.: Generalized telangiectasia: a clinical study, with special consideration of etiology and pathology. *Arch. Derm. & Syph., 14*:387, 1926.

78. BECKER, S. W. AND OBERMAYER, M. E.: Telangiectasia hemorrhagica hereditaria (Osler's Disease) and vitiligo. *Arch. Derm. & Syph., 44*:303, 1941.

79. BEEK, C. H.: Contribution to the histology of the disseminated papular telangiectasis and telangiectasis araneus. *Arch. Dermat. u. Syph., 175*:484, 1937.

80. BEERMAN, H.: Some aspects of dermatology in neurology. *Am. J. Med. Sc., 230*:441, 1955.

81. BEERMAN, H., STOKES, J. H., AND INGRAHAM, N. R. JR.: Pinta—a review of recent etiologic and clinical studies. *Am. J. M. Sc., 205*:611, 1943.

82. BELL, G. I.: Hereditary hemorrhagic telangiectasia. *Canad. M.A.J., 58*:279, 1948.

83. BELL, J.: *Principles of Surgery*. London, Tegg, 1826.

84. BENEDICT, E. B.: Hemorrhage from gastritis. *Am. J. Roentgenol., 47*:254, 1942.

85. BENKO, A.: Hemorrhagic disease in connection with hereditary hemorrhagic telangiectasis. *Wien. klin. Wchnschr., 59*:613, 1947.

86. BENNETT, I. L., JR.: A unique case of obstruction of the inferior vena cava. *Bull. Johns Hopkins Hosp., 87*:290, 1950.

87. BERK, J. E. AND GOLDBURGH, H. L.: The etiology and significance of hepatic changes in hyperthyroidism. *Internat. Clin., 4*:127, 1941.

88. BERKMAN, J.: The morphogeny of the capillary vascular lesions of diabetes. *Diabetes, 4*:265, 1955.

89. BERTHONG, M. AND SABISTON, D. C., JR.: Cerebral lesions in congenital heart disease. *Bull. Johns Hopkins Hosp., 89*:384, 1951.

90. BERWICK, G.: A new caustic for mother's marks. *Lancet, 2*:347, 1871.

91. BETTLEY, F. R.: Erythema nuchae. *Brit. J. Dermat., 52*:363, 1940.

92. BEVANS, M.: The arteriosclerotic lesions in diabetes. *Diabetes, 4*:259, 1955.

93. BEIGELMAN, P. M., GOLDNER, F., JR., AND BAYLES, T. B.: Progressive systemic sclerosis (scleroderma). *New Eng. J. Med., 249*:45, 1953.

94. BIER, A.: Hyperemia as a Therapeutic Agent. Chicago, Robertson, 1905.

95. BIERMAN, H. R., GILFILLAN, R. S., KELLY, K. H., KUZMA, O. T., AND NOBLE, M.: Studies on the blood supply of tumors in man. V. Skin temperatures of superficial neoplastic lesions. *J. Nat. Cancer Inst., 13*:1, 1952.

96. BIÖRCK, G., AXEN, O., AND THORSON, Å.: Unusual cyanosis in a boy with congenital pulmonary stenosis and tricuspic insufficiency. Fatal outcome after angiocardiography. *Am. Ht. J., 44*:143, 1952.

97. BIRD, R. M., HAMARSTEN, J. F., MARSHALL, R. A., AND ROBINSON, R. R.: A family reunion: a study of hereditary hemorrhagic telangiectasia. *New Eng. J. Med., 257*:105, 1957.

98. BISKIND, G. R.: The inactivation of estradiol and estradiol benzoate in castrate female rats. *Endocrinology, 28*:894, 1941.

99. BISKIND, M. S.: Nutritional deficiency in the etiology of menorrhagia, metorrhagia, cystic mastitis and premenstrual tension; treatment with vitamin B complex. *J. Clin. Endocrinol., 3*:227, 1943.

100. BISKIND, M. S. AND SHELESNYAK, M. C.: Effect of vitamin B complex deficiency on inactivation of ovarian estrogen in the liver. *Endocrinology, 30*:819, 1942.

101. BISKIND, M. S. AND BISKIND, G. R.: Effect of vitamin B complex deficiency on inactivation of estrone in the liver. *Endocrinology, 31*:109, 1942.

102. BISKIND, M. S. AND BISKIND, G. R.: Inactivation of testosterone propionate in the liver during vitamin B complex deficiency. Alteration of estrogen-androgen equilibrium. *Endocrinology, 32*:97, 1943.

103. BLACK, H. H. AND LANDAY, L. H.: Marfan's syndrome. *Am. J. Dis. Child., 89*:414, 1955.

104. BLANKENHORN, M. A. AND BEAN, W. B.: Vascular spiders. *Trans. Assn. Am. Phys., 61*:76, 1948.

105. BLIGH, W.: Note on a case of bleeding telangiectasis. *Lancet, 1*:506, 1907.

106. BLOODWORTH, J. M. B., JR., AND HAMWI, G. J.: Experimental diabetic glomerulosclerosis. *Diabetes, 5*:37, 1956.

107. BLOODWORTH, J. M. B., JR., AND HAMWI, G. J.: Histopathology of experimental glomerular lesions simulating human diabetic glomerulosclerosis. *Am. J. Path., 31*:167, 1955.

108. BLOOM, D.: Osler's disease (hereditary familial telangiectasia). *Arch. Derm. & Syph., 37*:678, 1938.

109. BLOOM, D.: Hereditary hemorrhagic telangiectasia. *Arch. Derm. & Syph., 45*:1180, 1942.

110. BLOOMFIELD, A. L.: The natural history of chronic hepatitis (cirrhosis of the liver). *Am. J. M. Sc., 195*:429, 1938.

111. BLUEFARB, S. N.: *Kaposi's Sarcoma.* Springfield, Thomas, 1957.

112. BLUMFELD, L.: Familial epistaxis. *Laryngoscope, 36*:573, 1926.

112a. BODER, E. AND SEDGWICK, R. P.: Ataxia-Telangiectasia: a familial syndrome of progressive cerebellar ataxia, oculo-cutaneous telangiectasia and frequent pulmonary infection. *U. So. Calif. Med. Bull., 9*:15, 1957.

113. VAN BOGAERT, L.: Sur l' angiomatose hémorragique héréditaire avec spleno hépatomegalie. *Bull. Soc. méd. Hôp. Paris, 49*:1572, 1933.

114. VAN BOGAERT, L., AND SCHERER, J. H.: Hémangiomatose familiale de Rendu-Osler et cirrhose hépatique; contribution à l' étude des cirrhoses familiales. *Ann. méd., 38*:290, 1935.

115. BOSTON, L. N.: Inherited epistaxis—associated with other arterial defects. *Med. Times, N. Y., 58*:68, 1930.

116. BOSTON, L. N.: Gastric hemorrhage due to familial telangiectasis. *Am. J. M. Sc., 180*:798, 1930.

330   VASCULAR SPIDERS AND RELATED LESIONS OF THE SKIN

117. BOTTEMA, C. W.: Morbus osler. Nederl tij. genees., 74:5560, 1930.
118. BOUCHARD, C. J.: Sur quelques altérations artérielles hémorragipares dans les cirrhoses. Rev. de méd., 22:837, 1902.
119. BOUCHARD, C. J.: Discussion of splenic enlargements other than luekemic (Osler). Br. Med. J., 2:1151, 1903.
119a. BOUCHARD, C. J.: Discussion on Osler, W.: Discussion of splenic enlargements other than luekemic. Brit. M. J., 2:1154, 1908.
120. BRAITHWAITE, J.: Leeds and West-Riding Medico-Chirurgical Society. Multiple aneurysm of pulmonary artery. Brit. M. J., 1:1223, 1897.
121. BRALEY, A. E.: Personal communication.
122. BRANDEL, E.: Recurring gastrointestinal hemorrhage in hereditary hemorrhagic telangiectasia (Osler). Acta medica Scand., 137:436, 1950.
123. BRANWOOD, A. W. AND BAIN, A. D.: Carcinoid tumor of small intestine with hepatic metastases, pulmonary stenosis, and atypical cyanosis. Lancet, 2:1259, 1954.
124. BRAYTON, D. AND NORRIS, W. J.: Gastrointestinal hemorrhage in infancy and childhood. J.A.M.A., 156:68, 1952.
125. BRICKNER, S. M.: Fibroma molluscum gravidarum: a new clinical entity. Am. J. Obst. & Gynec., 53:191, 1906.
126. BRICKNER, S. M.: The role of the glands of internal secretion in the genesis of fibroma molluscum gravidarum. Surg. Gynec. & Obst., 17:402, 1913.
127. BRINK, A. J.: Telangiectasia of the lungs with two cases of hereditary hemorrhagic telangiectasis with cyanosis. Quart. J. Med., 19:239, 1950.
128. BROAGER, B. AND HERTZ, H.: Cerebral complications in congenital heart disease. Acta Med. Scand., supp. 266:142, 293, 1952.
129. BROQ, L.: Les conséquences du décolletage permanent chez la femme (la dermatose du triangle sterno-claviculaire). Ann. dermat. et syph., 5 (6th series):113, 1916.
130. BUCHANAN, S.: The Doctrine of Signatures, A Plea for Theory in Medicine. New York, Harcourt, Brace & Co., 1938.
131. BULKLEY, L. D.: The Influence of the Menstrual Function on Certain Diseases of the Skin. New York, Rebman, 1906.
132. BURCHELL, H. B. AND CLAGETT, O. T.: The clinical syndrome associated with pulmonary arteriovenous fistulas, including a case report of a surgical cure. Am. Heart J., 34:151, 1947.
133. BURKE, J. P.: Angioma of the brain. Am. J. Clin. Path., 24:1276, 1954.
134. BURWELL, C. S. AND METCALFE, J.: Heart disease in pregnancy. Modern Concepts in Cardiovascular Disease, 23:250, 1954.
135. CABOT CASE 29301. New Eng. J. Med., 229:220, 1943.
136. CACCAMISE, W. C. AND WHITMAN, J. F.: Pulseless disease. Am. Heart J., 44:629, 1952.
137. CALENDA, D. G. AND URICCHIO, J. F.: Superior vena cava syndrome. A.M.A. Arch. Int. Med., 91:800, 1953.
138. CALVERT, R. J., NARDELL, S. G., AND RAEBURN, C.: Angiopathies in acrosclerosis. Angiology, 6:129, 1955.
139. CAMPANALE, R. P., ROBBINS, L. R., HOFFMAN, A. A., AND SHAW, R. R.: Arteriovenous fistula of the lung treated by segmental excision. U. S. Armed Forces Med. J., 5:1037, 1954.

140. CAMPBELL, A. M. G.: Hereditary familial telangiectasis with epistaxis and migraine. *Lancet, 2*:502, 1944.

141. CANTAROW, A., RAKOFF, A. E., PASCHKIS, K. E., HANSEN, L. P., AND WALKING, A. A.: Excretion of estrogen in bile. *Endocrinology, 31*:515, 1942.

142. CAPPON, D.: Hereditary hacmorrhagic telangiectasis. *Brit. M. J., 1*:440, 1945.

143. CAPRIGLIONE, L., BERARDINELLI, W., ET DA COSTA CRUZ, F.: Cirrhose hépatique et gynécomastie. *Presse méd., 42*:1419, 1934.

144. CARLETON, A., ELKINGTON, J. ST. C., GREENFIELD, J. G., AND ROBB-SMITH, A. H. T.: Maffucci's syndrome (Dyschrondoplasia with haemangeiomata). *Quart. J. Med., 11*:203, 1942.

145. CARTER, C. H., AGOSTAS, W. N., AND SYDENSTRICKER, V. P.: Rupture of an aortic aneurysm into the pulmonary artery. *Circulation, 5*:449, 1952.

146. CARTER, J.: Personal information concerning unreported studies.

147. CASTAIGNE, J., ET CHIRAY, M.: Manuel des maladies du foie et des voies biliares. *Masson et Cie,* Paris, 319, 1910.

148. CASTOR, C. W. AND BAKER, B. L.: The local action of adrenal cortical steroids on epidermis and connective tissue of the skin. *Endocrinology, 47*:234, 1950.

149. CHANDLER, F. G.: Bronchostaxis. *Brit. M. J., 1*:1227, 1937.

150. CHAPMAN, C.: Personal letter to the author.

151. CHARBON, B. C., ADAMS, W. E., AND CARLSON, R. F.: Surgical treatment of multiple arteriovenous fistulas in the right lung in a patient having undergone a left pneumonectomy seven years earlier for the same disease. *J. Thoracic Surg., 23*:188, 1952.

152. CHAUFFARD, M. A.: Hémophilie avec stigmates télangiectasiques. *Bull. Soc. méd. hôp. Paris, 13*:352, 1896.

153. CHEVALLIER, P.: Acquired essential telangiectases causing epistaxis and discovery by histologic examination. *Sang., 15*:146, 1942.

154. CHEVALLIER, P., MOUTIER, F., AND BERNARD, J.: Endoscopic diagnosis of gastric angioma in essential hemorrhagic telangiectasis of Rendu-Osler. *Sang., 17*:191, 1946.

155. CHIARI, O.: cited by Hanes, F. M. 1909. *Erfahrungen auf dem Gebiete der Hals und Nasenkrankheiten.* Wien, Tocplitz & Deuticke, 1887.

156. CHISHOLM, C.: The significance of cervical capillary markings. *Lancet, 1*:797, 1916.

157. CHVOSTEK, F.: Zur pathogenese der leberzirrhose. *Wien. klin. Wchnschr., 35*:381, 1922.

158. CHVOSTEK, F.: Zur pathogenese der leberzirrhose. *Wien. klin. Wchnschr., 35*:408, 1922.

159. ČIČOVAČKI, D.: Zur pathogenese der Oslerschen krankheit. *Wien. klin. Wchnschr., 53*:72, 1940.

160. ČIČOVAČKI, D.: Star-shaped cutaneous telangiectasis in hepatic cirrhosis and its diagnostic significance. *Wien. klin. Wchnschr., 53*:478, 1940.

161. ČIČOVAČKI, D. AND STOGER, R.: Ueber die Oslersche krankheit. *Wien. klin. Wchnschr., 52*:708, 1939.

162. CLARK, E. R. AND CLARK, E. L.: Observations on living arterio-venous anastomoses as seen in transplant chambers introduced into the rabbit's ear. *Am. J. Anat., 54*:229, 1934.

163. CLARK, E. R. AND CLARK, E. L.: The new formation of arterio-venous anastomoses in the rabbit's ear. *Am. J. Anat., 55*:407, 1934.

164. CLARK, W.: Infra-red photography. *J. Biol. Photographic A., 2:119* 1934,
165. CLARK, W. G. AND MACKAY, E. M.: The absorption and excretion of Rutin and related flavonoid substances. *J.A.M.A., 143*:1411, 1950.
166. CLIFFTON, E. E. AND WOLSTENHOLME, J. T.: Hypervolemia and associated changes in mice bearing a transplanted granulosa-cell tumor. *Cancer Research, 9*:331, 1949.
167. CLIFTON, J. A., ATKINSON, M., HENDRICKS, T. R. AND INGELFINGER, F. J.: The effect of 5-hydroxy tryptamine upon small intestinal motility in man. *Proc. Cent. Soc. Clin. Res., 29*:23, 1956.
168. CLUXTON, H. E. AND KRAUSE, L. A. M.: Acute lupus erythematosus disseminatus. *Ann. Int. Med., 19*:843, 1943.
169. COCHRANE, T. AND LESLIE, G.: Hereditary haemorrhagic telangiectasia. *Lancet, 1*:255, 1950.
170. COCKAYNE, E. A.: *Inherited Abnormalities of the Skin and its Appendages.* Oxford, Oxford University Press, 1933.
171. COE, J. W.: The treatment of purpuric conditions and hemophilia. *J.A.M.A., 47*:1090, 1906.
172. COFFIN, J. AND BASTENIE, P.: Angiomatose hémorrhagique héréditaire. *Bruxelles méd., 14*:577, 1934.
173. COMBES, F. C.: Hereditary hemorrhagic telangiectasia. *Arch. Derm. & Syph., 39*:754, 1939.
174. COMBES, F. C.: Hereditary hemorrhagic telangiectasia. *Arch. Derm. & Syph., 50*:143, 1944.
175. CONNOR, W.: Personal communication.
176. COOKE, W. T., CLOAKE, C. P. C., GOVAN, A. D. T., AND COLBECK, J. L.: Temporal arteritis: generalized vascular disease. *Q. J. Med., 39*:47, 1946.
177. COOPER, I. S. AND HOEN, T. I.: Gynecomastia in paraplegic males. *J. Clin. Endocrinology, 9*:457, 1949.
178. COPLEY, A. L.: The ecchymosis test for capillary hemorrhagic diathesis. *Science, 107*:201, 1948.
179. CORBETT, D.: Discussion. *Brit. J. Dermat., 26*:200, 1914.
180. CORDES, F. C. AND HOGAN, M. J.: Angiomatosis retinae (Hippel's disease): report of case in which roentgen therapy was used in an early stage. *Arch. Ophth., 23*:253, 1940.
181. COURSLEY, G., IVINS, J. C., AND BARKER, N. W.: Congenital arteriovenous fistulas in the extremities. *Angiology, 7*:201, 1956.
182. COX, H. T.: The cleavage lines of the skin. *Brit. J. Surg., 29*:234, 1941
183. CRAWFORD, M. G. AND LEEPER, R. W.: Diseases of the skin in pregnancy. *Arch. Dermat. & Syph., 61*:753, 1950.
184. CRITCHLEY, M. AND EARL, C. J. C.: Tuberose sclerosis and allied conditions. *Brain, 55*:311, 1932.
185. CROSS, W. G.: Gum tumors in pregnancy in gingivitis gravidarium. *Brit. Dent. J., 75*:85, 1943.
186. CURSCHMANN, H.: Üeber familiäeres nasenbluten als ausdruck einer pseudohäemophilie. *Klin. Wchnschr., 9*:677, 1930.
187. CURTIUS, F.: Untersuchungen uber das menschliche veneneystem. *Klin. Wchnschr., 7*:2141, 1928.
188. CUSHING, H.: *Pituitary Body, Hypothalmus, and Parasympathetic Nervous System.* Springfield, Thomas, 1932.

189. CUTLER, M. H.: Hereditary hemorrhagic telangiectasia. *Arch. Otolaryng., 40*:428, 1944.

190. DaCOSTA, S. M. AND CREMER, G.: Kaviarahnliche Korner unter der Zunge. *Dermat. Wchnschr., 91*:1206, 1930.

191. DAUGHERTY, G. W., MANGER, W. M., ROTH, G. M., FLOCK, E. V., CHILDS, D. S., JR. AND WAUGH, J. M.: Malignant carcinoid with hyperserotonemia occurring spontaneously or induced by palpation of the tumor or by intravenous histamine: report of a case. *Proc. Staff Meetings of the Mayo Clinic, 30*:595, 1955.

192. DAVIS, A.: Subcutaneous hemangio-endotheliomata associated with pregnancy. *J. Ob. & Gyn. of Br. Empire, 45*:667, 1938.

193. DAVIS, E.: Hereditary familial purpura simplex. *Lancet, 2*:1110, 1939.

194. DAVIS, E.: Hereditary familial purpura simplex. *Lancet, 1*:145. 1941.

195. DAWSON, J.: Pulmonary tuberous sclerosis. *Q. J. Med., 23*:113, 1954.

196. DAY, H. G. AND FOLLIS, R. H. JR.: Skeletal changes in rats receiving estradiol benzoate as indicated by histological studies and determinations of bone ash, serum calcium and phosphatase, *Endocrinology, 28*:83, 1941.

197. DeMORGAN, C.: *The Origin of Cancer Considered with Reference to the Treatment of the Disease.* London, Churchill, 1872.

198. DESBUQUES, M., ET CARROIS, J.: Hereditary familial angiomatosis in fatty hepatitis with hemorrhagic syndrome. *Bull. Soc. Med. Hôp. Paris, 3*:525, 1940.

199. DETERLING, R. A. AND BHONSLAY, S. B.: Use of vessel grafts and plastic prostheses for relief of superior vena cava obstruction. *Surgery, 38*:1008, 1955.

200. DIAS, J. F., JR.: Congenital arteriovenous aneyrysm of the retina. *U. S. Armed Forces Med. J., 6*:908, 1955.

201. DIGNAM, B. S.: Arteriovenous aneurysm of a branch of the pulmonary artery. *Am. Heart J., 41*:316, 1951.

202. DITZEL, J.: Morphologic and hemodynamic changes in the smaller blood vessels in diabetes mellitus. I. Considerations based on the literature. *New Eng. J. Med., 250*:541, 1954.

203. DITZEL, J. AND ROOTH, G.: The micro-angiopathy in diabetes mellitus. *Diabetes, 4*:474, 1955.

204. DITZEL, J. AND SAGILD, U.: Morphologic and hemodynamic changes in the smaller blood vessels in diabetes mellitus. II. The degenerative and hemodynamic changes in the bulbar conjunctiva of normotensive diabetic patients. *New Eng. J. Med., 250*:587, 1954.

205. DITZEL, J.: Angioscopic changes in the smaller blood vessels in diabetes mellitus and their relationship to aging. *Circulation, 14*:386, 1956.

206. DIXEY, J. R. B.: The "nape" naevus. *Brit. M. J., 1*:1032, 1955.

207. DOCKERTY, M. B.: Carcinoids of the gastrointestinal tract. *Am. J. Cl. Path., 25*:794, 1955.

208. DOCKERTY, M. B. AND SCHEIFLEY, C. H.: Metastisizing carcinoid: report of an unusual case with epiosodic cyanosis. *Am. J. Cl. Path., 25*:770, 1955.

209. DOENGES, J. P.: Treatment of hereditary hemorrhagic telangiectasia with rutin: a case report. *Bull. School Med. Univ. Maryland, 38*:142, 1953.

210. DOLOWITZ, D. A.: Hereditary hemorrhagic telangiectasia. *Am. Surgeon, 19*:776, 1953.

211. DOLOWITZ, D. A., RAMBO, O. N., JR., AND STEPHENS, F. E.: Hereditary hemorrhagic telangiectasia. *Ann. Oto. Rhino. & Laryn., 62*:642, 1953.

212. DORE, S. E.: Multiple familial telangiectases. *Proc. Roy. Soc. Med. (Sect. Derm)*, 20:1059, 1927.

213. DORMANDY, P. L.: Gastrointestinal polyposis with mucocutaneous pigmentation (Peutz-Jeghers syndrome). *New Eng. J. Med.*, 256:1093, 1141 and 1186, 1957.

214. DUNCAN, D., GARVEN, J. D. AND GIBBONS, J. L.: Argentaffin carcinoma of ileum with raised serum 5-hydroxytryptamine. *Br. Med. J.*, 2:1586, 1955.

215. DUNN, C. W.: Stilbestrol-induced gynecomastia in the male. *J.A.M.A.*, 115:2263, 1940.

216. EAST, C. F. T.: Familial facial telangiectases. *Proc. Roy. Soc. Med. (Clin. Sect.)*, 17:2, 1923.

217. EAST, C. F. T.: Familial telangiectasia. *Lancet*, 1:332, 1926.

218. EBERT, M. H.: Livido reticularis. *Arch. Derm. & Syph.*, 16:426, 1927.

219. EBERT, M. H.: Familial or hereditary hemorrhagic telangiectasia (Rendu-Osler-Weber syndrome). *Arch. Derm. & Syph.*, 51:350, 1945.

220. ECKSTEIN, J. W.: Unpublished observations.

221. EDEL, K., VAN GILSE, P. H. G., AND POSTMA, C.: Einige niederlandische familien mit erblichen teleangiektasien der schleimhaute der oberen luftund speisewege und der haut (sogen Osler' sche krankheit), gekennzeichnet durch recedivuren-des nasenbluten. *Acta oto-laryng.*, 13:525, 1929.

222. EDITORIAL: Argentaffinoma as endocrine tumour. *Lancet*, 2:1020, 1955.

223. EDMONSON, H. A., GLASS, S. J., AND SOLL, S. N.: Gynecomastia associated with cirrhosis of the liver. *Proc. Soc. Exper. Biol. & Med.*, 42:97, 1939.

224. EDWARDS, E. A. AND DUNTLEY, S. Q.: The pigments and color of living human skin. *Am. J. Anat.*, 65:1, 1939.

225. EDWARDS, E. A. AND DUNTLEY, S. Q.: Cutaneous vascular changes in women in reference to the menstrual cycle and ovariectomy. *Am. J. Ob. & Gyn.*, 57:501, 1949.

226. EDWARDS, E. A., FINKLESTEIN, M. A., AND DUNTLEY, S. Q.: Spectrophotometry of living human skin in the ultra violet range. *J. Invest. Dermat.*, 16:311, 1951.

227. EDWARDS, E. A., HAMILTON, J. B., AND DUNTLEY, S. Q.: Testosterone propionate as a therapeutic agent in patients with organic disease of the peripheral vessels. *New Eng. J. Med.*, 220:865, 1939.

228. EDWARDS, E. A., HAMILTON, J. B., DUNTLEY, S. Q., AND HUBERT, G.: Cutaneous vascular and pigmentary changes in castrate and eunuchoid men. *Endocrinology*, 28:119, 1941.

229. EHNI, G. AND CRAIN, E. L.: "Paradoxical" brain abscess—report of a unique case in association with Lutembacher's syndrome. *J.A.M.A.*, 150:1298, 1952.

230. EHRENBORG, G.: Five-year-old boy with telangiectatic skin changes of the face, left hand and legs. *Acta Paediat.*, 45:311, 1956.

231. ELAM, C.: *A Physician's Problems*. Boston, Fields, 1869.

232. ELKIN, D. C.: Arteriovenous aneurysm. *Mod. Conc. of Cardiovascular Disease*, 12: 1943.

233. ELKINS, D. C.: Arteriovenous aneurysm—the approach to the innominate vessels. *J.A.M.A.*, 129:26, 1945.

234. ELKIN, D. C.: Arteriovenous aneurysm. *Surg. Gynec. and Obst.*, 80:217, 1945.

235. ELKIN, D. C.: Traumatic aneurysm. The Matas operation—fifty-seven years after. *Surg. Gynec. and Obst.*, 82:1, 1946.

236. ELKIN, D. C.: Aneurysm following surgical procedures. *Ann. Surg.*, 127:769, 1948.

237. ELKIN, D. C.: Arteriovenous aneurysm of the phrenic vessels. *J.A.M.A., 141*:531, 1949.

238. ELKIN, D. C.: Diagnosis and treatment of aneurysms and arteriovenous fistulas. *Kentucky M. J., 50*:289, 1952.

239. ELKIN, D. C. AND BANNER, E. A.: Arteriovenous aneurysm following surgical operations. *J.A.M.A., 131*:1117, 1946.

240. ELKIN, D. C. AND HARRIS, M. H.: Arteriovenous aneurysm of the vertebral vessels. *Ann. Surg., 124*:934, 1946.

241. ELKIN, D. C. AND KELLY, R. P.: Arteriovenous aneurysm—exposure of the tibial and peroneal vessels by resection of the fibula. *Ann. Surg., 122*:529, 1945.

242. ELKIN, D. C. AND WARREN, J. V.: Arteriovenous fistulas—their effect on the circulation. *J.A.M.A., 134*:1524, 1947.

243. ELLER, J. J.: Multiple stellate telangiectases. *Arch. Derm. & Syph., 36*:892, 1937.

244. ELLIS, L. B., AND WEISS, S.: A study of the cardiovascular responses in man to the intravenous and intra-arterial injection of acetylcholine. *J. Pharm. & Exp. Therapeutics, 44*:235, 1932.

245. EMILE-WEIL, P.: Deux cas d'angiomatose hémorrhagique héréditaire. *Bull. Soc. méd. hôp. Paris, 50*:1135, 1926.

246. EMILE-WEIL, P.: Etude sur les angiomateux. *Sang., 1*:35, 1927.

247. EMILE-WEIL, P., AND LÉVY-FRANCKEL, A.: L hérédité dans les hémangiomes et dans la maladie d'Osler Rendu. *Sang., 10*:661,1936.

248. EPPINGER, H.: (Letter) *J.A.M.A., 85*:1573, 1925.

249. EPPINGER, H.: *Die Leberkrankheiten.* Vienna, Julius Springer, 1937.

250. EPSTEIN, F. H., POST, R. S., AND McDOWELL, M.: The effect of an arteriovenous fistula on renal hemodynamics and electrolyte excretion. *J. Clin. Investigation, 32*:233, 1953.

251. EPSTEIN, F. H., SHADLE, O. W., FERGUSON, T. B., AND McDOWELL, M. E.: Cardiac output and intracardiac pressures in patients with arteriovenous fistulas. *J. Clin. Investigation, 32*:543, 1953.

252. ERDHEIM, S.: Hereditary hemorrhagic telangiectasia: with a note on the age-incidence of the skin-lesions. *Br. J. Dermat. & Syph., 41*:55, 1929.

253. EVANS, J. P. AND McEACHERN, D.: The circulatory changes in cerebral vascular occlusion and in cerebral cicatrization. *Proc. of Assn. for Research in Nervous and Mental Disease, 18*:379, 1937.

254. EYLER, W. R., TESLUK, H., AND DRAKE, E. H.: Malignant argentaffinoma associated with cardiovascular abnormalities. *New Eng. J. Med., 254*:555, 1956.

255. FABRY, J.: Ein Beitrag zur Kenntniss der Purpura haemorrhagica Nodularis (Purpura papulosa haemorrhagica Hebrae). *Arch. f. derm., 43*:187, 1898.

256. FARBER, E. M. AND BARNES, V. R.: Livedo reticularis. *Stanford M. Bull., 13*:183, 1955.

257. FARBER, S. J., BECKER, W. H. AND EICHNA, L. W.: Electrolyte and water excretions and renal hemodynamics during induced congestion of the superior and inferior vena cava of man. *J. Clin. Investigation, 32*:1145, 1953.

258. FARBER, S. J. AND EICHNA, L. W.: An intracardiac catheter with inflatable balloon for producing increased venous pressures in the venae cavae of man. *J. Clin. Investigation, 32*:1140, 1953.

259. FEARNSIDES, E. G.: Telangiectases in children, in association with wasting and protracted diarrhea. *Brit. J. Dermat., 24*:35, 1912.

260. FELDAKER, M., HINES, E. A., JR., AND KIERLAND, R. R.: Livedo reticularis with summer ulcerations. *A.M.A. Arch. Derm., 72*:31, 1955.

261. FELDMAN, S.: A case for diagnosis (palmar eruption due to endocrine disturbance during pregnancy?). *Arch. Derm. & Syph., 39*:784, 1939.

262. FELDMAN, S.: A case for diagnosis (inflammatory papules or deep telangiectasia occurring during the course of pregnancy). *Arch Derm. & Syph., 40*:1024, 1939.

263. FELSON, B.: Personal communication.

264. FESSAS, P., WINTROBE, M. M., AND CARTWRIGHT, G. E.: Angiokeratoma corporis diffusum universale (Fabry). *A.M.A. Arch. Int. Med., 95*:469, 1955.

265. FIESSINGER, N.: La pathologie des capillaires chez les cirrhotiques. *Rev. gén. d. clin. et. d. thérap., 50*:241, 1936.

266. FIGI, F. A. AND WATKINS, C. H.: Hereditary hemorrhagic telangiectasia. Abstracted in *Prof. Staff Meet. Mayo Clin., 18*:418, 1943.

267. FIGI, F. A., AND WATKINS, C. H.: Hereditary hemorrhagic telangiectasia. *Ann. Otol. Rhin. & Laryng., 52*:330, 1943.

268. FINGERLAND, A. AND JANOUSEK, B.: Zur histologie der Oslerschen krankheit. *Arch. f. derm., 178*:54, 1938.

269. FISCHL, A. AND RUTHBERG, J.: Clinical implications of Marfan's syndrome. *J.A.M.A., 146*:704, 1951.

270. FISHER, M. M. AND RITZ, N. D.: Thrombosis of the inferior vena cava due to hypernephroma. *Arch. Int. Med., 81*:465, 1948.

271. FISHER, R. E. W.: Occupational skin cancer in a group of tar workers. *A.M.A. Arch. Indust. Hyg. & Occup. Med., 7*:12, 1953.

272. FITZHUGH, T., JR.: Splenomegaly and hepatic enlargement in hereditary hemorrhagic telangiectasia. *Am. J. M. Sc., 181*:261, 1931.

273. FITZHUGH, T., JR.: The importance of atavism in the diagnosis of hereditary hemorrhagic telangiectasia. *Am. J. M. Sc., 166*:884, 1923.

274. FITZWILLIAMS, D. C. L.: The etiology of naevi: nerve influence in their causation. *Brit. M. J., 2*:489, 1911.

275. FITZWILLIAMS, D. C. L.: Nevi in children and their treatment. *Practitioner, 107*:153, 1921.

276. FLANDIN, C. AND SOULIÉ, P.: Un cas d'angiomatose hémorragique héréditaire. *Bull. Soc. méd. Hôp. Paris, 52*:1781, 1928.

277. FLAVELL, G.: Reversal of pulmonary hypertrophic osteoarthropathy by vagotomy. *Lancet, 1*:260, 1956.

278. FOGGIE, W. E.: Hereditary haemorrhagic telangiectasia with recurring hematuria. *Edinburgh M. J., 35*:281, 1928.

279. FÖLDVARI, F.: Teleangiectasia haemorrhagica hereditaria. *Zentralb. f. haut., 35*:338, 1931.

280. FÖLDVARI, F.: Teleangiectasia haemorrhagica hereditaria. *Acta derm. ven., 14*:427, 1933.

281. FOLEY, W. T. AND WRIGHT, I. S.: The treatment of cerebral thrombosis and embolism with anticoagulant drugs: preliminary observations. *M. Clin. North America, 34*:909, 1950.

282. FOLKOW, B.: Nervous control of the blood vessels. *Physiol. Rev., 35*:629, 1955.

283. FOLSOME, C. E., HARAMI, T., LAVIETES, S. R., AND MASSELL, G. M.: Clinical evaluation of relaxin. *Ob. & Gyn., 8*:536, 1956.

284. FORDYCE, J.: Angiokeratoma of the scrotum. *J. Cut. Dis., 14*:81, 1896.

285. FORMAN, L.: Telangiectasia of the face, neck and arms associated with pregnancy. *Proc. Roy. Soc. Med., 27*:723, 1934.

286. FORMAN, L.: The skin manifestations of malignant diseases with special reference to vascular changes and dermatomyositis. *Brit. Med. J., 2*:911, 1952.

287. FOWLKES, R. W. AND PEPPLE, A. W.: Tumors of the glomus (glomangiomas or angiomyoneuromas). *South. M. J., 33*:269, 1940.

288. FOX, T. C.: A case of bilateral telangiectases of the trunk, with a history of marked epistaxis in childhood and recent rectal haemorrhage. *Brit. J. Dermat., 20*:145, 1908.

289. FRANCK, F. S.: Oral mucosa during pregnancy. *Dent. J. Austral., 17*:87, 1945.

290. FRANKE, H. AND BINDSEIL, W.: Genital form of Osler's disease. *Deut. med. Wchnschr., 67*:1012, 1941.

291. FRANKLIN, J. W., ZAVALA, D. C., AND RADCLIFFE ,C. E.: The detection of malignant melanoma by bone marrow aspiration. *Blood, 7*:934, 1952.

292. FRANKLIN, M., BEAN, W. B. AND HARDIN, R. C.: Fowler's solution as an etiologic agent in cirrhosis. *Am. J. Med. Sc., 219*:589, 1950.

293. FREEDMAN, M. J., HENSLER, N. M., AND POLLOCK, B. E.: Asymptomatic pulmonary arteriovenous fistula: report of two cases surgically treated. *Am. Heart J., 44*:594, 1952.

294. FREID, P. H., PERILSTEIN, P. K., AND WAGNER, B., JR.: A hormonal cause of the so-called varicose veins of pregnancy. *A.M.A. Arch. Surg., 72*:253, 1956.

295. FRIEDEN, E. H.: The effects of cysteine and other reducing agents upon relaxin. *Arch. Biochem., 30*:138, 1951.

296. FRIEDEN, E. H. AND HISAW, F. L.: The purification of relaxin. *Arch. Biochem., 29*:166, 1950.

297. FRIEDEN, E. H.: Chemical studies on relaxin. *Federation Proc., 10*:184, 1951.

298. FRIEDEN, E. H. AND HISAW, F. L.: The mechanism of symphyseal relaxation. The distribution of reducing groups, hexoseamine, and proteins in symphyses of normal and relaxed guinea pigs. *Endocrinology, 48*:88, 1951.

299. FRIEDEN, E. H., AND HISAW, F. L.: The mechanism of symphyseal relaxation changes in proteins of the guinea pig symphysis during pregnancy. *Endocrinology, 49*:119, 1951.

300. FREUDENTHAL, W.: Telangiectases of the face and mucous membranes of nose and throat associated with severe epistaxis. *New York J. Med., 113*:425, 1921.

301. FRICK, W.: An unusual case of dilated capillaries. *J. Cut. Dis., 30*:334, 1912.

302. FRIEDMAN, E. D.: An unusual hypophyseal syndrome. *New York J. Med., 114*:113, 1921.

303. FURTH, J. AND BOON, M. C.: Liver changes associated with a transplantable granulosa cell carcinoma in mice. *Proc. Soc. Exper. Biol. & Med., 58*:112, 1945.

304. GADDUM, J. H., HAMEED, K. A., HATHWAY, D. E., AND STEPHENS, F. F.: Qualitative studies of antagonists for 5-hydroxytryptamine. *Q. J. of Exp. Physiol., 40*:49, 1955.

305. GALLOWAY, J.: Visible signs of visceral disease. *Brit. M. J., 1*:665, 1908.

306. GALLOWAY, J.: Multiple cutaneous telangiectases of recent origin. *Proc. Roy. Soc. Med., 4*:42 (Clin. Sect.), 1911.

307. GAMBILL, E. E.: Recurring gastrointestinal hemorrhage in hereditary hemorrhagic telangiectasia. *Proc. Staff Meeting Mayo Clinic, 21*:157, 1946.

308. GARDNER, W. J. AND McCUBBIN, J. W.: Auriculotemporal syndrome. Gustatory sweating due to misdirection of regenerated nerve fibers. *J.A.M.A., 160*:272, 1956.

309. GARLAND, H. G. AND ANNING, S. T.: Hereditary hemorrhagic telangiectasia. *Brit. M. J., 1*:700, 1950.

310. GARLAND, H. G. AND ANNING, S. T.: Hereditary hemorrhagic telangiectasia: a genetic and bibliographic study. *Brit. J. Dermat., 62*:289, 1950.

311. GARLAND, J. G.: The discharging nipple. *The Jackson Clinic Bull., 16*:14, 1954.

312. GASCOYEN: *Trans. Path. Soc. London, 11*:267, 1860.

313. GEE, S. J.: *Medical Lectures and Clinical Aphorisms.* Oxford, Oxford University Press, 1908.

314. DEGENNES, L., DELARUE, J., AND DEVÉRICOURT, R.: Le syndrome endocrino-hépatocardiaque. *Presse méd., 44*:377, 1936.

315. GENTRY, R. W., DOCKERTY, M. B. AND CLAGETT, O. T.: Vascular malformations and vascular tumors of the gastrointestinal tract. *Surg., Gyn., & Ob., 88*:281, 1949.

316. GEOGHEGAN, T. AND MUELLER, E. J.: Diencephalic autonomic attacks: report of a case with predominantly sympathetic manifestations. *New Eng. J. Med., 247*:841, 1952.

317. GIAMPALMO, A.: The arteriovenous angiomatosis of the lung with hypoxaemia. *Acta Med. Scand., Supp. 248* (with Vol. 139), 1950.

318. GRIFFIN, H. Z.: Familial epistaxis without telangiectasia. *Am. J. M. Sc., 174*:690, 1927.

319. GILBERT, A. AND HERSCHER, M.: Des naevi artériels et capillaires dans les maladies du foie et des voies biliaires. *Compt. rend. Soc. de biol., 55*:167, 1903.

320. GILBERT, I.: Angioma venosum racemosum with angiomatous lesions of skin and omentum. *Brit. M. J., 1*:468, 1952.

321. GILBERT, N. C. AND deTAKATS, G.: Emergency treatment of apoplexy. *J.A.M.A., 136*:659, 1948.

322. GILFILLAN, R. S., FREEMAN, N. E., AND LEEDS, F. H.: A clinical estimation of the blood pressure in the minute vessels of the human skin by the method of elevation and reactive hyperemia. I. The treatment and prognosis of necrotic lesions of the foot. *Circulation, 9*:180, 1954.

323. GILMER, B. VON H.: The glomus body as a receptor of cutaneous pressure and vibration. *Psychol. Bull., 39*:73, 1942.

324. GILMER, B. VON H.: The relation of cold sensitivity to sweat duct distribution and the neuro-vascular mechanisms of the skin. *J. Psychol., 13*:307, 1942.

325. GILMER, B. VON H. AND HAYTHORN, S. R.: Cutaneous pressure-vibration spots and their underlying tissues. *Arch. Neurol. & Psychiat., 46*:621, 1941.

326. VAN GILSE, P. H. G. AND POSTMA, C.: Herhaalde hevige neusbloedingen als verschijnsel van erfelijke verwijding van eindbloedvaten van slijmvliezen en huid (Zietke van Osler). *Nederl. tij. genees., 72(II)*:2648, 1928.

327. GITLOW, S., AND FROSCH, H. L.: Multiple hemorrhagic telangiectasis (Rendu-Weber-Osler disease): report of four cases. *New York J. Med., 46*:635, 1946.

328. GJESSING, E.: Telangiectasia hereditaria haemorrhagica (Osler). *Dermat. Ztschr., 23*:193, 1916.

329. GLASS, S. J., EDMONDSON, H. D., AND SOLL, S. N.: Sex hormone changes associated with liver disease. *Endocrinology, 27*:749, 1940.

330. GLASS, W. H.: Rutin therapy in diffuse capillary bleeding: Ineffectiveness when fragility tests are normal. *Am. J. M. Sc., 220*:409, 1950.

331. GLUSHIEN, A. S. AND MANSUY, M. M.: Superior vena caval obstruction with survival after thirty-six years. *Angiology, 2*:210, 1951.

332. GOBLE, A. J., HAY, D. R., AND SANDLER, M.: 5-hydroxytryptamine metabolism in acquired heart disease associated with argentaffin carcinoma. *Lancet, 2*:1016, 1955.

333. GOETZ, R. H.: The pathology of progressive systemic sclerosis (generalized scleroderma) with special reference to changes in the viscera. *Clinical Proceedings, 4*:337, 1945.

333a. GOLDECK, H. AND STILLER, S.: Morbus Osler. *Med. Klin., 45*:1617, 1950.

333b. GOLDMAN, A.: Cavernous hemangioma of the lungs: secondary polycythemia. *Dis. of Chest, 9*:479, 1943.

333c. GOLDMAN, A.: Arteriovenous fistula of the lungs: its hereditary and clinical aspects. *Am. Rev. Tuber., 57*:266, 1948.

334. GOLDMAN, L. AND RICHFIELD, D. F.: Effect of corticotropin and cortisone on development of progress pigmented nevi. *J.A.M.A., 147*:941, 1951.

335. GOLDMAN, R., ASHER, L., AND WARE, E. R.: Hereditary hemorrhagic telangiectasis. *Gastroenterology, 12*:495, 1949.

336. GOLDSTEIN, H. I.: Hereditary hemorrhagic telangiectasia with recurring (familial) hereditary epistaxis: with a report of eleven cases in one family. *Arch. Int. Med., 27*:102, 1921.

337. GOLDSTEIN, H I.: Hereditary epistaxis, with and without hereditary (familial) multiple hemorrhagic telangiectasia (Osler's disease). *Internat. Clin., 40*:148, 1930.

338. GOLDSTEIN, H. I.: Hereditary epistaxis; with and without hereditary (familial) multiple hemorrhagic telangiectasia (Osler's disease). *Internat. Clin., 40*:253, 1930.

339. GOLDSTEIN, H. I.: Goldstein's heredofamilial angiomatosis with recurring familial hemorrhages. (Rendu-Osler-Weber's disease). *Arch. Int. Med., 48*:836, 1931.

340. GOLDSTEIN, H. I.: Goldstein's disease or Rendu-Osler-Weber's disease. *Acta. Derma. Ven., 13*:661, 1932.

341. GOLDSTEIN, H. I.: Hereditary multiple telangiectasia; Goldstein's heredofamilial angiomatosis with familial hemorrhages or Rendu-Osler-Weber's disease. *Arch. Derm. & Syph., 26*:282, 1932.

342. GOLDSTEIN, H. I.: Heredofamilial angiomatosis with recurring hemorrhages. *Trans. Amer. Therap. Soc., 47*:47, 1932.

343. GOLDSTEIN, H. I.: Heredofamilial angiomatosis (telangiectasia) with recurring hemorrhages. *Internat. Clin., 2*:43, 1934.

344. GOLDSTEIN, H. I.: Rendu-Osler-Weber's disease. *Brit. M. J., 1*:721, 1936.

345. GOLDSTEIN, H. I.: Familial haemoptysis of unusual aetiology. *Brit. M. J., 1*:1275, 1936.

346. GOLDSTEIN, H. I.: Unusual gastrorrhagia or hematemesis. *Med Rec., 146*:530, 1937.

347. GOLDSTEIN, H. I.: Unusual hematemesis or gastrorrhagia. *Amer. J. Dig. Dis., 5*:115, 1938.

348. GOLDSTEIN, H. I.: Unusual hemoptysis or bronchostaxis. *Med. World, 56*:385, 1938.

349. GOLDSTEIN, H. I.: Unusual (benign) hematemesis: gastric telangiectatic dysplasia; Rendu-Osler-Weber disease (Goldstein's hematemesis). *Rev. Gastroenterol.*, *14*:258, 1947.

350. GOLDSTEIN, H. I. AND GOLDSTEIN, H. Z.: Familial (hereditary) epistaxis. *M. Times*, *58*:331, 1930.

351. GOORWITCH, J. AND MADOFF, I.: Capillary hemangioma of the lung. *Dis. Chest*, *28*:98, 1955.

352. GORDON, H. W.: Telangiectasia: case for diagnosis. *Proc. Roy. Soc. Med.* (Sect. Derm.), *25*:1552, 1932.

353. GOTSCH, K.: Fall von Morbus Osler (Teleangiectasia hereditaria haemorrhagica). *Klin. Wchnschr.*, *11*:837, 1932.

354. GOUGERHOT, H. AND MEYER, J.: Télangiectasies périodiques, gravidiques et famiales, apparissant et disparaissant avec la grossesse. *Bull. Soc. franc. de derma. et Syph.*, *36*:1032, 1929.

355. GOYETTE, E. M. AND PALMER, P. W.: Cardiovascular lesions in arachnodactyly. *Circulation*, *7*:373, 1953.

356. GRAEF, I.: Medial hypertrophy of the renal arterioles in pregnancy. *Am. J. Path.*, *19*:121, 1943.

357. GRANT, R. T.: Observations on direct communications between arteries and veins in the rabbit's ear. *Heart, 15*:281, 1930.

358. GRANT, R. T. AND BLAND, E. F.: Observations on arteriovenous anastomoses in human skin and in the bird's foot with special reference to the reaction to cold. *Heart*, 15:385, 1931.

359. GRAVES, R. J.: *System of Clinical Medicine*. Dublin, Fannin and Co., 1843.

360. GRAY, F. D., JR., LURIE, P. R., AND WHITTEMORE, R.: Circulatory changes in pulmonary arterio-venous fistula. *Yale J. of Biol. and Med.*, *25*:107, 1952.

361. GREEN, R. E.: Rendu-Osler-Weber's disease. *U. S. Armed Forces Med. J.*, 5:1365, 1954.

362. GREY, H.: Telangiectasia (hereditary hemorrhagic). *Arch. Derm. & Syph.*, *25*:177, 1932.

363. GRIFFITH, J. Q., JR., COUCH, J. F., AND LINDAUER, M. A.: Effect of rutin on increased capillary fragility in man. *Proc. Soc. Exp. Biol. Med.*, *55*:228, 1944.

364. GRIGGS, D. E. AND BAKER, M. Q.: Hereditary hemorrhagic telangiectasia with gastrointestinal bleeding. *Am. J. Diges. Dis.*, *8*:344, 1941.

365. GUNDRUM, F. F.: Hereditary hemorrhagic telangiectases. *Calif. St. J. Med.*, *17*:78, 1919.

366. GUTTMAN, R. A.: Télangiectasie héréditaire et familiale avec hématémèses profuses ayant simulé un ulcère gastrique. *Presse méd.*, *40*:182, 1932.

367. GUY, W. H. AND AMSHEL, F.: Familial telangiectasia. *Arch. Derm. & Syph.*, *29*:778, 1934.

368. GWYN, N. B.: The clinical picture in spirochaetal jaundice, with notes on the detection of the parasite in the circulating blood. *Med. & Biol. Res.*, Dedicated to Sir William Osler, *1*:533, 1919.

369. HALPER, H. AND WEDLICK, L.: Maffucci's syndrome: with report of a case. *M. J. Australia, 1*:936, 1951.

370. HAMBERGER, C. A.: Telangiectasia haemorrhagica hereditaria (Osler). *Nord. Med.*, *4*:3472, 1939.

371. HAMWI, G. J.: Marfan's syndrome (arachnodactyly). *Am. J. Medicine, 11*:261, 1951.

419. HULTGREN, H. N. AND GERBODE, F.: Physiologic studies in a patient with a pulmonary arteriovenous fistula. *Am. J. Med., 17*:126, 1954.
420. HURLEY, H. J., JR. AND MESCON, H.: The cholinergic innervation of the digital arterial anastomoses of human skin. A histochemical localization of cholinesterase. *Am. J. App. Phys., 9*:82, 1956.
421. HURST, A. F., HAMPSON, A. C., PLUMMER, N. S., AND YATES, A. G.: Hereditary telangiectasia with haemorrhagic tendency. *Guy's Hosp. Rep., 82*:81, 1932.
422. HUTCHINSON, J.: On the spider-naevus. *Arch. Surg.* (Lond.), *4*:73, 1893.
423. HUTCHINSON, J.: *Archives of Surgery,* London, 1-11: 1889-1900.
424. HUTCHINSON, R. AND OLIVER, W. J.: Multiple telangiectases with epistaxis of the familial type. *Quart. J. Med., 9*:67, 1916.
425. HYDE, J. N.: Telangiectatic lesions of the skin occurring in the subjects of Graves' disease. *Brit. J. Dermat., 20*:33, 1908.
426. INGLIS, K.: The nature of neurofibromatosis and related lesions, with special reference to certain lesions of bones: illustrating the influence of intrinsic factors in disease when development of the body is abnormal. *J. Path. & Bact., 62*:519, 1950.
427. INGLIS, K.: Local gigantism (manifestation of neurofibromatosis): its relation to general gigantism and to acromegaly. *Am. J. Path., 26*:1059, 1950.
428. INGLIS, K.: The nature of agenesis and deficiency of parts: the influence of intrinsic factors in disease when development of the body is abnormal as illustrated by agenesis of the digits, facial hemiatrophy, and cerebral agyria and microgyria. *Am. J. Path., 28*:449, 1952.
429. INGLIS, K.: La nature du prétendu (adénome sébacé) de la sclérose tubéreuse. *La Semaine des Hopitaux de Paris (Archives d'Anatomie Pathologique), 30*: 26, 1954.
430. IRELAND, T. L. AND PASCUCCI, S. E.: Arachnodactyly (Marfan's syndrome) associated with rheumatic fever. *Bull. St. Francis Sanatorium, 10*:32, 1953.
431. ISRAEL, H. L. AND GOSFIELD, E., JR.: Fatal hemoptysis from pulmonary arteriovenous fistula. *J.A.M.A., 152*:40, 1953.
432. JACKSON, H. AND BALKIN, R.: Glomus tumors (angioneuromyomas). A clinical and pathologic report of an unusual case. *Arch. Surg., 53*:100, 1946.
433. JACOB, A.: Dépilation axillaire au cours des cirrhoses hépatiques. *Presse med., 42*:2076, 1934.
434. JACOBS, E. C.: Gynecomastia following severe starvation. *Ann. Int. Med., 28*: 792, 1948.
435. JACOBS, H. J., LEVY, L. II, CHASTANT, H., AND STRAUSS, H.: Angiocardiography in obstruction of the superior vena cava. *J.A.M.A., 147*:1051, 1951.
436. JACOBSON, P.: Spontaneous hemorrhage, a clinical entity with special reference to epistaxis. *A.M.A. Arch. Oto., 59*:523, 1954.
437. JANES, R. M.: Multiple cavernous haemangiomas of the lungs successfully treated by local resection of the tumours. *Brit. J. Surg., 31*:270, 1944.
438. JANEWAY, E. G.: Certain clinical observations upon heart disease. *Med. News, 75*:257, 1899.
439. JARVIS, F. J. AND KANAR, E. A.: Physiologic changes following obstruction of the superior vena cava. *J. Thoracic Surg., 27*:213, 1954.
440. JEFFORDS, J. V. AND KNISELY, M. H.: Concerning the geometric shapes of arteries and arterioles. A contribution to the biophysics of health, disease, and death. *Angiology, 7*:105, 1956.

441. JEGHERS, H.: Skin changes of nutritional origin. *New Eng. J. Med., 228*:714, 1943.

442. JEGHERS, H., McKUSICK, V. A., AND KATZ, K. H.: Generalized intestinal polyposis and melanin spots of oral mucosa, lips and digits: Syndrome of diagnostic significance. *New Eng. J. Med., 241*:993, and 1031, 1949.

443. JIMINEZ, D. C.: Aneurisma arteriovenosus pulmonar, con telangiectasis. *Rev. clín. Españ., 44*:1, 1952.

444. JOHNSEN, K.: Angiomatosis hereditaria (teleangiectasia hereditaria haemorrhagica (Osler). *Nord. Med., 14*:1413, 1942.

445. JOHNSON, R. M. AND HECHT, H. H.: Palmar erythema—its relationship to protein deficiency. *Am. J. M. Sc., 211*:79, 1946.

446. JOHNSON, W. M.: Hemiplegia during tetraethylthiuram disulfide (antabuse) therapy. *J.A.M.A. 149*:1014, 1952.

447. JOLLIFFE, N. AND JELLINEK, E. M.: Vitamin deficiencies and liver cirrhosis in alcoholism. *Quart. J. Stud. on Alcohol, 2*:544, 1941.

448. JOLLIFFE, N., ROSENBLUM, L. A., AND SAWHILL, J.: The effect of pyridoxine (vitamin B-6) on persistent adolescent acne. *J. Invest. Dermat., 5*:143, 1942.

449. JONES, E.: The demonstration of collateral venous circulation in the abdominal wall by means of infra-red photography. *Am. J. Med. Sc., 190*:478, 1935.

450. JONES, H. O. AND BREWER, J. I.: The arterial phenomena associated with uterine bleeding in tubal pregnancy. *Am. J. Obst. & Gynec., 38*:839, 1939.

451. JONES, J. C. AND THOMPSON, W. P.: Arterio-venous fistula of the lung: report of patient cured with pneumonectomy. *J. Thoracic Surg., 13*:357, 1944.

452. JONES, O. V.: Cyclical ulcerative vulvitis and stomatitis. *J. Ob. & Gyn., Br. Empire, 47*:557, 1940.

453. JUNIPER, K., JR.: Venous "spiders" in chronic lymphatic leukemia. *Am. J. Med., 16*:304, 1954.

454. JUNIUS, P.: Relationship between angiomatosis of the retina, exudative retinitis (Coat's) and Osler's disease. *Ztschr. f. Augenh., 84*:193, 1934.

455. KAHAN, A.: Spontaneous subarachnoid haemorrhage in children. *Brit. M. J., 1*:567, 1951.

456. KAHN, G. M.: The superior vena caval syndrome. *U. S. Armed Forces M. J., 1*:1455, 1950.

457. KAIJSER, R.: Uber Hamangiome des tractus gastrointestinales. *Archiv. fur klin chir., 187*:351, 1936-37.

458. KAPOSI, M., translated by Besnier, E. and Doyon, A.: *Pathology and Treatment of Skin Diseases.* Paris, Masson, 1891.

459. KARK, R. M., AITON, H. F., PEASE, E. D., BEAN, W. B., HENDERSON, C. R., JOHNSON, R. E., RICHARDSON, L. N.: Tropical deterioration and nutrition. Clinical and biochemical observations on troops. *Med., 26*:1, 1947.

460. KARK, R. M., MOREY, G. R., AND PAYNTER, C. R.: Re-feeding (nutritional) gynecomastia in cirrhosis of the liver: I. Clinical observations. *Am. J. Med. Sc., 222*:154, 1951.

461. KARSNER, H. T.: Gynecomastia. *Am. J. Pathology, 22*:235, 1946.

462. KEIL, H.: The rheumatic erythemas; a critical survey. *Ann. Int. Med., 11*:2223, 1938.

463. KELLER, P. D. AND NUTE, W. L., JR.: Cirrhosis of the liver in children. *J. Pediat., 34*:588, 1949.

464. KELLY, A. B.: Multiple telangiectases of the skin and mucous membranes of the nose and mouth. *Glasgow M. J., 65*:411, 1906.

465. KENNEDY, H. P.: Familial hemorrhagic telangiectasia with a note on use of oxidized cellulose as hemostatic agent in epistaxis. *New Eng. J. Med., 237*:180, 1947.

466. KESSEL, L.: Bleeding of benign origin. *J.A.M.A., 97*:1058, 1931.

467. KING, E. S. J.: Glomus tumor. *Australian and New Zealand J. Surg., 23*:280, 1954.

468. KING, G. AND SCHWARZ, G. A.: Sturge-Weber syndrome (encephalotrigeminal angiomatosis). *A.M.A. Arch. Int. Med., 94*:743, 1954.

469. KINNEY, T. W. AND FITZGERALD, P. J.: Lindau-von Hippel disease with hemangioblastoma of the spinal cord and syringomyelia. *Arch. Path., 43*:339, 1947.

470. KLATSKIN, G. AND RAPPAPORT, E. M.: Gynecomastia due to infectious hepatitis of the homologous serum type. *Am. J. Med. Sc., 214*:121, 1947.

471. KLATSKIN, G., SALTER, W. T., AND HUMM, F. D.: Gynecomastia due to malnutrition. I. Clinical Studies. *Am. J. Med. Sc., 213*:19, 1947.

472. KLAUDER, J. V.: Telangiectatic dysplasia of the Rendu-Osler-Weber type, with pigmentary changes. *Arch. Derm. & Syph., 42*:231, 1940.

473. KLAUDER, J. V.: Hereditary hemorrhagic telangiectasis treated with rutin. *Arch. Derm. & Syph., 57*:417, 1948.

474. KLEINSCHMIDT, W. H. AND SCHWARZ, S. O.: Familial hereditary hemorrhagic telangiectasia in the Negro. Report of a second case. *Ill. Med. J., 98*:298, 1950.

474a. KLUG, H.: Uber die ursache der teleangiektasien bei leberzirrhose und morbus Osler. *Wien. Ztschr. inn. Med., 30*:232, 1949.

475. KNAUER, J. G. AND MOYER, J.: Congenital familial hemorrhagic telangiectasis: case reports. *Bull. U. S. Army M. Dept., 8*:613, 1948.

476. KNISELY, M. H.: The histophysiology of peripheral vascular beds. *Blood, Heart and Circulation: Pub. No. 13,* A.A.A.S. Science Press, 1940.

477. KOCH, H. J., JR., ESCHER, G. C., AND LEWIS, J. S.: Hormonal management of hereditary hemorrhagic telangiectasia. *J.A.M.A., 149*:1376, 1952.

478. KOFLER, K.: Ein fall von "naevus Pringle" der haut mit teleangiektasien au den schleimhauten und wiederholten hamorrhagien aus denselben. *Wien. klin. Wchnschr., 21*:570, 1908.

479. KONRAD, E.: Essentielle teleangiektasien bei gravidität. *Centralbl. f. Haut. u. Geschlechtskr., 17*:275, 1925.

480. KOPP, K.: A case of multiple angiomata. *Arch. f. Derm., 38*:69, 1897.

481. KOSINER, R.: Uber familiare telangiektasie. *Klin. Wchnschr., 14*:713, 1935.

482. KRAMAR, J., MEYERS, V. W., SIMAY-KRAMAR, M., AND WILHELM J, C. M., JR.: Immediate capillary stress response. *Am. J. Phys., 184*:640, 1956.

483. KRAMAR, J., MEYERS, V. W., AND WILHELM J, C. M., JR.: Capillary stress response and species. *Proc. Soc. Exp. Biol. & Med., 89*:528, 1955.

484. KRAUSE, G. R.: Dyschondroplasia with hemangiomata (Maffucci's syndrome) case report. *Am. J. Roentgenol., 52*:620, 1944.

485. KROGH, A.: *The Anatomy and Physiology of Capillaries.* 2nd Ed., New Haven, Yale University Press, 1929.

486. KUGELMASS, I .N.: Clinical control of chronic hemorrhagic states in childhood. *J.A.M.A., 102*:287, 1934.

487. KUNO, Y.: *The Physiology of Human Perspiration.* London, Churchill, 1934.
488. KUNO, Y.: *Human Perspiration.* Springfield, Thomas, 1956.
489. KUSHLAN, S. D.: Gastrointestinal bleeding in hereditary hemorrhagic telangiectasia. *Gastroenterology, 7:*199, 1946.
490. KUSHLAN, S. D.: Incompatibility of rutin and sulfonamides. *J.A.M.A., 133:*716, 1947.
491. KUSHLAN, S. D.: Hereditary hemorrhagic telangiectasia with pulmonary arteriovenous aneurysm—possible etiology and prophylaxis. *Connecticut M. J., 16:* 505, 1952.
492. KUSHLAN, S. D.: Hereditary hemorrhagic telangiectasia, occurrence in the Negro. *Angiology, 4:*346, 1953.
493. KUZMA, J. F. AND KING, J. M.: Dyschrondroplasia with hemangiomatosis (Maffucci's syndrome) and teratoid tumor of the ovary. *Arch. Path., 46:*74, 1948.
494. LAFITTE, A.: La fonction vasculo-sanguine du foie en pathologie digestive. Thèse de Paris, Amédée Legrand, 1934.
495. LAFFONT, A.: Télangiectasie héréditaire hémorragique et angiomatose miliare. *Presse méd., 17:*763, 1909.
496. LAIGNEL-LAVASTINE, TROISIER J. AND BOQUIEN, Y.: Association de la cirrhose du foie à une dépilation plus ou moins complète et à une insuffisance thyroovarienne. *Bull. Soc. méd. hôp. Paris, 55:*829, 1931.
497. LAL, R. AND DAS GUPTA, A. C.: Investigations into the epidemiology of epidemic dropsy, part X. *Indian J. of Med. Research, 29:*157, 1941.
498. LAL, R. AND ROY, S. C.: Investigations into the epidemiology of epidemic dropsy, parts I and II. *Indian J. of Med. Research, 25:*163, 1937.
499. LANCEPLAINE, R.: *Télangiectasies Essentielles.* Paris Thesis, H. Jouve, 1904.
500. LANGMEAD, F.: A case of hereditary multiple telangiectases. *Proc. Roy. Soc. Med.* (Clin. Sect.), *3:*109, 1910.
501. LARRABEE, R. C. AND LITTMAN, D.: Hereditary hemorrhagic telangiectasia, with report of five cases in two families. *New Eng. J. Med., 207:*1177, 1932.
502. LATHEM, W., LESSER, G. T., MESINGER, W. J., AND GALDSTON, M.: Peripheral embolism by metallic mercury during arterial blood sampling. *A.M.A. Arch. Int. Med., 93:*550, 1954.
503. LAWLESS, T. K.: Telangiectasia (Hereditary hemorrhagic)? Osler's "recurring epistaxis with multiple telangiectases of the skin and mucous membranes"? *Arch. Derm. & Syph., 30:*295, 1934.
504. LAWTON, R. L., TIDRICK, R. T., AND BRINTNALL, E. S.: A clinico-pathological study of multiple congenital arteriovenous fistulae of the lower extremities. *Angiology, 8:*161, 1957.
505. LAZARUS, J. A. AND MARKS, M. S.: Benign intestinal tumors of vascular origin. *Surgery, 22:*766, 1947.
506. LEE, R. E.: Nutritional and metabolic factors in peripheral vasomotor reactions: vasocompensatory impairment induced by avitaminosis C. *Fed. Proc., 9:*76, 1950.
507. LEFTWICH, P.: Case of hereditary multiple telangiectasis (Rendu-Weber-Osler disease). *South African M. J., 14:*305, 1940.
508. LEGG, J. W.: A case of haemophilia complicated with multiple naevi. *Lancet, 2:*856, 1876.

509. LEHNER, E. AND KENEDY, D.: Further contributions to inflammations of the skin with reticulate or branched markings. Inflammatio cutis racemosa. *Arch. f. Dermat. u. Syph., 149*:387, 1925.

509a. LEHNER, E. AND KENEDY, D.: Inflammation of the skin with reticular or branched markings. *Archiv. f. Dermat. u. Syph., 141*:325, 1922.

510. LEINWAND, I., DURYEE, A. W., AND RICHTER, M. N.: Scleroderma, based on a study of over 150 cases. *Ann. Int. Med., 41*:1003, 1954.

511. LEITER, L.: The capillary vascular lesion in diabetes melitus. Its clinical manifestations and significance. *Diabetes, 4*:280, 1955.

512. LENSON, N.: Nevus unius lateralis. *New Eng. J. Med., 248*:757, 1953.

513. LEONARD, F. C. AND VASSOS, G. A., JR.: Congenital arteriovenous fistulation of the lower limb. *New Eng. J. Med., 245*:885, 1951.

514. LEQUIME, J. AND DENOLIN, H.: Circulatory dynamics in osteitis deformans. *Circulation, 12*:215, 1955.

515. LÉTIENNE, A. AND ARNAL, E.: Télangiectases multiples chez une basedowienne. *Arch. Gen de Méd., 1*:513, 1897.

516. LÉVI, L., AND DELHERM, L.: Un nouveau cas de télangiectases acquises généralisées. *Gaz. hebdomadaire de méd. et chir., 48*:13, 1901.

517. LEWIS, J. H., FERGUSON, J. H., FRESH, J. W. AND ZUCKER, M. B.: Primary hemorrhagic diseases. *J. Lab. & Clin. Med., 49*:211, 1957.

518. LEWIS, T.: Vascular reactions of the skin to injury. Part IV. An irresponsive condition of the vessels with special reference to the pathology of telangiectases and allied conditions. *Heart, 13*:153, 1926.

519. LEWIS, T.: *The Blood Vessels of the Human Skin and Their Responses.* London, Shaw & Sons, Ltd., 1927.

520. LIAN, P. C. AND COBLENTZ, B.: Le cathétérisme veineux au cours des compressions de la veine cave supérieure. *Arch. des Maladies du Coeru, 44*.634, 1951.

521. LIBMAN, E. AND OTTENBERG, R.: *Hereditary Hemoptysis.* Contributions to Medical and Biological Research Dedicated to Sir William Osler, Vol. I, p. 632, New York, Paul B. Hoeber, Inc., 1919.

522. LICHTMAN, S. S.: *Diseases of the Liver, Gall Bladder, and Bile Ducts.* 3rd ed., Philadelphia, Lea & Febiger, 1953.

523. LILLIAN, M.: Multiple pulmonary artery aneurysms. *Am. J. Med., 7*:280, 1949.

524. LINDE, L. M.: Diagnosis and management of dysautonomia. *Pediatrics, 18*:692, 1956.

525. LINDHEIMER, G. T., HINMAN, W. F., AND HALLIDAY, E. G.: Function and occurrence of citrin (Vitamin P). *J. Am. Dietet. A., 18*:503, 1942.

526. LISTER, W. A.: The natural history of strawberry naevi. *Lancet, 1*:1429, 1938.

527. LLOYD, C. W. AND WILLIAMS, R. H.: Endocrine changes associated with Laennec's cirrhosis of the liver. *Am. J. Med., 4*:315, 1948.

528. LOEPER, M., LOEW-LION, AND NETTER, A.: Les télangiectasies éruptives des hépatiques. *Le sang., 11*:677, 1937.

529. LOFGREN, R. C.: Erythema of the palms associated with pregnancy. *Arch. Derm. & Syph., 46*:502, 1942.

530. LUCAS, C. J. AND DAVIS, S.: Tuberous sclerosis with involvement of the cervical cord. *Lancet, 2*:1217, 1955.

531. LUKL, P.: Telangiecktasia hereditaria haemorrhagica (Oslerova choroba). *Cásopsis Lékaru Ceskych, 76*:1808, 1937.

532. LUNDBAEK, K.: Diabetic angiopathy, a specific vascular disease. *Lancet, 1*:377, 1954.

533. LYNN, R. B.: Chilblains. *Surg. Gynec. & Obst., 99*:720, 1954.

534. LYNN, R. B., STEINER, R. E., AND VAN WYK, F. A. K.: Arteriographic appearances of the digital arteries of the hands in Raynaud's disease. *Lancet, 1*:471, 1955.

535. LYONS, H. A. AND MANNIX, E. P., JR.: Successful resections for bilateral pulmonary arteriovenous fistulas. *New Eng. J. Med., 254*:969, 1956.

536. MACKAY, H. AND McKENTY, F. D.: Hereditary hemorrhagic telangiectasia. *Canad. M. A. J., 17*:65, 1927.

537. MACKENZIE, J. N.: Irritation of the sexual apparatus as an etiological factor in the production of nasal disease. *Am. J. M. Sc., 87*:360, 1884.

538. MACKLIN, M. T.: Heredity and the physician. *Scient. Monthly, 52*:56, 1941.

539. MADDEN, J. F.: Generalized angiomatosis (telangiectasia). *J.A.M.A. 102*:442, 1934.

540. MADDEN, J. F.: Hereditary hemorrhagic telangiectasia. *Arch. Derm. & Syph., 36*:675, 1937.

541. MADDEN, J. F.: Hereditary hemorrhagic telangiectasia. *Arch. Derm. & Syph., 44*:540, 1941.

542. MAGNUSON, H. J. AND RAULSTON, B. O.: The iron content of the skin in hemochromatosis. *Ann. Int. Med., 16*:687, 1942.

543. MAIER, H. C., HIMMELSTEIN, A., RILEY, R. L., AND BUNIM, J. J.: Arteriovenous fistula of the lung. *J. Thoracic Surg., 17*:13, 1948.

544. MAJOCCHI, D.: (Quoted by Harris, H. F.) *Pellagra*. New York, Macmillan, 1919.

545. MANDELBAUM, H., SPATT, S. D., AND FIERER, L. E.: Diencephalic epilepsy and the diencephalic syndrome. *Ann. Int. Med., 34*:911, 1951.

546. MANTCHIK, H.: Le traitement par les injections intratrachéales, technique et résultats. *Schweiz. med. Wchnschr., 3*:949, 1922.

547. MARCHAND, E. J., HEJTMANCIK, M. R., AND HERRMANN, G. R.: Extracardiac arteriovenous fistulas in the thorax. *Am. Heart J., 42*:682, 1951.

548. MARIE, A.: *Pellagra*. (Trans. by Lavinder, C. H. and Babcock, J. W.) State Co., Columbia, S. C., 1910.

549. MARKEE, J. E.: Relation of uterine regression to menstrual bleeding in intraocular endometrial transplants in the rhesus monkey. *Anat. Rec., 70* (Supp. 3):54, 1938.

550. MARKEE, J. E., DAVIS, J. H., AND HINSEY, J. C.: Uterine bleeding in spinal monkeys. *Anat. Rec., 64*:231, 1936.

551. MARKOFF, N.: Die rutin-behandlung der Oslerschen krankheit. *Schweiz. med. Wchnschr., 78*:984, 1948.

552. MARMIER, C. AND HITZIG, W. H.: Multiple arterio-venous lungenaneurysmen bei morbus Osler (Telangiectasia hemorrhagica hereditaria). *Radiol. Clin., 19*: 333, 1950.

553. MARONDE, R. F.: Brain abscess and congenital heart disease. *Ann. Int. Med., 33*:602, 1950.

554. MARSHALL, R. J.: On a case of multiple vascular naevi with subsequent disappearance of many of them. *Glasgow M. J., 39*:105, 1893.

555. MARTINI, G. A.: Lebercirrhose bei morbus Osler, cirrhosis hepatis teleangiectatica. *Gastronenterologia, 83*:157, 1955.

556. MARTINI, G. A. AND HAGEMANN, J. E.: Fingernail changes in cirrhosis of the liver due to changes in peripheral blood flow. *Klin. woch., 1*:25, 1956.

557. MARTINI, G. A. AND STAUBESAND, J.: The morphology of vascular spiders in the skin of patients with liver disease. *Virchow's Archiv., 324*:147, 1953.

558. MARTORELL, F.: Glomus tumors. *Angiology, 1*:451, 1950.

559. MASON, K. E.: Changing concepts of the antisterility vitamin (vitamin E). *Yale J. Biol. & Med., 14*:605, 1942.

560. MASON, K. E.: A hemorrhagic state in the vitamin E-deficient fetus of the rat. *Essays in Biol.,* U. of Calif. Press, 1943.

561. MASSON, P.: Le glomus neuromyo-arteriel des regions tactiles et ses tumeurs. *Lyon Chir., 21*:257, 1924.

562. MASSON, P.: Les glomus cutaneous de l'homme. *Bull. Soc. franc. dermat. et syph., 42*:1174, 1935.

563. MASSOPUST, L. C.: Infra-red photography. *Radiography and Clin. Photography, 10*:3, 1934.

564. MASSOPUST, L. C.: Infra-red photographic study of the changing pattern of the superficial veins in a case of human pregnancy. *Surg. Gynec. & Obst., 63*:86, 1936.

565. MASSOPUST, L. C.: Infra-red photography. *J. Biol. Photographic Assn., 13*:139, 1945.

566. MASSOPUST, L. C., SR.: *Infra-red Photography in Medicine.* Springfield. Thomas, 1952.

567. MASSOPUST, L. C. AND GARDNER, W. D.: Infrared photographic studies of the superficial thoracic veins in the female; anatomical considerations. *Surg. Gynec. & Obst., 91*:717, 1950.

568. MASSOPUST, L. C. AND GARDNER, W. D.: The infrared phlegogram in the diagnosis of breast complaints; an analysis of 1200 cases. *Surg. Gynec. & Obst., 97*:619, 1953.

569. MATIS, P., FUNFACK, H., AND ROCKSTROH, C.: Untersuchungen uber den einfluss des rutins die blutgerinming im hinblick auf die therapie und prophylaxie mit dicumarol bzw. Dicumarolderivaten. *Schweiz. med. Wchnschr., 80*:701, 1950.

570. McARTHUR, G. A. D.: Hereditary multiple telangiectasia, with the record of an affected Australian family. *M. J. Aust., 1*:780, 1937.

571. McCARTHY, L.: *Histopathology of Skin Diseases.* St. Louis, Mosby, 1931.

572. McCARTHY, W. D. AND PACK, G. T.: Malignant blood vessel tumors: a report of 56 cases of angiosarcoma and Kaposi's sarcoma. *Surg. Gyn. & Ob., 91*:465, 1950.

573. McDONOUGH, F. E., DRY, T. J., AND ROTH, G. M.: Hereditary telangiectasia with visceral involvement; Special studies of skin temperature: report of a case. *Mayo Clin. Proc. Staff Meet., 15*:593 and 624, 1940.

574. McEWAN, T.: Hereditary hemorrhagic telangiectasia: with report of a case. *Glasgow M. J., 29*:255, 1948.

575. McGIBBON, J. E. G. AND BAKER-BATES, E. T.: Direct bronchoscopic investigation in hemoptysis without physical or radiological manifestations. *Brit. M. J., 1*:109, 1937.

576. McGUINNESS, A. E., WATSON, L. C .A., LINDSELL, C. K., AND INGLIS, K.: Melorheostosis: Its relation to associated conditions and a case report. *Australian Ann. Med., 2*:84, 1953.

577. McIntire, F. T. and Sykes, E. M., Jr.: Obstruction of the superior vena cava: a review of the literature and report of two personal cases. *Ann. Int. Med., 30*:925, 1949.

578. McKhann, C. F., Belnap, W. D., and Beck, C. S.: Cervical arteriovenous anastomosis in treatment of mental retardation, convulsive disorders and cerebral spasticity. *Ann. Surg., 132*:162, 1950.

579. MacKenna, R. W.: *Diseases of the Skin.* 4th ed., Baltimore, Wood, 1937.

580. McKusick, V. A.: The cardiovascular aspects of Marfan's syndrome: a heritable defect of connective tissue. *Circulation, 11*:321, 1955.

581. McKusick, V. A.: *Heritable Disorders of Connective Tissue.* St. Louis. Mosby, 1956.

582. Meigs, J. V.: Endometriosis—its significance. *Ann. Surg., 114*:866, 1941.

583. Meikle, G. J.: A case of hereditary telangiectasia. *Lancet, 2*:863, 1933.

584. Mekie, E. C.: Hereditary haemorrhagic telangiectasia. *Brit. M. J., 1*:423, 1927.

585. Melbard, S. N.: Diagnostic value of capillaroscopy in pregnancy and in purpural sepsis. *Gyn. & Obst., 37*:200, 1938.

586. Memmesheimer, A. M.: Zur pathogenese der sogenannten essentiellen telangiektasien. *Dermat. Ztschr., 53*:399, 1928.

587. Mendlowitz, M.: Clubbing and hypertrophic osteoarthropathy. *Medicine, 21*: 269, 1942.

588. Mendlowitz, M.: *Digital Circulation.* New York, Grune & Stratton, 1954.

589. Meneely, J. K., Jr., and Bigelow, N. H.: Temporal arteritis—a critical evaluation of this disorder and a report of three cases. *Am. J. Med., 14*:46, 1953.

590. Merritt, H. H. and Aring, C. D.: The differential diagnosis of cerebral vascular lesions. *Proc. Assn. for Research in Nervous and Mental Dis., 18*:682, 1937.

591. Meyers, R.: Personal communication.

592. Mibelli: Una nuova forma di cheratosi, "angiokeratoma." *Gior. ital. d. mal. ven., 30*:285, 1889.

593. Michael, J. C. and Levin, P. M.: Multiple telangiectases of the brain; discussion of hereditary factors in their development. *Arch. Neurol. & Psychiat., 36*:514, 1936.

594. Milbradt, W.: Atypisches diffuse sklerodermie mit Oslerschem syndrome und leberstörung. *Dermat. Wchnsch., 99*:973, 1934.

595. Milian, G., Perin, L., and Langlois, L.: Angiomatose hémorragique familiale (Maladie de Rendu-Osler). *Bull. Soc. franc. Dermat. et Syph., 40*:846, 1933.

596. Millman, S.: Tricuspid stenosis and pulmonary stenosis complicating carcinoid of the intestine with metastasis to the liver. *Am. Heart J., 25*:391, 1943.

597. Mitchell, J. H.; Discussion of Madden, J. F.: Generalized angiomatosis, (telangiectasia). *J.A.M.A., 102*:448, 1934.

598. Mithoefer, J. and Bean, W. B.: Gynecomastia in cirrhosis of the liver. *Surgery, 25*:911, 1949.

599. Mohr, O. L. and Wriedt, C.: A new type of hereditary brachyphalangy in man. *Carnegie Inst. of Wash. Pub. 295,* 1919.

600. Morgan, H. W.: Personal letter to the author. 1953.

601. Morris, M.: Case. *Brit. J. Dermat., 14*:220, 1902.

602. Mortimer, H., Wright, R. P., Bachman, C. and Collip, J. B.: Effect of oestrogenic hormone administration upon nasal mucous membrane of the monkey (Macaca mulatta). *Proc. Soc. Exper. Biol. & Med., 34*:535, 1936.

603. Moses, M. F.: Aortic aneurysm associated with arachnodactyly. *Brit. M. J., 2:* 81, 1951.

604. Mosny and Malloizel: Un cas de télangiectases acquises généralizées chez un Saturnin. *Bull. et Mem soc méd de hôp. Paris,* 3rd series, 22:867, 1905.

605. Moyer, J. H. and Ackerman, A. J.: Hereditary hemorrhagic telangiectases associated with pulmonary arterio-venous fistula in two members of a family. *Ann. Int. Med., 29:*775, 1948.

606. Mufson, I., M.D.: An etiology of scleroderma. *Ann. Int. Med., 39:*1219, 1953.

607. Mullins, J. F. and Livingood, C. S.: Maffucci's syndrome (Dyschrondroplasia with hemangiomas): a case with early osseous changes. *Arch. Derm. & Syph., 63:*478, 1951.

608. Murison, A. R., Sutherland, J. W., and Williamson, A. M.: DeMorgan's spots. *Brit. M. J., 1:*634, 1947.

609. Murray, M. R. and Stout, A. P.: The glomus tumor. Investigation of its distribution and behavior, and the identity of its "epitheloid" cell. *Am. J. Path., 18:*183, 1942.

610. Murray, R. O.: Melorheostosis associated with congenital arterio-venous aneurysms. *Proc. Roy. Soc. Med.* (Ortho Scct.), *44:*473, 1951.

611. Naeceli, O.: Little known prodromes of progressive diffuse scleroderma (Eruptive telangiectases, purulent and diffuse pigmentation, urticarial erythema). *Scheweiz. med. Wchnschr., 65:*982, 1935.

612. Nardell, S. G.: Ollier's disease: dyschondroplasia. *Brit. M. J., 2:*555, 1950.

613. Neligan, G. A. and Strang, L. B.: A "harlequin" colour change in the newborn. *Lancet, 2:*1005, 1952.

614. Newman, B. A.: Discussion on Robinson, S. S.: Angioma serpiginosum. *Arch. Derm. & Syph., 45:*176, 1942.

615. Deleted in press.

616. Nickerson, J. L., Elkin, D. C., and Warren, J. V.: The effect of temporary occlusion of arteriovenous fistulas on heart rate, stroke volume, and cardiac output. *J. Clin. Investigation, 30:*215, 1951.

617. Nicoll, P. A. and Webb, R. L.: Vascular patterns and active vasomotion as determiners of flow through minute vessels. *Angiology, 6:*291, 1955.

618. Nielsen, A., Jackson, T., and Schreiber, F.: Brain abscess metastatic from pleuropulmonary disease—case report. *Harper Hosp. Bull., 8:*45, 1950.

619. Nightingale, J. A.: A case of pulmonary arteriovenous fistula. *Brit. M. J., 2:* 402, 1951.

620. Noble, J. F., Ferrin, A., and Merandino, K. A.: Pigmented nevus of the fingernail matrix. *Arch. Derm. & Syph., 65:*49, 1952.

621. Nödl, F.: The histopathology of hereditary hemorrhagic telangiectasia (Rendu-Osler). *Archiv. f. Klin u. Exper. Dermat., 204:*213, 1957.

622. Ober, W. B. and Lecompte, P. N.: Acute fatty metamorphosis of the liver associated with pregnancy. *Am. J. Med., 19:*743, 1955.

623. Obermayer, M. E., and Wilson, J. W.: Fascial hernias of the legs. *J.A.M.A., 145:*548, 1951.

624. Deleted in press.

625. O'Kane, G. H.: Hereditary multiple telangiectasis with epistaxis. *J.A.M.A., 111:*242, 1938.

626. Opie, L. H.: The pulmonary manifestations of generalized scleroderma (progressive systemic sclerosis). *Dis. of the Chest, 28:*665, 1955.

627. ORMSBY, O. S. AND MITCHELL, J. H.: Generalized telangiectasia. *Arch. Derm. & Syph.*, *5*:781, 1922.

628. OSLER, W.: On a family form of recurring epistaxis, associated with multiple telangiectases of the skin and mucous membranes. *Bull. Johns Hopkins Hosp.*, *12*:333, 1901.

629. OSLER, W.: On multiple hereditary telangiectases with recurring haemorrhages. *Quart. J. Med.*, *1*:53, 1907.

630. OSLER, W.: On telangiectasis circumscripta universalis. *Bull. Johns Hopkins Hosp.*, *18*:401, 1907.

631. PACK, G. T. AND DAVIS, J.: Moles and melanomas. *Modern Med.*, *24*:96, 1956.

632. PACK, G. T., LENSON, N., AND GERBER, D. M.: Regional distribution of moles and melanomas. *A.M.A. Arch. of Surg.*, *65*:862, 1952.

633. PACK, G. T. AND MILLER, T. R.: Hemangiomas, classification, diagnosis and treatment. *Angiology*, *1*:405, 1950.

634. PAGE, I. H.: A syndrome simulating diencephalic stimulation occurring in patients with essential hypertension. *Am. J. M. Sc.*, *190*:9, 1935.

635. PAGE, I. H.: Serotonin (5-hydroxytryptamine). *Physiol. Rev.*, *34*:563, 1954.

636. PAGNIEZ, P., PLICHET, A. AND RENDU, C.: Contribution à la connaissance de la maladie de Rendu-Osler (angiomatose hémorragique), à propos de deux cas anormaux (2). *Bull. Acad. Nat. Méd.*, *115*:742, 1936.

637. PAISSEAU, G. AND OUMANSKY, V.: Syndrome hypophysaire avec cirrhose du foie et splénomégalie. *Bull. Soc. méd. hôp. Paris*, *54*:267, 1930.

638. PARDO-CASTELLO, V. AND FARINAS, E. P.: Hereditary multiple telangiectasia (Rendu-Osler disease). *Arch. Derm. & Syph.*, *39*:1025, 1939.

639. PATEK, A. J., JR., POST, J. AND VICTOR, J. C.: The vascular "spider" associated with cirrhosis of the liver. *Am. J. M. Sc.*, *200*:341, 1940.

640. PATEK, A. J., JR., AND POST, J.: Treatment of cirrhosis of the liver by a nutritious diet and supplements rich in vitamin B complex. *J. Clin. Invest.*, *20*:481, 1941.

641. PAUL, O., SWEET, R. H., AND WHITE, P. D.: Coronary arteriovenous fistula. *Am. Heart J.*, *37*:441, 1949.

642. PAUL, S. N.: Hereditary angiomata (telangiectases) with epistaxis. *Brit. J. Dermat.*, *30*:27, 1918.

643. PAULA, F.: Gynäkomastie und Leberzirrhose. *Deutsches Archiv für klinische Medizin.*, *169*:83, 1930.

644. PAUTRIER, L. M., AND ULLMO, A.: Télangiectasies stellaires, acquises chez une femme enceinte, localisées au membre supérieur droit, sur le territoire du plexus cervical. *Bull. Soc. franc. dermat. et syph.*, *38*:309, 1931.

645. PEARSON: cited by Cockayne, E. A. (1933).

646. PECK, S. M.: Osler's hereditary familial telangiectases. *Arch. Derm. & Syph.*, *34*:1060, 1936.

647. PECK, S. M. AND ROSENTHAL, N.: Effect of moccasin snake venom (*ancistrodon pescivarus*) in hemorrhagic conditions. *J.A.M.A.*, *104*:1066, 1935.

648. PECK, S. M., ROSENTHAL, N. AND ERF, L.: Purpura—classification and treatment, with special reference to treatment with snake venom. *Arch. Derm. & Syph.*, *35*:831, 1937.

649. PELUSE, S.: Gingival hemorrhage with oral manifestations in hereditary hemorrhagic telangiectasis; successful control with sclerosing agent sylnasol; effect of vitamin P and nicotinic acid; role in case reported which was observed 5 years. *Arch. Otolaryng.*, *44*:668, 1946.

650. PENFIELD, W.: Diencephalic autonomic epilepsy. *Arch. Neurol. & Psychiat.,* 22:358, 1929.

651. PENFOLD, J. B. AND LIPSCOMB, J. M.: Elliptocytosis in man associated with hereditary hemorrhagic telangiectasis. *Quart. J. Med.,* 12:157, 1943.

652. PENROSE, L. S.: Some genetical problems in mental deficiency. *J. Ment. Sc.,* 84:693, 1938.

653. PERERA, G. A.: A note on palmar erythema (so-called liver palms). *J.A.M.A.,* 119:1417, 1942.

654. PERNET, G.: Symmetrical lividities of the soles of the feet. *Brit. J. Dermat.,* 37:123, 1925.

655. PERNOW, B., AND WALDENSTRÖM, J.: Paroxysmal flushing and other symptoms caused by 5-hydroxytryptamine and histamine in patients with malignant tumours. *Lancet,* 2:951, 1954.

656. PETCH, C. P.: Hereditary haemorrhagic telangiectasia. *Brit. M. J.,* 2:785, 1948

657. PETERKIN, G. A. G.: Malignant change in erythema ab igne. *Brit. M. J.,* 2:1599, 1955.

658. PETERS, G. A., PRICKMAN, L. E., KOELSCHE, G. A. AND CARRYER, H. M.: Smoking and asthma. *Proc. Staff Meet. Mayo Clin.,* 27:329, 1952.

659. PHILLIPS, S.: Multiple telangiectases. *Proc. Roy. Soc. Med.,* 1:64, 1908.

660. PICKERING, G. W.: Vascular spasm. *Lancet,* 2:845, 1951.

661. PIERQUIN, J., RICHARD, G. AND PIERQUIN, B.: Une méthode de traitment de la maladie de Rendu-Osler par la radiothérapie. *J. radiol. et électrol.,* 32:787, 1951.

662. PILLSBURY, D. M.: Multiple hereditary telangiectasia (Rendu-Weber-Osler syndrome). *Arch. Derm. & Syph.,* 32:145, 1935.

663. PILLSBURY, D. M., SHELLY, W. B. AND KLIGMAN, A. M.: *Dermatology.* Philadelphia, Saunders, 1956.

664. PINCUS, G. AND MARTIN, D. W.: Liver damage and estrogen inactivation. *Endocrinology,* 27:838, 1940.

665. PIPILAS, G. A. AND STAVRAKAS, B.: Acquired arteriovenous fistula. *Am. Heart J.,* 44:793, 1952.

666. PIULACHS, P. AND VIDAL-BARRAQUER, F.: Una nueva enfermedad vascular periferica: la isquemia cronica cutanea de las piernas. *Med. clin.,* 16:297, 1951.

667. PIULACHS, P. AND VIDAL-BARRAQUER, F.: Formas de comienzo de la ulcera en la isquemia cronica cutanea. *Med. Clin.,* 17:86, 1951.

668. PIULACHS, P. AND VIDAL-BARRAQUER, F.: Les ulcères de jambe au cours de la maladie de Raynaud. *Presse Méd.,* 59:1197, 1951.

669. PIULACHS, P., VIDAL-BARRAQUER, F., AND BIEL, J. M.: Considérations pathogéniques sur les varices de la grossesse. *Lyon Chir.,* 47:263, 1952.

670. PLATT, R.: Life (biological, not biographical). *Lancet,* 1:61, 1956.

671. PLUMMER, K., BURKE, J. O., AND WILLIAMS, J. P.: Hereditary hemorrhagic telangiectasia with intestinal bleeding. *Gastroenterology,* 12:988, 1949.

672. PLUNGIAN, M. B., MUNCH, J. C., AND WOLFFE, J. B.: Effect of rutin on coagulation time of rat blood. *J. Pharmacol. & Exper. Therap.,* 93:383, 1948.

673. POLAYES, S. H. AND NEVINS, T. F.: Fatal hemorrhage from an angiomatous polyp of the ileum complicating pregnancy. *Am. J. Ob. & Gyn.,* 50:207, 1945.

674. POPOFF, N. W.: The digital vascular system. *Arch. Path.,* 18:295, 1934.

675. POTTER, J. M.: Carotid-cavernous fistula. *Brit. M. J.,* 2:786, 1954.

676. POWELL, E.: Cerebral malnutrition and its diagnosis. *Internat. Clin., 1*:101, 1941.
677. POYNTON, F. J. AND WYLLIE, W. G.: Hepatic cirrhosis in children with special reference to the biliary forms. *Arch. Dis. in Childhood, 1*:1, 1926.
678. PRASIL, K.: Clinical diagnosis of pulmonary arteriovenous areurysm in the course of Rendu-Osler's disease. *Casop. lék. česk., 89*:838, 1950.
679. PRICE, J. H.: Angiokeratoma corporis diffusum. *Brit. J. Dermat., 67*:105, 1955.
680. PROCTOR, W. H., JR.: Arteriovenous fistula of the aortic arch. *J.A.M.A., 144*:818, 1950.
681. PROPPE, A.: Zur Kasuistik der Oslerschen Teleangiektasia haemorrhagica hereditaria. *Dermat. Wchnschr., 106*:233, 1938.
682. PUGSLEY, H. E. AND JANES, R. M.: Arteriovenous aneurysm of the lung. *Dis. Chest., 20*:177, 1951.
683. PUSEY, W. A.: Discussion of Lane, J. E. Erythema palmare hereditarium. *Arch. Derm. & Syph., 20*:447, 1929.
684. RAASCHOU, F.: Et tilfaelde af teleangiectasia hereditaria haemorrhagica (Rendu-Osler) med stamtavle. *Nord. Med., 11*:2743, 1941.
685. RADSCHOW, M. AND BRODECKER, H.: The significance of vascular spiders in the diagnosis of liver disease. *Neue Med. Welt., 1*:1439, 1950.
686. RAPPORT, M. M., GREEN, A. A. AND PAGE, I. H.: Crystalline serotonin. *Science, 108*:329, 1948.
687. RATNOFF, O. D., AND PATEK, A. J., JR.: The natural history of Laennec's cirrhosis of the liver; an analysis of 386 cases. *Medicine, 21*:207, 1942.
688. RAVETTA, M.: Su di un caso di angiomatosi imonagica familiare (malattia Rendu-Osler). *Minerva med., Roma, 2*:332, 1937.
689. RAVINA, A.: Hereditary hemangiomatosis and arterio-venous aneurysm of the lung. *Presse méd., 57*:776, 1949.
690. RAYER, P.: *Traité des maladies de la peau.* Paris, 1835.
691. REINIGER, A.: Uber die teleangiectasia hereditaria haemorrhagica. *Wien. med. Wchnschr., 81*:1590, 1931.
692. REITZEL, R. J. AND BRINDLEY, P.: Spontaneous intracranial hemorrhage from a vascular tumor. *Am. J. M. Sc., 178*, 689, 1929.
693. RENAUT, JOSEPH-LOUIS: *Traité de l'Histologie Pratique,* Tom. I. Fascic. I. Paris, Lecrosnier and Babe, 1889.
693a. RENDU, H.: Epistaxis répétées chez un sujet porteur de petits angiomes cutanés et muqueux. *Bull. Soc. méd. hôp. Paris, 13*:731, 1896.
694. RENON, L. AND MIGNOT: Naeva vasculaires confluents de la face à la période prodromique de la cirrhose de Laennec. *Bull. Soc. méd. hôp. Paris, 39*:661, 1915.
695. RENSHAW, J. F.: Multiple hemorrhagic telangiectasis with special reference to gastroscopic appearance. *Cleveland Clinic Q., 6*:226, 1939.
696. REYNOLDS, S. R. M.: Essential features of ovarian and uterine blood flow in visceral circulation. *Ciba Foundation Symposium*, Boston, Little, Brown & Co. 1953.
697. REYNOLDS, S. R. M., HAMILTON, J. B., DIPALMA, J. R., HUBERT, G. R., AND FOSTER, F. I.: Dermovascular change: dermovascular actions of certain hormones in castrate, eunuchoid, and normal men. *J. Clin. Endocrinology, 2*:228, 1942.
698. REYNOLDS, S. R. M. AND FOSTER, F. I.: Peripheral vascular action of estrogen observed in the ear of the rabbit. *J. Pharmacol. & Exper. Therap., 68*:173, 1940.

699. REYNOLDS, R. P., OWEN, C. I. AND CANTOR, M. O.: Arteriovenous aneurysm of uterine artery and vein. *J.A.M.A., 141*:841, 1949.
700. RICE, L., FRIEDEN, J., KATZ, L. N., ELISBERG, E. I., AND ROSENBERG, E.: A case of spontaneous thrombosis of the superior vena cava with some observations on the mechanism of edema formation. *Am. Heart J., 43*:821, 1952.
701. RICE-OXLEY, J. M., AND COOKE, A. M.: Temporal arteritis. *Lancet, 1*:89, 1951.
702. RICHARDSON, H. B.: Familial epistaxis; a case report. *Am. J. M. Sc., 154*:95, 1917.
703. RICHINS, C. A.: Use of the freezing-drying technique for study of vasomotor activity. *Science, 107*:25, 1948.
704. RICKHAM, P. P.: A case of hemangiomatosis of the small intestine. *Br. J. Surg., 39*:462, 1952.
705. RILEY, C. M., DAY, R. L., GREELEY, D. M. AND LANGFORD, W. S.: Central autonomic dysfunction with defective lacrimation. *Pediatrics, 3*:468, 1949.
706. RIVIERE, C.: The significance of cervical capillary markings. *Lancet, 1*:697, 1916.
707. RIVOLTA, F.: Arteriosclerosi precoce tramautica. *Il Policlinico, 14*:108, 1907.
708. ROBB, G. P., AND GOTTLIEB, C.: Report of a case of pulmonary arteriovenous fistula in the left lower pulmonary field. *Exper. Med. & Surg., 9*:431, 1951.
709. ROBERTS, J. C.: A case of bronchostaxis. *Brit. M. J., 1*:1069, 1937.
710. ROBINSON, L. S.: The collateral circulation following ligation of the inferior vena cava. *Surgery, 25*:329, 1949.
711. ROBINSON, S. S. AND TASKER, S.: Angiomas of the scrotum (angiokeratoma, Fordyce). *Arch. Derm. & Syph., 54*:667, 1946.
712. RODBARD, S., TEITELMAN, S. L., AND ZIMMERMAN, L. M.: Physical factors in the dilation of vessels. *Angiology, 7*:309, 1956.
713. RODES, C. B.: Cavernous hemangiomas of the lung with secondary polycythemia. *J.A.M.A., 110*:1914, 1938.
714. ROE, D. S. A., HODGES, C., INNES, G. S., AND POPE, L. I.: Radiophosphorus in the treatment of capillary naevi. *Lancet, 2*:1111, 1955.
715. ROLES, F. C.: A case of multiple telangiectasis with splenomegaly. *St. Barth. Hosp. J., 36*:19, 1928.
716. ROLLESTON, H. D.: *Diseases of the Liver, Gall-bladder and Bile Ducts.* 2nd ed., London, Macmillan, 1912.
717. ROLLESTON, H.: Diseases of the liver. *Oxford Med., 3*:303, 1933.
718. ROMAN, B.: Acute yellow atrophy of the liver. *Arch. Path., 4*:399, 1927.
719. RONCHESE, F.: Hemangiomas. Should treatment be expectant or active? *Rhode Island M. J., 29*:658, 1946.
720. RONCHESE, F.: The spontaneous involution of cutaneous vascular tumors. *Am. J. Surg., 86*:376, 1953.
721. RONCHESE, F.: The fluorescence of ulcerated epidermoid carcinoma under the Wood light. *Med. Radiography and Photography, 29*:6, 1953.
722. RONCHESE, F. AND KERN, A. B.: Kaposi's sarcoma (angioreticulomatosis). *Postgraduate Medicine, 14*:101, 1953.
723. RONCHESE, F. AND KERN, A. B.: Bone lesions in Kaposi's sarcoma. *A.M.A. Arch. Derm. & Syph., 70*:342, 1954.
724. RONCHESE, F. AND KERN, A. B.: Kaposi's sarcoma and diabetes mellitus. *A.M.A. Arch. Derm. & Syph., 67*:95, 1953.

725. RONDELL, P. A., KEITZER, W. F., AND BOHR, D. F.: Distribution of flow through capillaries and arteriovenous anastomoses in the rabbit ear. *Am. J. Phys.*, *183*:523, 1955.

726. ROSE, W. McI.: Survival period of patients with cerebral haemorrhage dying in hospital. *Lancet, 2*:561, 1948.

727. ROSEN, D. A., MAENGWYN-DAVIES, G. D., BECKER, B., STONE, H. H., AND FRIEDENWALD, J. S.: Xanthurenic acid excretion studies in diabetics with and without retinopathy. *Proc. Soc. Exper. Biol. & Med.*, *88*:321, 1955.

728. ROSENBLOOM, S. E.: Superior vena cava obstruction in primary cancer of the lung. *Ann. Int. Med.*, *31*:470, 1949.

729. ROSENKRANTZ, H., MILHORAT, A. T., FARBER, M. AND MILMAN, A. E.: Purification and identification of the antistiffness factor. *Proc. Soc. Exp. Biol. & Med.*, *76*:408 1951.

730. ROSENKRANTZ, J. A., WOLF, J., AND KAICHER, J. J.: Paget's disease (osteitis deformans). *Arch. Int. Med.*, *90*:610, 1952.

731. ROSENTHAL, F.: Oslersche Krankheit. *Zentralbl. f. Haut—u. Geschlechtskr.*, *40*:720, 1932.

732. ROSENTHAL, F., AND UNNA, P.: Uber das wesen der Oslerschen krankheit. *Klin. Wchnschr., 12*:865, 1933.

733. RÖSSLE, R.: Entzundungen der Leber. *Henke-Lubarsch's Handbuch der Speziellen Anatomie und Pathologie, 5*:27, 1930.

734. ROSWIT, B., KAPLAN, G., AND JACOBSON, H. G.: The superior vena cava obstruction syndrome in bronchogenic carcinoma. *Radiology, 61*:722, 1953.

735. ROTHMAN, S.: *Physiology and Biochemistry of the Skin.* U. of Chicago Press, 1954.

736. ROUSSAK, N. J. AND HEPPLESTON, J. D.: Obstruction of the inferior vena cava by a leiomyosarcoma. *Lancet, 2*:853, 1950.

737. RUITER, M.: Angiokeratoma corporis diffusum. *A. M. A. Arch. Dermat. & Syph.*, *68*:21, 1953.

738. RULISON, R. H.: Multiple hereditary hemorrhagic telangiectasia. *Arch. Derm. & Syph., 34*:522, 1936.

739. RUMBALL, J. M.: Multiple hemorrhagic telangiectasia (Rendu-Osler-Weber disease): case with visceral involvement. *Mil. Surgeon, 105*:53, 1949.

740. RUNDLES, R. W.: Hemorrhagic telangiectasia with pulmonary artery aneurysms: case report. *Am. J. M. Sc., 210*:76, 1945.

741. RUNSTROM, G. AND SIGROTH, K.: Two cases of vascular anomalies in the lung. *Acta. med. Scandinav.*, supp. *246*:176, 1950.

742. SAHS, A. H.: Personal communication.

743. SAKSELA, N. AND HALONEN, P. I.: Liver cirrhosis in Finland. *Ann. med. int. Fenniae, 35*:7, 1946.

744. SALINE, M. AND BAUM, G. L.: Triethylene melamine in bronchogenic carcinoma with vena caval obstruction. *J.A.M.A., 156*: 1493, 1954.

745. SALTER, W. T., KLATSKIN, G., AND HUMM, F. D.: Gynecomastia due to malnutrition. II. Endocrine studies. *Am. J. Med. Sc., 213*:31, 1947.

746. SANCETTA, S. M. AND ZIMMERMAN, H. A.: Congenital heart disease with septal defects in which paradoxical brain abscess causes death. *Circulation, 1*:593, 1950.

747. SCARFF, G. R.: Familial multiple telangiectases of skin and mucous membranes. *Bristol. Med. Chir. J., 50*:113, 1933.

748. SCHECHTER, M. M. AND ZISKIND, M. M.: The superior vena cava syndrome. *Am. J. Med., 18*:561, 1955.

749. SCHEDL, H. P., BEAN, W. B., STEVENSON, B. N. AND SCHUMACHER, E. R.: Correction for color differences between standards in urine extracts and their ketonic fractions in the Callow-Zimmerman reaction. *J. Lab. & Clin. Med., 45*:191, 1955.

750. SCHEDL, H. P., DITTO, K., AND BEAN, W. B.: Corticosteroid excretion in liver disease. *J. Lab. & Clin. Med., 42*:116, 1953.

751. SCHILLER, A. A.: Mechanism of action of vitamin P flavonoid (rutin) on the cutaneous circulations. *Am. J. Physiol., 165*:293, 1951.

752. SCHMITT, H.: Zur frage der erblichkeit, erkennung und behandlung der Osler-schen krankheit (Telangiectasia hereditaria haemorrhagica). *Ztschr. Laryng. Rhin. Otol., 22*:28, 1931.

753. SCHOEN, R.: Familiäre teleangiectasie mit habituellen nasenbluten. *Deutsches Arch. klin. Med., 166*:156, 1930.

754. SCHOLL, P. R., AND BLACK, B. M.: Superior vena caval syndrome resulting from lymphocytic thyroiditis. *Proc. Staff Meet. Mayo Clin., 29*:259, 1954.

755. SCHOLTE, A. J.: A case of angioma teleangiectaticum cutis with chronic endocarditis and malignant carcinoid of small intestine. *Beitrag. Path. Anat., 86*:440, 1931.

756. SCHREINER, G. E., FREINKEL, N., ATHENS, J. W., AND STONE, W.: Cardiac output, central volume and dye injection curves in traumatic arteriovenous fistulas in man. *Circulation, 7*:718, 1953.

757. SCHROEDER, H. A. AND GOLDMAN, M. L.: Test for the presence of "hypertensive diencephalic syndrome" using histamine. *Am. J. Med., 6*:162, 1949.

758. SCHÜPBACH, A.: Teleangiektasiebildung und Leberkrankheiten. *Schweiz med. Wchnschr., 24*:1186, 1943.

759. SCHUSTER, N. H.: Familial hemorrhagic telangiectasia associated with multiple aneurysms of the splenic artery. *J. Path. & Bact., 44*:29, 1937.

760. SCHWARTZ, V. J.: Hereditary hemorrhagic telangiectasia. *Minnesota Med., 8*:551, 1925.

761. SCHWARTZ, S. O. AND ARMSTRONG, B. E.: Familial hereditary hemorrhagic telangiectasia in the Negro. *New Eng. J. Med., 239*:434, 1948.

762. SCHWARTZ, S. O. AND BLUMENTHAL, S. A.: Exogenous hemochromatosis resulting from blood transfusions. *Blood, 3*:617, 1948.

763. SEAMAN, W. B. AND GOLDMAN, A.: Roentgen aspects of pulmonary arteriovenous fistula. *Arch. Int. Med., 89*:70, 1952.

764. SEELEY, S. F., HUGHES, C. W., COOK, F. N. AND ELKIN, D. C.: Traumatic arteriovenous fistulas and aneurysms in war wounded. *Am. J. Surg., 83*:471, 1952.

765. SELYE, H.: The alarm reaction and the diseases of adaptation. *Ann. Int. Med., 29*:403, 1948.

766. SELYE, H. AND RICHER, C. L.: A syndrome of multiple telangiectases produced by a transplantable fibrosarcoma. *Cancer Research, 16*:856, 1956.

767. SEQUEIRA, J. H.: A case of multiple telangiectases. *Brit. J. Dermat., 25*:154, 1913.

768. SEQUEIRA, J. H.: Multiple telangiectases. *Proc. Roy. Soc. Med.,* (Derm. Sect.) *6*:128, 1913.

769. SETTELEN, M. E.: Osler'sche Krankheit. *Pract. Oto-rhino-laryng., 8*:537, 1946.

770. SÉZARY, A. AND CUVEREAUX, M.: Forme douloureuse de l'angiomatose hemorragique familiale. *Ann. de dermat. et syph., 2*:507, 1942.

771. Sézary, A., Lefèvre, P., and Horowitz, A.: Angiomatose hereditaire familiale (maladie de Rendu Osler). *Bull. Soc. franc. dermat. et syph., 43*:990, 1936.

772. Shafar, J. and Doig, A.: The "nape nevus". *Brit. M. J., 1*:913, 1955.

773. Shaffer, J. M.: Disease of the liver in hyperthyroidism. *Arch. Path., 29*:20, 1940.

773a. Shambron, E.: Personal communication.

774. Shanks, G. and De, M. N.: The pathology of epidemic dropsy. *Indian J. M. Res., 19*:469, 1931.

775. Sharpe, O.: A "harlequin" colour change in the newborn. *Lancet, 2*:1180, 1952.

775a. Shefts, L. M.: Personal communication.

776. Shelmire, B.: Certain diseases of the oral mucous membrane and vermillion borders of the lips. *Sou. Med. J., 21*:169, 1928.

777. Shenkin, H. A., Cabieses, F., and Van Den Noordt, G.: The effect of bilateral stellectomy upon the cerebral circulation of man. *J. Clin. Invest., 30*:90, 1951.

778. Shennan, T.: Histologically non-malignant angioma, with numerous metastases. *J. Path. & Bact., 19*:139, 1914.

779. Shepherd, J. A.: Angiomatous conditions of the gastrointestinal tract. *Brit. J. Surg., 40*:409, 1953.

780. Sherber, D. A.: The control of bleeding. *Am. J. Surg., 86*:331, 1953.

781. Sibley, W. K.: Bilateral telangiectasis (naevus araneus). *Brit. J. Dermat., 26*:197, 1914.

782. Silberberg, M. and Silberberg, R.: The difference in the response of skeletal tissues to estrogen in mice of various ages. *Anat. Rec., 80*:347, 1941.

783. Silberberg, M. and Silberberg, R.: Further investigations concerning the influence of estrogen on skeletal tissues. *Am. J. Anat., 69*:295, 1941.

784. Silverman, J. J. and Littman, D. S.: The cardiologist looks at the hand. *New Eng. J. Med., 249*:839, 1953.

785. Silvestini, R.: La reviviscenza mammaria vel'como affetto da cirosi del Laennec. *Riforma med., 42*:701, 1926.

786. Singer, K. and Wolfson, W. Q.: Hereditary hemorrhagic telangiectasia: an analysis of capillary heredopathies. *New Eng. J. Med., 230*:637, 1944.

787. Sirota, J. H.: Spontaneous perforation of an aortic aneurysm into the superior vena cava with survival for 136 days. *Am. Heart J., 39*:782, 1950.

788. Sklarz, E.: Telangiectatic ("nape") naevi. *Brit. M. J., 1*:1221, 1955.

789. Sloper, J. C. and Storey, G.: Aneurysms of the ascending aorta due to medial degeneration associated with arachnodactyly (Marfan's disease). *J. Clin. Path., 6*:299, 1953.

790. Smirk, F. H.: Observations on the capillary permeability in cases of nephritis and of hepatic cirrhosis with hypoproteinaemia. *Clin. Sc., 2*:57, 1935.

791. Smith, A. H.: Treatment of hereditary telangiectasia. *Clin. J., 69*:120, 1940.

792. Smith, H. L. and Horton, B. T.: Arteriovenous fistula of the lung associated with polycythemia vera: report of a case in which diagnosis was made clinically. *Am. Heart J., 18*:589, 1939.

793. Smith, J. H. and Evans, J. P.: Diagnosis of epidural and subdural hematomata. *J. Med., 20*:16, 1939.

794. Smith, J. L. and Lineback, M. I.: Thrombocytopenia and thrombocytomegaly in Rendu-Osler's disease. *J. M. A. Georgia, 42*:418, 1953.

795. SMITH, J. L. AND LINEBACK, M. I.: Hereditary hemorrhagic telangiectasia: 9 cases in one Negro family with special reference to hepatic lesions. *Am. J. of Med., 17*:41, 1954.

796. SMITH, P. H., ALBRIGHT, F. AND DODGE, E.: (Method of Klinefelter, Albright, and Griswold) Modifications in methods for precipitation and assay of increased amounts of pituitary gonadotropic substances in the urine. *J. Lab. & Clin. Med., 28*:1761, 1943.

797. SNELL, E. S., CRANSTON, W. I., AND GERBRANDY, J.: Cutaneous vasodilatation during fainting. *Lancet, 1*:693, 1955.

798. SNOW, P. J. D., LENNARD-JONES, J. E., CURZON, G., AND STACEY, R. S.: Humoral effects of metastasising carcinoid tumours. *Lancet, 2*:1004. 1955.

799. SNYDER, L. H.: *The Principles of Heredity.* 2nd ed. Boston, Heath, 1940.

800. SNYDER, L. H. AND DOAN, C. A.: Studies in human inheritance: is the homozygous form of multiple telangiectasia lethal? *J. Lab. & Clin. Med., 29*:1211, 1944.

801. SOBEL, H. AND FURTH, J.: Hypervolemia in mice bearing granulosa-cell growths; time of onset and some associated physiological and chemical changes. *Endocrinology, 42*:436, 1948

802. SOLEM, J. H.: Cutaneous arterial spiders following use of adreno-cortitrophic hormone. *Lancet, 2*:1241, 1952.

803. SOLIS-COHEN, S.: Vasomotor ataxia: a contribution to the subject of idiosyncrasies. *Am. J. Med. Sc., 107*:130, 1894.

804. SORNBERGER, C. F. AND SMEDAL, M. I.: The mechanism and incidence of cardiovascular changes in Paget's disease (osteitis deformans). *Circulation, 6*:711, 1952.

805. SPAIN, D. M.: Association of gastrointestinal carcinoid tumor with cardiovascular abnormalities. *Am. J. Med.., 19*:366, 1955.

806. SPALTEHOLZ, W.: *Blutgefässe der Haut.* Handb. d. haut u. Geschlechstkr. Bd. 1, Th. 1, Berlin, Springer, 1927.

807. SPENCER, R. P.: Malignant melanoma. *New Eng. J. Med., 253*:18, 1955.

808. STABINS, S. J., THORNTON, J. J., AND SCOTT, W. J. M.: Changes in the vasomotor reaction associated with glomus tumors. *J. Clin. Invest., 16*:685, 1937.

809. STANDER, H. J. AND CADDEN, J. F.: Acute yellow atrophy of the liver in pregnancy. *Am. J. Obst. & Gynec., 28*:61, 1934.

810. STANLEY, M. M.: Gonococcic peritonitis of the upper part of the abdomen in young women. *Arch. Int. Med., 78*:1, 1946.

811. STAUFFER, H. M., ARBUCKLE, B. K., AND AEGERTER, E. E.: Polyostotic fibrous dysplasia with cutaneous pigmentation and congenital arteriovenous aneurysms. *J. Bone & Joint Surg., 23*:323, 1946.

812. STEINBERG, I. AND McCLENAHAN, J.: Pulmonary arteriovenous fistula. *Am. J. Med., 19*:549, 1955.

813. STEINER, L. AND VOERNER, H.: Angiomatosis Miliaris—"An idiopathic disease of the blood vessels.: *Deutsches Archiv klin Med., 96*:105, 1909.

814. STEINER, W. R.: Hereditary hemorrhagic telangiectasia. *Arch. Int. Med., 19*:194, 1917.

815. STEINMANN, J.: Des étoiles vasculaires chez les cirrhotiques. *Rev. méd. chir. de mal. du foie., 10*:149, 1935.

816. STEINMANN, J.: Hémorrhagies et étoiles vasculaires chez un cirrhotique. *J. d. Praticiens, 50*:854, 1936.

817. STELLAR, L. I.: Hereditary telangiectasis: report of a case. *New Eng. J. Med.,* 226:336, 1942.
818. STERMAN, M. M., AND SCAL, J. C.: Familial telangiectasia with recurring epistaxis. *New York J. Med., 37*:287, 1937.
819. STEVENSON, F. H.: Infected arteriovenous fistula in the lung. *Lancet, 1*:626, 1953.
820. STILLIANS, A. W.: Telangiectasia (Familial). *Arch. Derm. & Syph., 12*:568, 1925.
821. STOCK, M. F.: Hereditary hemorrhagic telangiectasia (Osler's disease): a review of the literature and report of cases. *Arch. Otolaryng., 40*:108, 1944.
822. STOKES, W.: *Diseases of the Heart and the Aorta.* Dublin, Hodges and Smith, 1854.
823. STOREY, W. E. AND AKAMATSU, G. T.: Multiple hereditary hemorrhagic telangiectasia; case report with pathologic study. *South. M. J., 34*:934, 1941.
824. STOUT, A. P.: Solitary cutaneous and subcutaneous leiomyoma. *Am. J. Cancer, 29*:435, 1937.
825. STOUT, A. P. AND CASSEL, C.: Hemangiopericytoma of the omentum. *Surgery, 13*:578, 1943.
826. STOUT, A. P. AND MURRAY, M. R.: Hemangiopericytoma. A vascular tumor featuring Zimmermann's pericytes. *Ann. Surg., 116*:26, 1942.
827. STRACHAN, H.: Malarial multiple peripheral neuritis. *Annual of the Universal Medical Sciences (Sajou's Annual), 1*:139, 1888.
828. STRANG, C. AND RANNIE, I.: Dyschondroplasia with hemangiomata (Maffucci's Syndrome): report of a case complicated by intracranial chondrosarcoma. *J. Bone & Joint Surg., 32B*:376, 1950.
829. STRAYHORN, D. AND WELLS, E. B.: Arachnodactyly with aneurysmal dilatation of the aorta. *Trans. of Am. Clin. and Climat. Assn., 59*:205, 1947.
830. SUCQUET, J. P.: *D'une Circulation dérivative dans les Membres et dans la tete chez l'Homme.* Paris, 1862.
831. SUTTON, H. G.: Epistaxis as an indication of impaired nutrition and degeneration of the vascular system. *Med. Mirror, 1*:769, 1864.
832. SYMMERS, D.: Cutaneous angiomata and their significance in the diagnosis of malignant disease: a statistical study based upon the observation of nearly four hundred cases. *Med. News, 81*:1207, 1902.
833. SYMMERS, D.: Telangiectatic splenomegaly. *J.A.M.A., 77*:2019, 1921.
834. TALBOT, N. B.: The inactivation of endogenous estrogen by the liver. *Endocrinology, 25*:601, 1939.
835. TALBOT, T. J., AND SILVERMAN, J. J.: Asymptomatic arteriovenous fistula of the lung. *Arch. Int. Med., 90*:569, 1952.
836. TEAHAN, W. W.: Hereditary hemorrhagic telangiectasis occurring in six generations. *Ann. Int. Med., 13*:535, 1939.
837. TEMPLETON, H. J.: Multiple hemorrhagic familial telangiectasia of the skin and mucous membrane. *Arch. Derm. & Syph., 34*:143, 1936.
838. TEMPLETON, H. J.: Hereditary hemorrhagic telangiectasia (Osler). *Arch. Derm. & Syph., 38*:498, 1938.
839. TENNENT, E. C. AND HARMAN, J. W.: A study of factors affecting the prognosis of cerebral vascular accident. *Am. J. M. Sc., 218*:361, 1949.
840. TERRY, R.: White nails in hepatic cirrhosis. *Lancet, 1*:757, 1954.
841. THEORIN, S.: Eine familie aus norrland mit morbus Rendu Osler. *Acta med. Scandinav., Supp. 123*:268, 1941.

842. THOMSON, M. S.: An hitherto undescribed familial disease. *Brit. J. Dermat.,* 35:455, 1923.

843. THORSON, Ä., BIÖRCK, G., BJÖRKMAN, G., AND WALDENSTRÖM, J.: Malignant carcinoid of the small intestine with metastases to the liver, valvular disease of the right side of the heart (pulmonary stenosis and tricuspid regurgitation without septal defects), peripheral vasomotor symptoms, bronchoconstriction, and an unusual type of cyanosis. *Am. Heart J., 47*:795, 1954.

844. TIWISINA, T.: Dyschondroplasie (Ollier) mit multiplen Haemangiomen und ortlicher maligner Entartung (Chondrosarkom). *Beitr. klin. Chir., 188*:8, 1954.

845. TOBIN, J. R., JR., BAU, E. B., AND HUMPHREYS, E. M.: Marfan's syndrome in the adult. *Arch. Int. Med., 80*:475, 1947.

846. TOBIN, J. R. AND WILDER, T. C.: Pulmonary arteriovenous fistula associated with hereditary hemorrhagic telangiectasis: a report of their occurrence in a father and son. *Ann. Int. Med., 38*:868, 1953.

847. TOURAINE, A., LORTAT-JACOB, E. AND BOSC: Angiomatose hémorragique héréditaire. *Ann. Derm. Syph., 5*:295, 1945.

848. TRAISMAN, H. S. AND JOHNSON, F. R.: Arachnodactyly associated with aneurysm of the aorta. *Am. J. Dis. Children, 87*:156, 1954.

849. TRAUB, E. F.: The pigmented, hairy and warty nevi and their relationship to malignancy. *South. M. J., 40*:1000, 1947.

850. TRAUB, E. F.: Early recognition of possibly dangerous nevi (moles) and the best procedure to avoid development of malignant melanomas (nevocarcinoma). *New York J. Med., 49*:1661, 1949.

851. TRAUB, E. F.: Nevi. *Med. Clin. No. Am., 35*:301, 1951.

852. TRAUB, E. F.: Prognosis and treatment of nevi. *Postgrad. Med., 10*:153, 1951.

853. TRAUB, E. F. AND KYLE, H.: The "common mole": its clinical pathologic relations and the question of malignant degeneration. *Arch. Dermat. & Syph., 41*:214, 1940.

854. TROSTLER, L. S.: Erythema of the extremities in tuberculosis. *Am. Rev. Tuberc., 47*:168, 1943

855. TROUSSEAU, A.: *Clinical Medical Lectures.* Trans. from the 3rd enlarged edition by Cormack, J. R. and Baziere. Philadelphia, Blakiston, 1882.

856. ULLMANN, K.: Uber Begriff und Krankheitsbilder der Angiomatosis. *Wien. klin. Wchnschr., 43*:1538, 1930.

857. ULLMANN, K.: Angiomatosis and Osler's disease. *Urol. & Cutan. Rev., 37*:619, 1933.

858. ULRICH, H. L.: Personal communication.

859. UMANSKY, A. L.: Dyschondroplasia with hemangiomata (Maffucci's Syndrome): early case with mild osseous manifestations. *Bull. Hosp. Joint Dis., 7*:59, 1946.

860. URBACH, E.: Essentielle telangiecktasien. *Zentralbl. f. Haut—u. Geschlechtskr., 18*:339, 1925.

861. VAN WAGENEN, C. D.: Multiple hereditary telangiectasis of the tongue, turbinates, and septum with recurring hemorrhages. *Med. Rec., 81*:109, 1912.

862. VENNING, E. H.: Adrenal function in pregnancy. *Endocrinology, 39*:203, 1946.

862a. VENNING, E. H. AND BROWNE, J. S. L.: Excretion of glycogenic corticoids and of 17-ketosteroids in various endocrine and other disorders. *J. Clin. Endocrinology, 7*:79, 1947.

863. VEREL, D.: Telangiectasia in Raynaud's disease. *Lancet, 1*:914, 1956.
863a. VIGNES, H., HANOUN, F., AND VIAL, G.: *Maladies des femmes enceintes. Vol. III. Affections de la peau.* Masson et Cie. Paris, 1937.
864. VISCHER, W.: Teleangiectasia haemorrhagica hereditaria: pathologic and anatomical findings and blood group research. *Acta haemat., 5*:168, 1951.
865. VOGLER, E. AND GOLLMANN, G.: The significance of the terminal circulation in the development of vascular disease and disturbances of blood flow: vasographic studies. *Angiology, 6*:540, 1955.
866. VON WILLEBRAND, E. A.: Hereditary pseudohemophilia: description; previously observed cases. *Finska lak.-sallsk. handl., 68*:87, 1926.
867. VOYLES, G. Q. AND RITCHEY, J. O.: Hereditary hemorrhagic telangiectasia: report of two cases. *Ann. Int. Med., 22*:730, 1945.
868. WAGGETT, E. B.: A case of multiple telangiectases. *Proc. Roy. Soc. Med. (Laryng. Sect.), 1*:70, 1908.
869. WAGNER, G.: Zur altershaufigkeit der disseminierten papulosen teleangiektasien, sogenannten "senilen angioma")—the age incidence of the disseminated papulous teleangiectases (so-called senile angiomas). *Sonderdruck aus Zeitschrift für Haut—und Geschlechtskrankheiten,* Vol. 14, No. 1, 1953.
870. WALDMANN, E. B., MARTIN, W. J., AND FERRIS, D. O.: Carcinoid tumors of the small intestine: possible confusion of their manifestations with primary pancreatic or hepatic disease. *Proc. Staff Meet. Mayo Clinic, 30*:127, 1955.
871. WALLER, J. V.: Hemorrhagic telangiectasia treated with stilbestrol. *Ann. Int. Med., 44*:204, 1956.
872. WALSH, E. N. AND BECKER, S. W.: Erythema palmare and naevus-araneus-like telangiectases. *Arch. Derm. Syph., 44*:616, 1941.
873. WARD, E.: Multiple pigmented warts in pregnancy. *Brit. J. Dermat., 25*:153, 1913.
874. WARREN, J. V., ELKIN, D. C. AND NICKERSON, J. L.: The blood volume in patients with arteriovenous fistulas. *J. Clin. Invest., 30*:220, 1951.
875. WARREN, J. V., NICKERSON, J. L., AND ELKIN, D. C.: Cardiac output in patients with arteriovenous fistulas. *J. Clin. Invest., 30*:210, 1951.
876. WATSON, C. J.: Regurgitation jaundice. *J.A.M.A., 114*:2427, 1940.
877. WATSON, J.: Observations on the nature and treatment of telangiectasis, or that morbid state of the blood vessels which gives rise to naevus and aneurism from anastomosis. *Am. J. M. Sc., 24*:24, 1839.
878. WATSON, W. L. AND MCCARTHY, W. D.: Blood and lymph vessel tumors. *Surg. Gynec. & Obst., 71*:569, 1940.
879. WEBER, F. P.: A note on cutaneous telangiectases and their etiology: comparison of the etiology of hemorrhoids and ordinary varicose veins. *Edinburgh M. J., 15*:346, 1904.
880. WEBER, F. P.: Multiple hereditary developmental angiomata (telangiectases) of the skin and mucous membranes associated with recurring hemorrhages. *Lancet, 2*:160, 1907.
881. WEBER, F. P.: Remarks on small subcutaneous and cutaneous growths. *Brit. J. Dermat., 20*:313, 1908.
882. WEBER, F. P.: The significance of cervical capillary markings. *Lancet, 1*:589, 1916.
883. WEBER, F. P.: Developmental telangiectatic hemorrhage and so-called "telangiectasia"—familial and non-familial. *Brit. J. Child. Dis., 21*:198, 1924.

884. WEBER, F. P.: "De Morgan's spots." *Brit. M. J.*, *2*:693, 1936.

885. WEBER, F. P.: Inborn and familial tendency to the development of hepatic cirrhosis. *Lancet, 1*:305, 1936.

886. WEBER, F. P.: Haemorrhagic telangiectasia of the Osler type—"telangiectatic dysplasia". An isolated case with discussion of multiple pulsating telangiectases and other striking hemangiectatic conditions. *Brit. J. Dermat., 48*:182, 1936.

887. WEBER, F. P.: Telangiectasia of the Rendu-Osler type with camptodactylia and muscular atrophy in the hands. *Proc. Roy. Soc. Med.* (Sect. Derm.), *31*:258, 1938.

888. WEBER, F. P.: A pulsating stellate naevus (naevus arachnoides). *Brit. J. Dermat. & Syph., 50*:31, 1938.

889. WEBER, F. P.: Telangiectatic dysplasia of the Rendu-Osler type and De Morgan spots. *Proc. Roy. Soc. Med., 32*:1393, 1939.

890. WEBER, F. P.: Some telangiectatic and other anomalous vascular groups, especially those of dysplastic origin. *M. Press, 210*:219, 1943.

891. WEBER, F. P.: *Rare Diseases and Some Debatable Subjects.* London, Staples Press, Ltd., 1946.

892. WEBER, F. P.: Encephalo trigiminal angiomatosis. *Brit. M. J., 1*:726, 1955.

893. WEBER, F. P.: Nuchal-bulbar hemangiomatosis and encephalo-facial hemangiomatosis. *Lancet, 2*:981, 1955.

894. WEBER, F. P. AND HELLENSCHMIED, R.: Telangiectasia macularis eruptiva perstans. *Brit. J. Dermat., 42*:374, 1930.

895. WEBSTER, J. R.: The identification and management of the more common nevi. *M. Clin. North America, 33*:219, 1949.

896. WEGELIN, C.: Stellate telangiectases of the skin in hepatic cirrhosis. *Schweiz. Ztschr. f. Path. u. Bakt., 5*:374, 1942.

897. WEISS, J. A.: Radium therapy for recurrent epistaxis in hereditary hemorrhagic telangiectasia. *Laryngoscope, 48*:865, 1938.

898. WEISS, S., ROBB, G. P. AND BLUMGART, H. L.: The velocity of blood flow in health and disease as measured by the effect of histamine on the minute vessels. *Am. Heart J., 4*:604, 1929.

899. WELLS, E. B.: Hereditary hemorrhagic telangiectasia. *Am. J. M. Sc., 211*:577, 1946.

900. WERNER, M.: Oslersche Krankheit und Leberveränderungen (zugleich ein Beitrag zur Cerebralen Form der Teleangiectasia haemorrhagica hereditaria). *Deutsches Arch. klin. Med., 189*:214, 1942.

901. WETZEL, N. C. AND ZOTTERMAN, Y.: On the differences in the skin coloration in various regions of the normal skin. *Heart, 13*:358, 1926.

902. WHEELER, C. E., CAWLEY, E. P., GRAY, H. T., AND CURTIS, A. C.: Gynecomastia: A review and an analysis of 160 cases. *Ann. Int. Med., 40*:985, 1954.

903. WHEELER, C. E., CAWLEY, E. P., GRAY, H. T., AND CURTIS, A. C.: Occurrence of gynecomastia in conjunction with dermatologic disorders. *A.M.A. Arch. Dermat. & Syph., 68*:685, 1953.

904. WHITAKER, W.: Cavernous haemangioma of the lung. *Thorax, 2*:58, 1947.

905. WHITE, J. M.: Case of diffuse spreading superficial naevus. *Scottish Med. and Surg. J., 1*:312, 1897.

906. WHITFIELD, A. G. W., ARNOTT, W. M., AND STAFFORD, J. L.: "Myocarditis" and aortic hypoplasia in arachnodactyly. *Lancet, 1*:1387, 1951.

907. WHITTAKER, S. R. F. AND SHEEHAN, J. D.: Dissecting aortic aneurysm in Marfan's syndrome. *Lancet, 2*:791, 1954.

908. WHITTLE, C. H.: Haemorrhagic telangiectasia of Rendu-Osler-Weber. *Brit. J. Dermat., 59*:63, 1947.

909. WIGLEY, J. E. M. AND HEGGS, G.: Osler-Rendu-Weber familial telangiectases in association with Raynaud's disease. *Brit. J. Dermat., 46*:230, 1934.

910. WIGLEY, J. E. M. AND HEGGS, G.: Osler-Rendu-Weber familial telangiectasia. *Brit. J. Dermat., 47*:125, 1935.

911. WILLIAMS, C. D., JR., HEIPLE, K. G., AND EBERT, R. H.: The effect of cortisone on vascular reactivity: *in vivo* observations using the rabbit ear chamber technique. *J. Lab. & Clin. Med., 44*:210, 1954.

912. WILLIAMS, C. F. AND FLINK, E. B.: Hereditary hemorrhagic telangiectasia in association with cerebral manifestations and pulmonary arteriovenous aneurysm. *J. Lab. & Clin. Med., 32*:1401, 1947.

913. WILLIAMS, C. M.: Hereditary hemorrhagic telangiectasia. *Arch. Derm. & Syph., 14*:1, 1926.

914. WILLIAMS, D. H. AND SNELL, A. M.: Pulsating angioma (generalized telangiectasia) of the skin associated with hepatic disease. *Arch. Int. Med., 62*:872, 1938.

915. WILLIAMS, G. A. AND BRICK, I. B.: Gastrointestinal bleeding in hereditary hemorrhagic telangiectasia. *A.M.A. Arch. Int. Med., 95*:41, 1955.

916. WILLIAMS, M. H.: Traumatic arteriovenous aneurysm associated with streptococcic septicemia. *J.A.M.A., 148*:726, 1952.

917. WILLIAMS, R. H.: *Textbook of Endocrinology.* Philadelphia, Saunders, 1950.

918. WILSON, E.: *Healthy Skin. A Popular Treatise on the Skin and Hair, Their Preservation and Management.* 2nd Am. ed., Philadelphia, Blanchard and Lea, 1854.

919. WILSON, E.: Eruptive angiomata. *J. Cutan. Med. & Dis. of Skin, 3*:198, 1869.

920. WILSON, G. M.: Peripheral circulatory changes associated with arteriovenous aneurysms. *Brit. Heart J., 13*:334, 1951.

921. WILSON, M. J. AND SILVERSTEIN, M. E.: Paget-Schroetter syndrome. *Arch. Int. Med., 88*:507, 1951.

922. WINTERNITZ, M. C. AND BOGGS, T. R.: A unique coincidence of multiple subcutaneous hemangio-endothelioma, multiple lymphangio-endothelioma of the intestinal tract and multiple polypi of the stomach undergoing malignant changes; associated with generalized vascular sclerosis and cirrhosis of the liver. *Bull. Johns Hopkins Hosp., 21*:203, 1910.

923. WINTROBE, M. M.: *Clinical Hematology.* 3rd ed., Philadelphia, Lea & Febiger, 1951.

924. WISSMAN, J. AND TAGNON, H. J.: The syndrome of hemangioma and thrombocytopenic purpura in infants. *A.M.A. Arch. Int. Med., 92*:523, 1953.

925. WITTKOWER, E. AND RAREY, B.: Beitrag zur Oslerschen Krankheit (Teleangiektasia hereditaria haemorrhagica). *Ztschr. klin. Med., 124*:41, 1933.

926. WODEHOUSE, G. E.: Hemangioma of the lung: a review of 4 cases including two not previously reported, one of which was complicated by brain abscess due to influenza. *Gen. Thor. Surg., 17*:408, 1948.

927. WOLFSON, H.: Hereditary familial telangiectasia. *Lancet, 2*:581, 1944.

928. WOOD, W.: Painful subcutaneous tubercle. *Edinburgh Med. J., 8*:283, 1812.

929. Wood, W.: Observations on painful subcutaneous tubercle with cases and histories of the disease. *Trans. Medico-Chirurg. Soc. Edinburgh, 3*:317, 1829.

930. Yater, W. M., Finnegan, J., and Giffin, H. M.: Pulmonary arteriovenous fistula (varix). *J.A.M.A., 141*:581, 1949.

931. Yde, A. and Olesen, M.: Angiomatosis hereditaria (Osler's disease): to danske familier. *Hospitalstid., 77*:1010, 1934.

932. Ytrehus, O.: Teleangiectasia haemorrhagica hereditaria og levercirrhose. *Nord. Med., 38*:730, 1948.

933. Zakon, S. J.: Rendu-Osler-Weber disease. *Arch. Derm. & Syph., 57*:470, 1948.

934. Zarrow, M. X.: Relaxin content of blood, urine and other tissues of pregnant and postpartum guinea pigs. *Proc. Soc. Exper. Biol. & Med., 66*:488, 1947.

935. Zarrow, M. X.: The antidiuretic action of relaxin-containing preparations. *Proc. Soc. Exper. Biol. & Med., 71*:705, 1949.

936. Zarrow, M. X.: The role of the steroid hormones in the relaxation of the symphysis pubis of the guinea pig. *Endocrinology, 42*:129, 1948.

937. Zavodny, F.: Arterio-venous aneurysm of lungs in Rendu-Osler's disease diagnosed clinically. *Casop. lěk. česk., 88*:741, 1949.

938. Zeisler, E. F.: Telangiectasia associated with syphilis and pregnancy. *Arch. Derm. & Syph., 5*:781, 1922.

939. Zimmermann, K. W.: Der feinere Bau der Blutcapillaren. *Ztschr. Anat., 68*:29, 1923.

940. Ziskin, D. E.: The effect of hormone treatment on the gums and mucosa of women. *J. Dent. Res., 16*:367, 1937.

941. Ziskin, D. E.: Pregnancy gingivitis: history, classification and etiology. *Amer. J. Ortho. and Oral Surg., 32*:390, 1946.

942. Zweifach, B. W. and Metz, D. B.: Selective distribution of blood through the terminal vascular bed of mesenteric structures and skeletal muscle. *Angiology, 6*:282, 1955.

943. Zweifach, B. W. and Metz, D. B.: Relation of blood-borne agents acting on mesenteric vascular bed to general circulatory reactions. *J. Clin. Invest., 34*: 653, 1955.

ADDITIONAL REFERENCES

Introductory Comment

Repeated checking of the references has reduced mistakes to a minimum. No doubt some errors remain. In the text I have called attention to a reference by number if there was likelihood of ambiguity; otherwise they are to be found as listed in alphabetical order. This facilitates the use of the references for further study. I have not included several hundred references to articles I have read, mostly because they added nothing new to the subject I was discussing. Indeed, some of those listed here have been included rather casually.

To provide a further use for the references I have made this listing of major references which deal with particular topics to facilitate the task of those who wish to read further. General discussions and text books are not included in this list.

List of Major Subjects

367

INDEX